Feminist Bioethics

Feminist Bioethics

At the Center, on the Margins

Edited by

Jackie Leach Scully, Ph.D.

Laurel E. Baldwin-Ragaven, M.D.C.M.

Petya Fitzpatrick, M.A.

The Johns Hopkins University Press

Baltimore

© 2010 The Johns Hopkins University Press
All rights reserved. Published 2010
Printed in the United States of America on acid-free paper

2 4 6 8 9 7 5 3 1

The Johns Hopkins University Press
2715 North Charles Street
Baltimore, Maryland 21218-4363
www.press.jhu.edu

Library of Congress Cataloging-in-Publication Data

Feminist bioethics : at the center, on the margins / edited by Jackie Leach Scully,
Laurel E. Baldwin-Ragaven, and Petya Fitzpatrick.
p.; cm.
Includes bibliographical references and index.
ISBN-13: 978-0-8018-9424-4 (hardcover : alk. paper)
ISBN-10: 0-8018-9424-7 (hardcover : alk. paper)
ISBN-13: 978-0-8018-9425-1 (pbk. : alk. paper)
ISBN-10: 0-8018-9425-5 (pbk. : alk. paper)
1. Medical ethics.   2. Bioethics.   3. Feminist ethics.   I. Scully, Jackie Leach.
II. Baldwin-Ragaven, Laurel.   III. Fitzpatrick, Petya, 1975–
[DNLM: 1. Bioethics.   2. Feminism.   3. Bioethical Issues. WB 60 F329 2010]
R724.F396 2010
174'.957—dc22   2009024468

A catalog record for this book is available from the British Library.

*Special discounts are available for bulk purchases of this book. For more information,
please contact Special Sales at 410-516-6936 or specialsales@press.jhu.edu.*

The Johns Hopkins University Press uses environmentally friendly book materials,
including recycled text paper that is composed of at least 30 percent post-consumer
waste, whenever possible. All of our book papers are acid-free, and our jackets and
covers are printed on paper with recycled content.

CONTENTS

JENNIFER BAKER, Ph.D., is an Indigenous senior lecturer in the Unaipon School, Indigenous College of Education and Research at the University of South Australia, and a regular contributor to Indigenous and women's health forums in South Australia. Postcolonial settings and the impacts on health and well-being for Indigenous women and men are an ongoing area of interest for her.

LAUREL E. BALDWIN-RAGAVEN, M.D.C.M., is a physician, educator, and activist. The former Henry R. Luce Professor of Health and Human Rights at Trinity College in Hartford, Connecticut, she now teaches and sees patients at the Asylum Hill Family Practice Residency Training Program affiliated with the University of Connecticut and is a visiting professor at the University of Cape Town Faculty of Health Sciences School of Public Health and Family Medicine in South Africa.

LORI D'AGINCOURT-CANNING, Ph.D., is an ethicist and codirector of the Clinical Ethics Service, Children's and Women's Health Centre of British Columbia, Vancouver, Canada. She has a joint appointment as clinical assistant professor in the Department of Pediatrics, Faculty of Medicine, University of British Columbia, and adjunct professor in the UBC School of Nursing. Her current research focuses on feminist ethics, social justice, and access to health care.

ANNE DONCHIN, Ph.D., is Emerita Professor of Philosophy and Women's Studies at Indiana University, Indianapolis, an affiliated research scholar at Mt. Sinai School of Medicine (New York City), and a founding "mother" of the International Network on Feminist Approaches to Bioethics (FAB). She is an associate editor of the journal *Bioethics* and a member of the editorial board of the *International Journal of Feminist Approaches to Bioethics*. She is coeditor of two volumes based on FAB conference papers and author of numerous essays on feminism and bioethics.

TERRY DUNBAR, B.B.B.S., M.P.E.&T., is an Indigenous senior research fellow and Ph.D. candidate in the Faculty of Education, Health and Science at the Charles Darwin University, Northern Territory, Australia, and a member of the National Health and Medical Research Council of Australia, Australian Health Ethics Committee. Her current research interests include: investigation of the historical aspects to legislation; development of social policy for Aboriginal and Torres Strait Islander peoples in the Northern Territory and assessment of the context and impact through ethical lenses; exploration of ways to best translate improved understanding of research and research ethics with Indigenous communities; consideration of how to produce useful resources for human research ethics committees; and examination of ways to articulate Indigenist methodologies.

PETYA FITZPATRICK, M.A., is a health researcher interested in the lived experience of illness and disability, women's health, and morality in health and illness. Previously located at the Menzies Centre at the University of Tasmania, Hobart, Australia, she is now studying toward her doctorate at Australian National University, Australian Capital Territory, Australia.

INA MAY GASKIN, M.A., C.P.M., is founder and director of the Farm Midwifery Center, located near Summertown, Tennessee. Author of *Spiritual Midwifery* (1975, revised 2002) and *Ina May's Guide to Childbirth* (2003), she promotes ecstatic birth, maintenance of breech delivery skills, and recognition of certain ingenious skills and techniques used by indigenous midwives of Mexico and Brazil. She initiated and coordinates the Safe Motherhood Quilt Project.

RUTH GROENHOUT, Ph.D., is professor of philosophy at Calvin College, Grand Rapids, Michigan. Her book *Connected Lives* (2004) traces the account of human nature found in an ethics of care. Other recent publications include *Philosophy, Feminism, and Faith* (2002), coedited with Marya Bower, as well as essays on liberal feminism, bioethics and care theory, and nurse/client relationships.

AL-YASHA ILHAAM, Ph.D., is a women's health activist specializing in ecofeminist theory, HIV/AIDS advocacy, and reproductive justice. She is an associate professor of philosophy in the Department of Philosophy and Religious Studies at Spelman College in Atlanta, Georgia, and she was a Fulbright Scholar at the University of Buea in Cameroon, Central Africa, in 2008–09.

CATRIONA MACKENZIE received her Ph.D. from the Australian National University and is currently professor of philosophy at Macquarie University, Sydney, Australia. Her main areas of research are moral psychology, applied ethics, and feminist philosophy. She is coeditor of *Relational Autonomy: Feminist Perspectives on Autonomy, Agency and the Social Self* (2000) and of *Practical*

Identity and Narrative Agency (2008). In 2007, she was awarded the Australian Museum Eureka Prize for Research in Ethics.

MARY B. MAHOWALD, Ph.D. (philosophy), is a professor at the University of Chicago (Illinois) in the MacLean Center for Clinical Medical Ethics and the Department of Obstetrics and Gynecology. Her books in feminist philosophy and bioethics include *Philosophy of Woman: Classical to Current Concepts* (3rd ed., 1994); *Women and Children in Health Care: An Unequal Majority* (1993, reprinted 1996); *Genes, Women, Equality* (2000), and *Bioethics and Women: Across the Life Span* (2006).

JANICE MCLAUGHLIN, Ph.D., is the executive director of the Policy, Ethics and Life Sciences Research Centre in the School of Geography, Politics and Sociology at Newcastle University, Newcastle upon Tyne, United Kingdom. Her current empirical research focuses on disability in childhood, drawing on a range of theoretical perspectives, including feminist theory and disability studies.

JESSICA PRATA MILLER, Ph.D., is an associate professor of philosophy at the University of Maine and clinical ethicist at Eastern Maine Medical Center, a four-hundred-bed tertiary-care facility in Bangor, Maine.

JING-BAO NIE, Ph.D., is an associate professor at the Bioethics Centre, University of Otago, New Zealand, and honorary adjunct/visiting professor in several Chinese universities. He is the author of *Behind the Silence: Chinese Voices on Abortion* (2005), *Medical Ethics in China: A Cross-cultural Interpretation* (forthcoming), and more than seventy journal articles and book chapters on bioethics and the history of medicine. He is finishing a coedited volume and a book monograph on Japanese wartime medical atrocities. Another major project of his current research is the ideology and ethics of China's birth control program.

MARY C. RAWLINSON, Ph.D., is a professor of philosophy at Stony Brook University, New York, and the coeditor of *Thinking with Irigaray* (forthcoming), *The Voice of Breast Cancer in Medicine and Bioethics* (2006), and *Derrida and Feminism* (1997). She has been the editor of five issues of the *Journal of Medicine and Philosophy*, including *Foucault and the Philosophy of Medicine*, *The Future of Psychiatry*, and *Feminist Bioethics*. Her publications include articles on Hegel, Proust, literature and ethics, bioethics, and contemporary French philosophy. She is the editor of the *International Journal of Feminist Approaches to Bioethics* as well as the codirector of the Irigaray Circle.

CHRISTOPH REHMANN-SUTTER, Ph.D., is a philosopher with initial training in molecular biology. He is currently a professor of theory and ethics of the life sciences at the University of Lübeck, Germany. Since 2008, he has been a visiting professor at BIOS, London School of Economics and Political Science, and from 2001 to 2009 he was chair of the Swiss National Advisory Commission on Biomedical Ethics. His research interests include philosophy and ethics of genetics and stem cell research, end-of-life care, governance issues, and methodology of bioethics from a hermeneutic perspective.

MARGARET SCRIMGEOUR, Ed.D., is a lecturer in the School of Education at the University of South Australia. She has a background in Indigenous education and Indigenous research methodology and ethics. Identifying barriers to the implementation of changed approaches to engagement with Indigenous peoples over research issues and transferring these findings into practice is her main research interest. Recent projects include qualitative data collection and analysis relating to Aboriginal and Torres Straits Islander health-sector accreditation, and improving housing responses to Indigenous patterns of mobility.

JACKIE LEACH SCULLY, Ph.D., is a reader in social and bioethics in the School of Geography, Politics and Sociology, and director of research at the Policy, Ethics and Life Sciences Research Centre, Newcastle University, Newcastle upon Tyne, United Kingdom. Her current research interests include genetic and reproductive technologies, disability, assistive technologies, and the formation of moral opinion.

RICHARD TWINE, Ph.D., is a senior research associate at the Economic and Social Research Council (ESRC-UK) Center for Economic and Social Aspects of Genomics (Cesagen), Lancaster University, United Kingdom. His writings span diverse areas, including critical bioethics, ecofeminism, posthumanism, and the social, economic, and ethical questioning of human/animal relations in the context of biotechnologies.

FIONA UTLEY received her Ph.D. from the University of New England, Australia, and is currently an honorary associate with the School of Arts at UNE. She previously worked in the field of women's health with a family-planning NGO for 10 years and taught communications for women's advocacy groups and vocational courses for 15 years.

In the early twenty-first century, we as feminist bioethicists experience a mixture of pride in how far we have come, concern about what we have not yet achieved, and fear about what we might be turning into. The aim of this volume is to bring together writers who in different ways reflect on the positioning of feminist bioethics. Some directly address the history of feminist bioethics, its epistemological and methodological foundations, and the tools it has developed for bioethical work. Others use these tools to contribute to the exploration of old and new bioethical questions. Yet others explicitly reflect on feminist bioethics' current relationship to the mainstream(s) of bioethical work and the intersection between feminism and other marginalities that are of growing importance in bioethics, conceptually and practically.

In part I, three authors examine the development of feminist bioethics and consider its contributions to mainstream bioethical debate. Anne Donchin's chapter provides a background context for this collection: she reviews the origins of feminist bioethics with a particular focus on the achievements of the International Network on Feminist Approaches to Bioethics (FAB). She outlines "where we [may be] going," identifying some of the directions in which feminist bioethical enquiry is headed in the twenty-first century.

Next Christoph Rehmann-Sutter provides a commentary on "where we have been" indicating how "the mainstream" has benefited from contributions from feminist bioethics. Using prenatal diagnosis as a case study, he performs content analysis on three successive entries in a standard work to trace how mainstream thinking on this issue has changed over the past 25 years. From his position as a sympathetic observer, he suggests that feminist bioethics could profit from reconceptualizing what is understood by "mainstream bioethics."

Richard Twine's chapter challenges the reader to "reflect on the *types* of feminism" that shape bioethics. He argues we should strengthen our relationship with feminist philosophy of science and science studies and engage with the emerging field of "critical bioethics." He also questions feminist bioethics' neglect of environmental issues and the impact of biotechnology on animals and the environment.

Part II explores the ways in which feminists have engaged with the philosophical foundations of bioethics. Three authors apply feminist analyses to provide unique perspectives on current issues in bioethics. These contributions demonstrate the flexibility and scope of feminist bioethical theory.

Catriona Mackenzie's contribution clearly sets out the feminist objections to the dominant conception of autonomy in Euro-American bioethics literature. She argues that this "maximal choice" conception of autonomy, in failing to consider the relational nature of the self and the powerful social and political forces that affect the availability of individual choice, is ultimately inadequate. She illustrates this by outlining how the maximal-choice view of autonomy is applied to some key topics in bioethics and goes on to demonstrate the value of a relational conception of autonomy in these debates.

The second chapter of this section moves to a different but equally rich area for moral inquiry: the notion of trust. Jessica Prata Miller wonders why feminist bioethicists have yet to develop an account of trust as a moral category other than within care theory. This delay is surprising because bioethicists, feminist or otherwise, are concerned with unequal power relationships between social groups or individuals, and trust (or distrust) must be an integral component of these relations. While feminist ethicists such as Annette Baier and Margaret Urban Walker have been active in foregrounding trust as a moral good and as a lens through which feminist morality in unequal relations can be viewed, bioethics has tended to view both trust and distrust as unproblematic. Miller argues for a feminist reconceptualization of trust in bioethics to capture its potential to challenge ontological and epistemological assumptions of dominant bioethics frameworks.

While the chapters by Mackenzie and Miller challenge and rework the ontological foundations of bioethics, Mary C. Rawlinson addresses epistemological concerns. Taking the 2005 United Nations Educational Scientific and Cultural Organization (UNESCO) *Universal Declaration on Bioethics and Human Rights* as her point of departure, she argues that Euro-American bioethics' invocation of universal rights is undermined by their failure to engage critically with the concept of universality. Following Luce Irigaray, she critiques the discourse of human rights, exposing the problematic conceptual underpinnings that sustain it, and argues for gendered rights that can begin to undermine bioethics' commitment to the "universal man."

Following Part II's demonstration that feminist theory provides new perspectives on the theoretical underpinnings of bioethical thinking, Part III focuses on uniquely feminist ways of *doing ethics*. While methodologies that can be identified as feminist vary widely (and indeed, are not always overtly recognized as such), for bioethics to be feminist it must be informed explicitly by the experiences of women. Unsurprisingly then, feminist bioethicists were among the first to use empirical methods in bioethics.[1] Lori d'Agincourt-Canning's chapter illustrates the requirement to base ethical work in everyday moral experience. Drawing from women's narratives of hereditary breast cancer, she considers the particularity of knowledge construction and from this, provides a feminist exploration of the harms and benefits of genetic testing.

Fiona Utley next takes up the problem of the public/private divide by addressing an issue not usually seen as within bioethics' remit. The chapter broadens our understanding of narrative to include *bodily* narratives that reveal shortcomings in the public response to traumatic events such as rape. Her analysis offers a perspective of post-traumatic stress disorder as a "normal" rather than pathological response to trauma, removing the onus of responsibility for recovery from the individual and placing it within the realm of social reform.

Janice McLaughlin's contribution is an interesting twist on the "disability critique" (Parens and Asch 1999) of prenatal genetic testing. Her chapter considers the case for parental selection for sexual orientation, defended by a number of bioethicists on the grounds of reproductive liberty. She argues against the privileging of liberal approaches in ethical debates on assisted reproductive technologies by using an analytic methodology that uncovers the false presumptions of equality and freedom to choose that underpin the liberal framework. To safeguard a fair and just society and enable different versions of the "good life" to flourish, McLaughlin also argues against the reinforcement of boundaries between public and private life. The methodological presumptions backing her analysis are an acknowledgement that the private choices of individuals have social significance, and thus that individual decisions to use prenatal screening cannot be separated from social and cultural values, which include values that are fundamentally homophobic.

In the final contribution to this section, Al-Yasha Ilhaam and Ina May Gaskin demonstrate the practice of collaboration between disciplines, which is relatively common in feminism and other disciplines but rarer in philosophical ethics. It could be argued that bioethics is always a collaborative enterprise, because philosophers and medical practitioners have together produced a substantial amount of foundational theory in mainstream bioethics. However, the tendency to see bioethics as existing to service professional medicine compromises the power of bioethical critique, while the habit of physicians to posit the "doctor-patient rela-tionship" as the locus of decision making dynamics risks reproducing patriarchal assumptions inherent in the traditionally male-dominated disciplines of medi-cine and philosophy. As Ilhaam and Gaskin show, nurses and midwives, being more intimately involved in the care of the patient but occupying low status within deeply hierarchical working environments, are in a position to impart a different professional perspective.

Part IV considers the possibility of forging relationships between feminist and other "marginal" groups in bioethics. The four contributions in this section can roughly be categorized as addressing issues of "race" and "ability." Each chap-ter explores the potential for collaboration between feminist and other social groupings.

Feminism is one of the post-Enlightenment streams of thought that has long grappled with how to account for differences between human individuals. Bio-medicine and bioethics also struggle, though in rather different ways than femi-nism, to integrate difference within a fundamentally universalizing conceptual framework. One key area of bioethics that stands to benefit from a model for incorporating pluralism is public health research ethics. Integrating difference into the understanding of health and disease requires a radical revision of domi-nant public health ethical frameworks, which largely follow traditional biomedi-cal ethics in emphasizing individualist human existence, abstract reasoning, and personal autonomy divorced from social context. Ruth Groenhout examines the political issues at stake in incorporating difference into public health research, with a focus on the inclusion of minority populations. Arguing for an ethics-of-care perspective in research, she uses the example of BiDil, the first medication to be approved for use in a racially exclusive way to treat heart failure in Afri-can Americans, to tease out the complexities of how racial and ethnic categories can cut both ways and to explore what is ethically acceptable in accommodating difference.

Jennifer Baker, Terry Dunbar, and Margaret Scrimgeour consider the possi-bilities of a collaboration between Australian Indigenous activism and feminist bioethics to facilitate reform of health care research that involves Indigenous Australians or Indigenous interests. Aware of the unpromising history of en-counter between the feminist movement and Indigenous peoples in Australia, they ask, "What sort of sisterhood can be constructed when we begin from un-equal positions within a politics that defines our racial difference yet masks its own?" Ethics and bioethics are not discernible distinct entities in Aboriginal cul-tures; rather, they are "woven through." Nevertheless, the authors identify some unexpected commonalities between care ethics and understandings of "community" in Aboriginal culture. Baker, Dunbar, and Scrimgeour sketch out the benefits and difficulties of using such commonalities to forge alliances between Indigenous and feminist bioethics.

China's birth-control program, directed towards improving the living standards of people in China, is widely touted as a success by the Chinese government. Jing-Bao Nie's chapter explores the effects the one-child policy has had on Chinese society, in particular on Chinese women. Even though more than one-fifth of women in the world are directly affected by the policy, it has so far received little attention from Western feminists or feminist bioethics. In critically examining this issue, Nie draws on feminist and Confucian insights and uses empirical and narrative methodologies to analyze the practical consequences of the policy.

The final contribution in this section provides a different example of intersection between feminist theory and the marginal experience of disability. Mary B. Mahowald draws from virtue ethics, feminist standpoint theory, and disability theory to defend a human-flourishing account of disability in place of the function-based account that dominates mainstream bioethics. Every human being has different capabilities for human flourishing that "may or may not be fostered by social circumstance." Mahowald argues that policies can be tested for the extent to which they promote equality by applying feminist standpoint theory to establish whether and how they promote human flourishing.

We came together as editors with the initial idea of inviting contributions that explore the place and positioning of contemporary feminist bioethics. Given the enormous range of topics and approaches that this embraces, and the limits of space and time, we had to make difficult decisions about focusing our attention. Thus, the result is far from an exhaustive survey, but rather a look at some dynamic growing points of the discipline of feminist bioethics today. One of our regrets is that we have not been able to include more work by feminist bioethicists from Africa, Asia, and Latin America: in the end, we realized that this is a rich area for another book. Recognizing that many readers may be new to feminist bioethics and hence unable to navigate easily through this diverse collection, we have included "bridging commentaries" between each substantive section. These attempt to link the preceding and subsequent chapters, give some historical orientation, and highlight the conceptual threads that are shared by the breadth of contributions. As editors, we have tried throughout the collection and our commentaries to underscore the internally self-reflective and self-critical nature of feminist inquiry, believing that this, as much as any theoretical feature, distinguishes feminist from other bioethical approaches.

NOTE

1. Many bioethicists have long resisted the potential of sociology to make important contributions to bioethics; however, there has been a move in recent years toward the use of empirical data to develop bioethical theory, and a body of work using sociological and other methods of gathering empirical data has developed. For examples, see note 1 in the introduction to part I.

REFERENCE

Parens, E., and A. Asch 1999. The disability rights critique of prenatal genetic testing: Reflections and recommendations. *Hastings Center Report* 29 (5): S1–22.

Our first thanks go to the International Network on Feminist Approaches to Bioethics (FAB), whose Congress in Sydney in 2004 was the catalyst for this collection. We are immensely grateful to all the contributing authors of this volume for their efforts, solidarity, and patience. Special thanks to Wendy Harris and Emma Sovich at the Johns Hopkins University Press and to Monica Buckland for organizational and editorial help in preparing the manuscript. The editors gratefully acknowledge the financial support of the Unit for Ethics in the Life Sciences, University of Basel, Switzerland, for the preparation of the index.

PART ONE

Introduction to Feminist Bioethics

PETYA FITZPATRICK, M.A., AND
JACKIE LEACH SCULLY, PH.D.

Feminist bioethics is at a defining point in its 20-year history: positioned in the tension between becoming part of mainstream bioethical thought and remaining, as it has been, a marginal voice overtly challenging a central consensus. In this collection we explore some of the insights and difficulties of that position and consider where feminist bioethics might go next. Knowing that not all readers will be familiar with the background of feminist bioethics, in this introduction we offer a basic overview of bioethics' and feminist bioethics' interwoven history and current relationship and the stance of feminist bioethics to the viewpoints from other "margins."

What Is Bioethics?

an ethics founded in and reflective of life

M. C. Rawlinson, 2001

Bioethics as a discipline emerged in the late 1960s and early 1970s and encompasses various fields of enquiry, including medical ethics, research ethics, clinical ethics, and biomedical ethics (Hedgecoe 2004). Bioethics is both practical and theoretical, responding to ethical problems arising from the practice of modern medicine, but identifiable as well by significant contributions to philosophical and moral theory. Now that bioethics is well established within academia and in the world of policy making, particularly in Anglo-European countries, there is also a growing public awareness of bioethics as a contributor to cultural life, as evidenced by a proliferation of popular literature and media on topics such as the ethics of cloning, stem cell research, transhumanism, and abortion.

Developing at a time when patient advocacy, civil rights, and human rights groups were also finding a voice (Wolf 1996), bioethics has inevitably had a strong focus on the relationships between patients and professionals in the medical and life sciences. As a result, it has been called on to provide guidelines for the protection of research subjects or for scrutinizing the tensions inherent in the physician-patient dyad. In the process, patient autonomy and justice have emerged as preeminent principles in both the bioethics literature and clinical practice.

However, the application of ethical theory in bioethics is not restricted to the realm of patient-clinician interactions. Bioethical issues, as Susan Wolf (1996) notes in her book *Feminism and Bioethics: Beyond Reproduction*, arise everywhere: in interactions between health professionals, family members, researchers, re-search participants, patients at a fertility clinic, staff at a women's shelter, aid workers in a developing country, beyond the consulting room or hospital bed to the home, the courts, and the medical laboratory. Furthermore, the focus of con-cern extends beyond patients (or clients) to individuals not currently receiving a service or even to individuals not yet in existence. The multidisciplinarity of bioethics reflects this wide range of concerns. Broadly construed, today's bioeth-ics is not solely the province of philosophers: its practitioners come from a vari-ety of professional backgrounds. They include doctors, nurses, genetic counsel-ors, lawyers, environmental scientists, life scientists, anthropologists, social scientists, and theologians. Some would also include the "ordinary bioethicists" (Scully, Banks, and Shakespeare 2006), that is, the lay public in its encounters with bioethical issues.

Despite this breadth of scholarly involvement, bioethics has frequently been criticized for failing to draw on an adequately wide range of resources to de-velop bioethics theory. What has generally become known as "mainstream bio-ethics" has been largely shaped by the theoretical and methodological frame-works dominant in the analytic traditions of Western moral philosophy: primarily Kantian deontology or utilitarianism, or the practice-oriented princi-plism of Beauchamp and Childress (1994). In response to the perceived short-comings of these frameworks in tackling bioethical problems, other theories and methods have emerged. These include a revival of Aristotelian virtue ethics, moral sentiment theory, pragmatism, narrative, and communitarian ethics. Moreover, the social sciences have brought their voice to discussions on shaping bioethics theory, calling for more empiricism in bioethics.[1] Among the strongest of the innovative strands within bioethics, both substantively and numerically, is feminist bioethics.

What Is Feminist Bioethics?

Feminist bioethics starts from the premise that dominant ways of doing bioethics are *fundamentally* gendered and that they thus contribute to culturally inscribed oppressive practices. Feminist bioethicists claim that mainstream ways of doing bioethics marginalize women's interests and relegate women (and other socially and politically vulnerable people) to a position of moral inferiority. This occurs in two ways. First, the *subject matter* of bioethics often reflects, wittingly or not, masculine experience and masculine priorities. Second, the *ontological and epistemological foundations* of bioethics currently privilege ways of being and knowing that are culturally masculine, and thus inherently devalue that which is (culturally constructed as) feminine.

The most plainly visible feminist work in bioethics has dealt with issues related to women's health: abortion, surrogacy, and assisted reproductive technologies (Warren 1985; Overall 1987; Rowland 1987; Warren 1988; Dodds and Jones 1989; Anderson 1990). However, from the earliest days, other issues such as end-of-life decision making, genetic and embryo research, sexuality, and violence also appeared in feminist writings. More recently, intimate relationships, the emotions, the experience of embodiment, childrearing, caring for the sick and elderly, and other topics that have tended to be dismissed from serious consideration by mainstream bioethics are now established as important and worthy of analysis by feminist scholars.

Feminist inquiry in bioethics is also political: its attempts to address fundamental questions about the nature of knowledge, philosophical method, and subjectivity are with the aim of improving women's lives in the real world. Hence, it makes explicit, and critiques, oppressive and exclusionary practices in mainstream bioethics and seeks to provide nonoppressive, nonexclusionary alternatives. Where mainstream bioethics has been skilled at analyzing particular kinds of power differentials, notably in the asymmetry between doctor and patient, feminist bioethics has been able to spot the nuances of gendered or raced relationships—between different kinds of patient or doctor—and how social positioning inflects the ethics of their interactions. Feminist bioethics has made it a priority to move the analytic gaze beyond the clinic or laboratory to consider the social and political contours of moral responsibility.

To practice bioethics in a feminist fashion is thus to deliberately engage with power relations inherent in ways of knowing and being in philosophical thought. As Lorraine Code (1991) noted, philosophy "oppresses women in ways which feminists are still learning to understand." Any systems of philosophical knowledge, including bioethics and feminist bioethics, must then, by extension, be treated with suspicion. Feminist bioethics is therefore explicitly self-reflexive and self-critical, engaged in an internal dialogue that creates richness and complexity, as well as tensions and divisions.

Such tensions and divisions reflect feminist bioethics' internal heterogeneity. There are many different approaches within feminist bioethics to both theory and practice. These might be loosely classified under headings such as liberal, socialist, "feminine" (for example, the work of Nel Noddings or Sara Ruddick), or postmodern (for example, Margrit Schildrick), but even this categorization does not convey adequately the diversity of scholarship. While it can be said that most feminists are united in their dissatisfaction with current emphasis on abstract principles or claims to universal objectivity, their means of addressing feminist concerns vary tremendously. Some writers have devoted their energies to reformulating nonexclusionary bioethical principles, in particular, autonomy (Donchin 1995; Sherwin 1998; Mackenzie and Stoljar 2000), justice (Okin 1989; Young 1990), and trust (Baier 1986; McLeod 2002). Others (Nelson 1997) have explored the potential for innovative methodologies, such as narrative ethics, to convey the subtleties of ethical dilemmas. Care theory is perhaps the best known of distinctly feminist theories in bioethics, sharing many features with virtue ethics (Groenhout 2004). Often explained as an alternative to "justice-oriented" theories (Held 1995; Walker 1998), care ethics and related theories emphasize the (inter)connectedness of moral actors and the importance in moral decision making of intimate relationships.[2]

Despite these overlaps, however, many women have not seen themselves or their interests as being represented by feminist bioethics and have wholly or partly disassociated themselves from "western, white, middle-class feminism" (Lugones and Spelman 1983). Race, class, sexuality, ability, religion, and age must affect gender-based analyses, and it has become apparent that feminism, despite claims to the contrary, often represents only a narrow group of Anglo-Saxon, educated, middle-class women. Similarly, feminist bioethics is accused of presuming a commonality of moral experience, identity, and knowledge among women, and in doing so has marginalized or excluded that which does not fit white Western ways of being and knowing. This has hitherto reinforced oppressive social structures by allowing the most privileged to direct the feminist bioethical agenda. These criticisms of feminism and feminist bioethics are an uncomfortable echo of those directed by feminists toward mainstream bioethics itself.

Because of the differences among women about what feminism is, what feminism should do, and, indeed, the meaning of "you," "us," and "them" in feminism, many recent writers have begun to speak circumspectly of "feminisms," explicitly or implicitly to avoid representing their perspective as a universal, monolithic theory.

The Mainstream and Feminist Bioethics: From the Outside Looking In

Standard bioethics texts of 10 or 20 years ago rarely, if at all, mentioned feminist bioethics, and feminist approaches are still not considered an integral part of the mainstream as indicated by bioethics anthologies published within the last decade. Yet, feminism is increasingly regarded as offering legitimate *alternative* or *additional* perspectives and analyses. Kuhse and Singer's *Companion to Bioethics* (2001) and *Bioethics: An Anthology* (1999), for example, both include single chapters by feminist bioethicists; the fifth edition of Beauchamp and Childress's *Principles of Biomedical Ethics* (2001), while not addressing feminist bioethics per se, does contain a section on the ethics of care; the third edition of the *Encyclopedia of Bioethics* (Post 2003) contains entries on feminism and women; the online *Stanford Encyclopedia of Philosophy* (Zalta 2007) contains 137 entries relating to feminist branches of philosophy, including an entry on feminist ethics and a separate entry on feminist bioethics; and a recent collection, *Case Analysis in Clinical Ethics* (Ashcroft et al. 2005), contains one chapter on feminist care ethics, out of eleven dealing with a range of approaches.

Represented, however, as an "alternative" viewpoint, the inclusion of feminist perspectives can seem like tokenism. In bioethics texts, the feminist perspective on philosophical problems is still too often consigned to a chapter entitled something like, "The Feminist View"; and feminist bioethicists are often called on to comment on "women's matters," such as surrogacy and prenatal testing. So it seems that, within mainstream ethics, there is still little understanding of what feminist bioethics is. By way of illustration, care ethics is often taken to be synonymous with feminist ethics (as, for example, in the Ashcroft et al. volume mentioned above). Yet in reality, while some feminist ethicists are proponents of care ethics, others have leveled strong criticism against it, arguing that it is "feminine" rather than "feminist" ethics (Tong 1993). Misrepresentations such as this, in combination with simple lack of exposure, mean that there remains little awareness among mainstream bioethicists of the sophistication and complexity of feminist bioethical theories and methodologies.

Feminist Bioethics and the "Mainstream": From the Inside Looking Out

On the other hand, it must also be recognized that some feminist critics have tended to treat the theories and practices of mainstream bioethics as more mono-lithic than they really are. "Mainstream bioethics" is an ill-defined entity. The term is often used as shorthand to indicate a particular kind of secular and liberal-based bioethics, although it could also refer to more communitarian-oriented theories. In general, "mainstream" loosely refers to prevailing theories and practices in bioethics that are not feminist and that are therefore felt to be oppressive of women and other marginalized groups in their foundations. Clearly, there are difficulties involved in such diffuse and oversimplified labeling. Nevertheless, it is useful to retain this terminology in a pragmatic sense to indicate those modes of doing bioethics that are rooted in more traditional philosophical viewpoints and whose moral language is less able to articulate feminist concerns.

Notwithstanding these barriers, misperceptions, and exclusions, the work of feminist bioethicists is appearing more frequently in nonfeminist publications; collaboration goes on between feminist and nonfeminist bioethicists; and non-feminist bioethicists are acknowledging and using feminist theories. Insofar as the feminist goal of widespread consciousness-raising outside of its own circle is concerned, feminist bioethics appears to be on the right path. However, such growing acceptance is accompanied by fears that the critique provided by feminism's "radical edge" will be blunted as it becomes part of the bioethical es-tablishment. A key concern is that feminist insights, priorities, theories, and methodologies will thereby be diluted, because (it is argued) at least some of the analytical force of feminist bioethics stems from its intellectual and political loca-tion on the margin. At the same time, there is a complementary fear of feminist bioethics' ghettoization if it remains so marginal. This is entangled with the com-plex problem of self-definition: if feminist bioethics remains on the margins, identified with a group of radical outsiders, must its self-understanding always be defined over and against those modes of bioethics it critiques, paradoxically bound to the language and structures that it seeks to transform?

Feminism and "Other Margins"

Others, located like women in the social interstices of power, have added their voices to bioethical debate. Indeed, feminist bioethics sometimes overlaps with other social and cultural margins, such as disability, sexual orientation, and race;

much more is said about this in part IV. Ultimately, feminist bioethics must continually renegotiate its engagement with the mainstream, including an accommodation of the latter's growing pluralism. Often this provides opportunities for creative partnerships and collaborations, while also challenging feminist theory's commitment to continual reevaluation as its relationship with mainstream bioethics and with other "marginal voices" changes.

With this background to hand, then, we begin by looking at recent developments in feminist bioethics, focusing first on its history and then on two examinations of its relationship with canonical bioethics and with another new field shaped by feminist thought: science and technology studies.

NOTES

1. For examples of contributions to the development of bioethical theory from social scientists, see De Vries (2004), Hedgecoe (2004), Lopez (2004), Sugarman (2004), and Hoeyer (2006).

2. A concern among some feminists is that care theory pays insufficient attention to the political dimensions of morality, and theorists are now attempting to reconcile care ethics with attention to unequal power relations.

REFERENCES

Anderson, E. S. 1990. Is women's labor a commodity? *Philosophy and Public Affairs* 19 (1): 71–92.

Ashcroft, R., A. Lucassen, M. Parker, M. Verkerk, and G. Widdershoven. 2005. *Case studies in clinical ethics*. Cambridge: Cambridge University Press.

Baier, A. 1986. Trust and anti-trust. *Ethics* 96:231–60.

Beauchamp, T. L., and J. F. Childress. 2001. *Principles of biomedical ethics,* 5th ed. New York: Oxford University Press.

Code, L. 1991. *What can she know?* Ithaca, N.Y.: Cornell University Press.

De Vries, R. 2004. How can we help? From "sociology in" to "sociology of" bioethics. *Journal of Law, Medicine and Ethics* 32 (2): 279–92.

Dodds, S., and K. Jones 1989. Surrogacy and autonomy. *Bioethics* 3 (1): 1–17.

Donchin, A. 1995. Reworking autonomy: Toward a feminist perspective. *Cambridge Quarterly of Healthcare Ethics* 4 (1): 44–55.

Frye, M. 1991. A response to lesbian ethics: Why ethics? In *Feminist ethics,* ed. C. Card, 52–59. Lawrence: University of Kansas Press.

Groenhout, R. E. 2004. *Connected lives: Human nature and the ethics of care.* Lanham, Md.: Rowman & Littlefield.

Hedgecoe, A. M. 2004. Critical bioethics: Beyond the social science critique of applied ethics. *Bioethics* 18 (2): 120–43.

Held, V. 1995. *Justice and care: Essential readings in feminist ethics.* Boulder, Colo.: Westview.

Hoagland, S. L. 1988. *Lesbian ethics.* Palo Alto, Calif.: Institute of Lesbian Studies.

Hoeyer, K. 2006. The power of ethics: A case study from Sweden on the social life of moral concerns in policy processes. *Sociology of Health and Illness* 28 (6): 775–801.

Kittay, E. F. 1999. *Love's labor: Essays on women, equality, and dependency.* New York: Routledge.

Kittay, E. F., and E. Feder 2002. *Theoretical perspectives on dependency and women.* Lanham, Md.: Rowman & Littlefield.

Kuhse, H., and P. Singer, eds. 1999. *Bioethics: An anthology.* Blackwell Philosophy Anthologies. Oxford: Blackwell.

———. 2001. *A companion to bioethics.* Blackwell Companions in Philosophy. Oxford: Wiley Blackwell.

Lopez, J. 2004. How sociology can save bioethics… maybe. *Sociology of Health and Illness* 26 (7): 875–96.

Lugones, M., and E. Spelman 1983. Have we got a theory for you! Feminist theory, cultural imperialism, and the demand for "the woman's voice." *Women's Studies International Forum* 6 (6): 573–81.

Mackenzie, C., and N. Stoljar, eds. 2000. *Relational autonomy: Feminist perspectives on autonomy, agency and the social self.* Oxford: Oxford University Press.

McLeod, C. 2002. *Self-trust and reproductive autonomy.* Cambridge: MIT Press.

Mendus, S. 1993. Recent work in feminist philosophy. *Philosophical Quarterly* 43 (173, Special issue: Philosophers and philosophies): 513–19.

Nelson, H. L. 1997. *Stories and their limits: Narrative approaches to bioethics.* New York: Routledge.

Okin, S. M. 1989. *Justice, gender, and the family.* New York: Basic Books.

Overall, C. 1987. *Ethics and human reproduction: A feminist analysis.* Boston: Allen & Unwin.

Post, S. G., ed. 2003. *Encyclopedia of bioethics.* Andover: Gale Cengage Learning.

Rowland, R. 1987. Making women visible in the embryo experimentation debate. *Bioethics* 1 (2): 179–88.

Scully, J. L., S. Banks, and T. Shakespeare. 2006. Chance, choice and control: Lay debate on prenatal social sex selection. *Social Science and Medicine* 63:21–31.

Sherwin, S. 1998. A relational approach to autonomy in health care. In *The politics of women's health: Exploring agency and autonomy,* ed. Feminist Health Care Ethics Research Network, 19–47. Philadelphia: Temple University Press.

Sugarman, J. 2004. The future of empirical research in bioethics. *Journal of Law, Medicine and Ethics* 32 (2): 226–31.

Tong, R. 1993. *Feminine and feminist ethics.* Belmont, Calif.: Wadsworth.

Walker, M. U. 1998. *Moral understandings: A feminist study in ethics.* New York: Routledge.

Warren, M. A. 1985. *The case for freedom of choice. Gendercide: The implications of sex Selection.* Totowa, N.J.: Rowman & Allanheld.

———. 1988. IVF and women's interests: An analysis of feminist concerns. *Bioethics* 2 (1): 37–57.

Wendell, S. 1996. *The rejected body: Feminist philosophical reflections on disability.* New York: Routledge.

Wolf, S. M. 1996. Introduction: Gender and feminism in bioethics. In *Feminism and bioethics: Beyond reproduction,* ed. S. M. Wolf, 3–43. New York: Oxford University Press.

Young, I. M. 1990. *Justice and the politics of difference.* Princeton, N.J.: Princeton University Press.

Zalta, E. N., ed. 2007. *The Stanford encyclopedia of philosophy.* http://plato.stanford .edu/archives/win2003/entries/davidson.

CHAPTER ONE

The Expanding Landscape

Recent Directions in Feminist Bioethics

ANNE DONCHIN, PH.D.

My aim in this chapter is to look both backward and forward, to review the background against which feminist bioethics emerged, draw together the accomplishments of the International Network for Feminist Approaches to Bioethics (FAB), and anticipate future feminist bioethics scholarship and activism.

Historical Origins of Feminist Bioethics

By way of preface, I would like to acknowledge the debt feminist bioethicists owe to those generations of women who preceded them—reaching back to the health care activists who predate the 1960s resurgence of feminism. Women have a long history of interest in health care issues. This history antedates the seizure of control of the practices of midwifery and nursing by the medical profession.[1] These influences fostered the protest movements of the 1960s. That revival reinvigorated and extended longstanding concerns and directed attention to areas of health care where women's interests were most severely neglected—access to birth control and abortion, pregnancy, and representations of female sexuality. Then increasing medicalization and commodification of women's bodily functions intensified the need for vigilance and called attention to the sexist biases in medical research and practice. Protest against the widespread exclusion of women from clinical trials in the United States swelled momentum still further. Feminists in many countries campaigned for increased breast cancer research, more convenient and cheaper contraceptive methods, research on the physiology of menopause, and elimination of unnecessary surgical interventions, particularly hysterectomies, cesarean sections, and radical mastectomies. Advocacy groups struggled to raise public awareness of women's health issues, influence health policy, and act as a counterforce to organized medicine and the pharmaceutical industry.

Feminist scholars began to complement the agendas of health care activists, and some straddled both scholarly and activist communities. They documented the erosion of abortion access, presumably secured by the 1973 *Roe v. Wade* Supreme Court decision, and critiqued childbirth practices that sacrifice the interests of the birthing woman to the convenience of her obstetrician and the allegedly independent "right" of her fetus. By the 1980s, feminist bioethics scholarship was being widely circulated in feminist publications (e.g., Holmes, Hoskins, and Gross 1980, 1981; Corea 1985a). A sprinkling of this effort was surfacing in bioethics journals (e.g., Whitbeck 1981; Young 1984). Feminist commentary on innovative reproductive interventions was burgeoning (e.g., Arditti, Klein, and Minden 1984; Corea 1985b; Stanworth 1987). Bioethics courses were proliferating and increasing the market for bioethics texts, but few included articles by feminists. Editors had a growing body of feminist literature on which to draw, but stereotypes persisted. Feminist approaches were often mistakenly assumed to address "women's concerns"—a special ethics for women. Feminist contributions to the leading texts were confined principally to treatment of reproductive issues—abortion, maternal-fetal relations, and reproductive technologies. Interconnections between these issues and more pervasive bioethical concerns tended to be ignored (Wolf 1996).

Against this background, FAB was founded at the initial conference of the International Association of Bioethics in 1992. FAB has sought to provide a congenial home for feminists working in marginalized areas of bioethics, to encourage international cross-fertilization, and to influence the agenda of mainstream bioethics. FAB has worked to foster development of a more inclusive theory of bioethics at both the academic and the grassroots levels, to integrate into bioethical theory concerns about race, class, ethnicity, and gender; to reexamine the guiding principles of bioethics; and to create new strategies and methodologies that are responsive to the positions of socially marginalized people. FAB's central focus includes adaptation of the theoretical grounding of bioethics to more fully reflect key components of moral life that structure physician-patient and researcher-subject relationships, power differences that mark these relationships, and cross-cultural perspectives on bioethical issues that reflect intersections between specific technologies and the social, political, and economic structures in which they are embodied.

The founding of FAB coincided with the appearance of a critical mass of feminist bioethics scholarship. In 1992 a collection of articles previously published in the journal *Hypatia* was brought out as *Feminist Perspectives in Medical Ethics,* edited by Helen Bequaert Holmes and Laura Purdy. Susan Sherwin published *No Longer Patient: Feminist Ethics and Health Care,* the first book-length treatment of feminist bioethical theory (1992). In this groundbreaking work, Sherwin expanded feminist bioethics in new directions that circumvented the prevalent theoretical approaches of the dominant bioethics framework and demonstrated its shortcomings. Volumes by Susan Bordo (1993) and Mary Mahowald (1993) critiqued medical and cultural attitudes toward women's bodies. Susan Wendell's *The Rejected Body* (1996) pressed this theme further, showing how cultural attitudes toward the body contribute to the stigma of disability and denial of the body's inevitable weaknesses.

Soon bioethics think tanks and journals began to recognize feminist approaches. Several journals featured special issues by feminist scholars spanning a cluster of topics including AIDS, reconfiguration of the principle of autonomy, gender issues in psychiatry, and global dimensions of feminist bioethics. Bioethics conferences in a number of countries began to schedule sessions that explicitly addressed feminist bioethics, and more feminists were gaining inclusion in the general program. In 1994 bioethicists in China held the first of a series of conferences featuring feminist approaches. However, the dearth of feminist representation on governmental panels formulating public policy, particularly in English-speaking countries, changed remarkably little. A group of Canadian feminists addressed this omission from the perspective of their own efforts to influence government policy. In an illuminating collection of essays, they related their frustrations following the completion of projects funded by Canadian governmental agencies. They enumerated obstacles to implementation of published reports that hinder policy reforms and revamped practices (Sherwin et al. 1998).

FAB Publications

The present volume brings to five the number of anthologies that have grown out of presentations at former FAB conferences. The initial volume (Donchin and Purdy 1999) calls attention to the traditional mind/body dualism, specifically its tendency to delegitimize women's cognitive and emotional lives by focusing only on representations of women's bodily functions. Contributors to the second volume (Tong, Anderson, and Santos 2001) seek to transcend the usual dichotomies dividing the contemporary world into developed/developing economies and technological/nontechnological societies to address a broad array of concerns that pave new ground where feminist work intersects global features of the human condition.

The 2004 volume (Tong, Donchin, and Dodds) draws on and extends human rights discourse affecting global health and amplifies debate about global ethics. It takes account of a number of considerations that are infrequently addressed in the bioethics literature, including the economic, social, and political effects of globalized capitalism and the need to negotiate tensions between cultural imperialism and cultural relativism. Contributors demonstrate the ability of explicitly feminist approaches to transcend meta-ethical conflicts between essentialism and relativism and extend feminist analysis to the needs of marginalized people across diverse economies. Some articles examine the ways in which national policy, innovative reproductive therapies, and international trade and foreign policy shape women's reproductive choices and alternatives. Others explore the possibilities and risks of developments in genetic research, critically assessing the effects of patents that extend private property rights over human genetic material. They assess the benefits to private corporations from exclusive rights and privileged access to peoples' common genetic inheritance. And they show how people, especially in developing economies, will be excluded from the diagnostic benefits of genetic screening programs. Other contributors address the human rights challenges confronting health-policy makers in the face of HIV/AIDS.

All of these volumes are the fruit of collaboration between feminist bioethicists in the advanced industrialized countries and their colleagues in transitional areas of the world. They document the ways dominant Western technological practices are crossing geographical boundaries and leading developing economies to mimic morally dubious Western technological practices, thereby diverting scarce resources from efforts to extend basic health care services and rein in preventable morbidity and mortality. Of particular concern are the problematic moral consequences for those who lack the power to alter externally imposed conditions that control their lives.

To encourage more work in feminist bioethics and disseminate it more widely, FAB has established its own journal, the *International Journal of Feminist Approaches to Bioethics (IJFAB)*. The initial issue appeared in spring 2008. *IJFAB* carries forward and extends the themes developed in prior collections based on papers delivered at FAB conferences. The journal provides a new forum within bioethics for feminist thought and debate. *IJFAB* considers papers approaching any problem or topic in bioethics from the resources of feminist scholarship and encourages proposals for special thematic issues.

Further Developments in Feminist Bioethics

FAB publications overlap and complement other feminist contributions to the bioethical literature. A particularly active area of feminist interest concerns the rapid pace of genetic research and the need to counterbalance the effusive claims of enthusiasts who extol the rosy future that expanding genetic knowledge will bring to humankind. The scope of feminist interest ranges over a broad array of issues, including sex-selection techniques, genetic ties to children, disabilities, genetic testing and screening, abortion, discrimination in health insurance and employment, and human cloning. Of immediate concern are two issues: the burdens genetic interventions impose on women to use prenatal techniques to produce only "perfect" children, and intensified stigma if future children happen to be born with disabilities. Many of these issues overlap concerns feminists have voiced in other contexts, such as the impact of caregiving responsibilities on the caregiver and the bearing of economic policies on marginalized groups. They offer proposals to minimize the threat of intensified inequalities, such as including within policy making bodies representatives of affected groups (e.g., people with disabilities and breast cancer survivors). Some are expanding into interrelated fields such as public health ethics (Rogers 2006) and international bioethics policy (Rawlinson and Donchin 2005; Eckenwiler et al. 2008).

The search for a more compatible grounding for bioethics theory has led in several directions. Some favor dispensing with principles entirely and reconstituting bioethics through narrative case-specific interpretation. Others, taking their cues from Continental feminist thought, emphasize the masculine markings of the supposedly generic human subject. Still others deploy poststructuralist and postmodern theory to discredit universal claims and build a more particularist feminist framework. Yet many remain persuaded that a framework incorporating universal principles at some level of generality should constitute one dimension of an adequate bioethical theory provided its principles are formulated in nonexclusionary terms and reflect the relational contexts of individual and group life. They draw on two themes in feminist theory. The first stems from attention to an ethics of care and the second from reflections on the sources of women's subordination in patterns of domination and oppression.

Out of these multiple, sometimes clashing, perspectives, a new orientation has been emerging that draws on debates about care and justice. Initially, care theorists distrusted traditional moral principles and pressed for an ethics that stresses alternative values such as love, care, and responsibility that capture contextual subtleties and relational bonds. In their judgment, principle-oriented frameworks are too abstract to encompass such perspectives. But others voiced doubts about the adaptability of a care ethic to some of the concerns of feminist bioethics. Susan Sherwin pointed to connections between care ethics and a long academic tradition that views women as having a distinctively different character than men. This orientation, she observed, lacks an explicit political perspective toward patterns of domination and oppression that affect women (Sherwin 1992, 42–49). Many now share this concern. They do not wholly reject an ethics that encompasses caring relationships but stress the need to complement it with a framework that includes considerations of justice suitably reconfigured to circumvent the tendency to abstract generalization that has been so pronounced within the dominant bioethics framework.

Feminist bioethicists who have been responsive to this criticism have looked to cues from feminist theorists such as Sara Ruddick (1989), Virginia Held (1993, 1995, 2005), and Joan Tronto (1993). Their work exemplifies the tendency to modify and extend features of a care ethic beyond resolution of interpersonal problems to the social and political issues that require more generalized principled treatment. Rosemarie Tong emphasizes the extent to which justice and care are intertwined on a practical level (1997). She points out that caring values count heavily in providing high-caliber health care. Yet, as Virginia Warren (1992) so cogently observes, the caring tasks of medicine have been demeaned as mere "housekeeping issues" that garner little interest and even less remuneration, while "crisis issues" dominate attention and reward their practitioners handsomely.

More recent work seeks to bring increased attention to this situation, particularly insofar as it affects those who require extended care. Both Jennifer Parks's *No Place Like Home: Feminist Ethics and Home Health Care* (2003) and Rosalind Ladd and her coauthors' *Ethical Issues in Home Health Care* (Ladd, Pasquerella, and Smith 2002), address an issue of alarming proportions for the welfare of the aging and homebound. They bring to their task much recent feminist work on both justice and care. Several other feminist bioethicists have joined the growing company of disability scholars who adapt features of care ethics conjoined with issues of justice to a range of themes intersecting disability (see, for example, Silvers, Wasserman, and Mahowald 1999; Parens and Asch 2000).[2]

Other care-related work branches off in further directions. Ruth Groenhout's *Connected Lives: Human Nature and the Ethics of Care* (2004) combines a care perspective with virtue theory. She teases out structural similarities between an ethics of care and bioethical theory to support a feminist bioethics that attends to the holistic nature of human persons, their particular social contexts, and the centrality of emotional responses in ethical reasoning. She insists that actions should not be judged apart from the lived narrative that confers meaning on them and the contexts, social locations, and power imbalances that influence the provision of care.

A related stream of feminist theorizing centers around the advantages of retaining a conception of autonomy within bioethics that is framed more robustly than the narrow conception common in the mainstream bioethics literature. Susan Sherwin and Susan Dodds point out several respects in which the dominant conception fails to fit good medical practice. First, the traditional view of autonomy directs no attention to the details of personal experience, so individuals are treated as interchangeable. Sherwin emphasizes that "if we are to effectively address these concerns, we need to move away from the familiar Western understanding of autonomy as self-defining, self-interested, and self-protecting, as if the self were simply some special kind of property to be preserved" (Sherwin et al. 1998, 35). Dodds (2000) points more specifically to a consequence of the tendency among bioethicists and physicians to reduce autonomy to informed consent and restrict its exercise in medical practice to a patient's selection of choices from a restricted set of options. This formulation of the principle fails to take adequate account of background conditions that patients bring to their medical experience and is insensitive to institutional power relationships that influence their health care options.[3] Both the options available and patient preferences are constrained by multiple pressures including physician authority, power hierarchies within families, economic disparities, and other inequitable social arrangements. Once the influence of such constraints is recognized, the need for a more nuanced conception of autonomy becomes obvious.

A number of suggestions have been put forward to reconceive autonomy in ways that would give fuller consideration to the agency of patients. Virginia Warren (2001) argues that the concept needs to be supplemented by an ethics of empowerment that gives patients access to a broader informational network that includes the perspectives of feminist activists. Others would overhaul the conception more extensively and tailor other leading bioethical principles accordingly. They emphasize the importance of encouraging patient development of autonomy capacities to balance disparities in education and prestige that distort physician-patient communication. Autonomy ought not to be viewed solely as a proficiency possessed by all competent adults, but also as an aspiration that requires moral development, social cooperation, and supportive institutions.[4] An adequate conception would make visible the ways social norms and pressures condition the choices offered to patients and stress the obligations of both health care providers and insurers to actively support patient autonomy.

This perspective shares with care theory the conviction that human agents are not fundamentally single-minded, rational, self-interested choice makers but social beings whose selfhood is constituted and maintained within overlapping relationships and communities. Recognizing the complexity of connection among individuals, their social milieu, and their cultural matrix, some feminists are now calling for adoption of a relational model of autonomy that stresses the web of interconnected (and sometimes conflicting) relationships that shape and support individuality. They point out how oppressive social environments, illness, or trauma impair autonomy and how repair depends on supportive family and community relationships. In an insightful book, *Aftermath: Violence and the Remaking of the Self*, Susan Brison (2001), drawing on her own rape experience, views the loss of connection experienced by trauma survivors as a serious threat to their autonomous selfhood. Like trauma, serious illness endangers these interconnections and thwarts autonomous pursuits. The body one has trusted to pursue one's plans and projects is shown to be vulnerable, fragile, and unprotected (Donchin 2000).

This direction of inquiry has been resourcefully extended by Carolyn McLeod (2002). She elucidates a novel conception of self-trust within a feminist theoretical framework, thereby adding a new dimension to projects that aim to reframe the dominant conception of personal autonomy in a way that illuminates its relational character. Drawing her illustrations principally from reproductive contexts including miscarriage, infertility treatment, and prenatal diagnosis, she shows how encounters with health care providers may undermine women's self-trust, thereby threatening their autonomy. She suggests how providers might reduce barriers to self-trust and why respect for patient autonomy obligates providers to be attentive to their power to influence the trust patients place in their own capacities. Her insightful analysis and well-chosen case histories invite extension of her conceptual innovations to further health care contexts.

Conclusion

Through a shared vision and cross-fertilization of theoretical orientations, feminist bioethicists have brought fresh perspectives to bioethical theory and virtually all the major topics in bioethics. Their contributions are distinctive insofar as treatment of these topics is grounded in feminist scholarship that draws on background norms and prevailing conditions that shape health options. They have disputed the adequacy of abstract universal norms and the framework of allegedly universal moral principles that have dominated bioethical theory. They point out how the reigning approach, by focusing on a generic subject, privileges the perspective of an elite, mostly male group, justifying the prevailing status quo and inhibiting consideration of constructive social change. They look toward a future when feminist thought has a more profound influence on bioethics, when the voices of the socially marginalized are fully recognized, and the needs of all social groups are integrated into a system of health care justice that is responsive to the diverse needs of humans across the globe. The overriding vision of feminist bioethics is a nonhierarchical human community committed to optimizing everyone's health and well-being.

ACKNOWLEDGMENTS

This chapter borrows from my article in the online *Stanford Encyclopedia of Philosophy* and my commentary in the initial issue of the *International Journal of Feminist Approaches to Bioethics* (Donchin 2008). Of course, it could not have been written without the enduring support of my many FAB colleagues.

NOTES

1. For a more comprehensive review of this history and references to the extensive literature on the women's health movement, see Dresser (1996).

2. Note also the symposium on Feminism and Disability in *Hypatia* 16 (4): 2001.

3. Laura Purdy (2006) describes in detail a situation where a medical institution allowed women to opt for prenatal reduction of three or more fetuses to two but not reduction to just one.

4. Mackenzie and Stoljar (2000) include in their anthology a comprehensive introduction that sorts out feminist critiques of autonomy and constructive reformulations in more detail.

REFERENCES

Arditti, R., R. D. Klein, and S. Minden. 1984. *Test-tube women: What future for motherhood?* London: Routledge & Kegan Paul.

Bordo, S. 1993. *Unbearable weight: Feminism, Western culture, and the body*. Berkeley: University of California Press.

Brison, S. J. 2001. *Aftermath: Violence and the remaking of the self*. Princeton, N.J.: Princeton University Press.

Corea, G. 1985a. *The hidden malpractice: How American medicine mistreats women*, 2nd ed. New York: Harper & Row.

———. 1985b. *The mother machine: Reproductive technologies from artificial insemination to artificial wombs*. New York: Harper & Row.

Dodds, S. 2000. Choice and control in feminist bioethics. In *Relational autonomy: Feminist perspectives on autonomy, agency, and the social self*, ed. C. Mackenzie and N. Stoljar, 213–35. New York: Oxford University Press.

Donchin, A. 2000. Autonomy and interdependence: Quandaries in genetic decision making. In *Relational autonomy: Feminist perspectives on autonomy, agency, and the social self*, ed. C. Mackenzie and N. Stoljar, 236–58. New York: Oxford University Press.

———. 2008. Commentary: Remembering FAB's past, anticipating our future. *International Journal of Feminist Approaches to Bioethics* 1 (1): 145–60.

Donchin, A., and L. M. Purdy. 1999. *Embodying bioethics: Recent feminist advances*. Lanham, Md.: Rowman & Littlefield.

Dresser, R. 1996. What bioethics can learn from the women's health movement. In *Feminism and bioethics: Beyond reproduction*, ed. S. M. Wolf. Oxford: Oxford University Press.

Eckenwiler, L. A., and F. G. Cohn, eds. 2007. *The ethics of bioethics: Mapping the moral landscape*. Baltimore: Johns Hopkins University Press.

Eckenwiler, L. A., D. Feinholz, C. Ells, and T. Schonfeld. 2008. The Declaration of Helsinki through a feminist lens. *International Journal of Feminist Approaches to Bioethics* 1 (1): 161–77.

Groenhout, R. 2004. *Connected lives: Human nature and the ethics of care*. Lanham, Md.: Rowman & Littlefield.

Held, V. 1993. *Feminist morality*. Chicago: University of Chicago Press.

———. 1995. *Justice and care: Essential readings in feminist ethics*. Boulder, Colo.: Westview Press.

———. 2005. *The ethics of care: Personal, political, and global*. New York: Oxford University Press.

Holmes, H. B., B. B. Hoskins, and M. Gross. 1980. *Birth control and controlling birth*. Clifton, N.J.: Humana Press.

———. 1981. *The custom-made child? Women-centered perspectives*. Clifton, N.J.: Humana Press.

Holmes, H. B., and L. M. Purdy. 1992. *Feminist perspectives in medical ethics*. Bloomington: Indiana University Press.

Ladd, R. E., L. Pasquerella, and S. Smith. 2002. *Ethical issues in home health care*. Springfield, Ill: C. C. Thomas.

Mackenzie, C., and N. Stoljar. 2000. *Relational autonomy: Feminist perspectives on autonomy, agency, and the social self*. New York: Oxford University Press.

Mahowald, M. B. 1993. *Women and children in health care: An unequal majority.* London: Oxford University Press.

McLeod, C. 2002. *Self-trust and reproductive autonomy.* Cambridge, Mass.: MIT Press.

Parens, E., and A. Asch. 2000. *Prenatal testing and disability rights.* Washington, D.C.: Georgetown University Press.

Parks, J. A. 2003. *No place like home: Feminist ethics and home health care.* Bloomington: Indiana University Press.

Purdy, L. M. 2006. Women's reproductive autonomy: Medicalization and beyond. *Journal of Medical Ethics* 32:287–91.

Rawlinson, M. C., and A. Donchin. 2005. The quest for universality: Reflections on the Universal Draft Declaration on Bioethics and Human Rights. *Developing World Bioethics* 5 (3): 258–66.

Rogers, W. A. 2006. Feminism and public health ethics. *Journal of Medical Ethics* 32:351–54.

Ruddick, S. 1989. *Maternal thinking: Toward a politics of peace.* Boston: Beacon Press.

Salles, A. L. F., and M. J. Bertomeu, eds. 2002. *Bioethics: Latin American perspectives.* New York: Rodopi.

Sherwin, S. 1992. *No longer patient: Feminist ethics and health care.* Philadelphia: Temple University Press.

Sherwin, S., and the Feminist Health Care Ethics Research Network. 1998. *The politics of women's health: Exploring agency and autonomy.* Philadelphia: Temple University Press.

Silvers, A., D. Wasserman, and M. B. Mahowald. 1999. *Disability, difference, discrimination: Perspectives on justice in bioethics and public policy.* Lanham, Md.: Rowman & Littlefield.

Stanworth, M. 1987. *Reproductive technologies: Gender, motherhood, and medicine.* Minneapolis: University of Minnesota Press.

Tong, R. 1997. *Feminist approaches to bioethics: Theoretical reflections and practical applications.* Boulder, Colo.: Westview Press.

Tong, R., G. Anderson, and A. Santos. 2001. *Globalizing feminist bioethics: Women's health concerns worldwide.* Boulder, Colo.: Westview Press.

Tong, R., A. Donchin, and S. Dodds. 2004. *Linking visions: Feminist bioethics, human rights, and the developing world.* Lanham, Md.: Rowman & Littlefield.

Tronto, J. 1993, *Moral boundaries: A political argument for an ethic of care.* New York: Routledge.

Warren, V. L. 1992. Feminist directions in medical ethics. In *Feminist perspectives in medical ethics*, ed. H. B. Holmes and L. M. Purdy, 32–45. Bloomington: Indiana University Press.

———. 2001. From autonomy to empowerment: Health care ethics from a feminist perspective. In *Bioethics, justice, and health care*, ed. W. Teays and L. Purdy, 49–53. Belmont, Calif.: Wadsworth.

Wendell, S. 1996. *The rejected body: Feminist philosophical reflections on disability.* New York: Routledge.

Whitbeck, C. 1981. A theory of health. In *Concepts of Health and Disease*, ed. A. L. Caplan, H. T. Engelhardt, and J. McCartney, 611–26. Reading, Mass.: Addison-Wesley.

Wolf, S. 1996. *Feminism and bioethics: Beyond reproduction.* New York: Oxford University Press.

Young, I. M. 1984. Pregnant embodiment: Subjectivity and alienation. *Journal of Medicine and Philosophy* 9:45–62.

CHAPTER TWO

"It Is Her Problem, Not Ours"

Contributions of Feminist Bioethics to the Mainstream

CHRISTOPH REHMANN-SUTTER, PH.D.

In some 35 years as a distinctive discourse (Jonsen 1998), bioethics has gone through many processes of mainstreaming, diversification, and re-mainstreaming. Feminist critics of "mainstream bioethics" have not only disturbed its concepts, methods, and practice, but also contributed significantly to what we would describe today as "the mainstream" in bioethics. What are these significant contributions? How has the (old) mainstream been transformed? And what is the ethical and social relevance of this transformation: its "genealogy" in the Foucauldian sense of the word? In this chapter I tackle these questions using a text sample from the three editions of the *Encyclopedia of Bioethics* that cover the 26 years from 1978 to 2004. As the *topos* for comparison, I have chosen prenatal diagnosis. The analysis will demonstrate the depth of the changes in how these texts conceptualize the ethical problems of this area of biomedical practice. The changes are traceable to influences from feminist ethics. However, the texts are not labeled as either "nonfeminist" or "feminist," nor are they explicitly bound to or detached from the ethical theory of liberal individualism that some feminist scholars have identified as "the mainstream" approach within bioethics. The *Encyclopedia* has been chosen as one of the most frequently used standard references for bioethical work and can therefore be seen to represent a well-accepted mainstream of argumentative resources, using "mainstream" in a discursive sense.

An Introduction to the "Mainstream"

In a review of *Gender and Bioethics*, Jan Crosthwaite wrote in 1998: "Bioethics in the 1990s is increasingly aware of the need to include the perspectives and experiences of marginalized social groups, and frequently includes feminist commentaries in its discussion of issues. However, merely presenting such perspectives is not yet integrating them into the framework of bioethics" (39). The process she describes is that of bioethicists including feminist perspectives as a result of external pressure, more or less *contre coeur*, without integrating them into those theoretical structures of bioethics that are trusted to lead to philosophically defensible resolutions of moral issues. In the 1990s, according to Crosthwaite, the theoretical framework of mainstream bioethics remained unchanged.

Bioethics' difficulty with feminism can be attributed to its early embrace of liberal individualism as the leading moral vision (see also Wolf 1996, 5):

> Liberal individualism gives priority to respect for individual self-determination or autonomy. It sees fairness and equality of treatment as requiring the impartial application of universal principles which abstract essential commonalities from the messy specificities of real individuals as fundamentally autonomous agents, aware of their own preferences and values, and motivated by rational self-interest (though not necessarily selfish). Their connections to one another are primarily through voluntary contractual relationships mediated by reason-determined codes of rights and obligations. (Crosthwaite 1998, 37)

Such an idealistic approach has difficulty in recognizing the complex relationships between individuals in the real historical world, including the deep-rooted gendered asymmetry in the distribution of power and entitlements. In Crosthwaite's characterization of liberal individualism, we recognize the basic traits of Carol Gilligan's ethic of justice that is juxtaposed with her feminist model of an ethic of care (Gilligan 1982; Kittay 2006). In criticizing mainstream ethics, feminist (bio)ethics was critically addressing liberal individualism as a theoretical framework that is structurally inhospitable to concerns about gender. A second reason for liberal individualism's difficulties with feminist bioethics lies in the claim of impartiality: an ethical solution of a moral issue requires an impartial application of universal principles. By contrast, feminist (bio)ethics explicitly adopted a standpoint and did not argue in the required impartial way.

Objections to feminist approaches to ethics, however, were unjustified for at least two reasons. First, the asymmetric distribution of power and privileges that feminism criticizes is deeply unjust by the standards of liberal individualism itself. The premise of systematically addressing one dominant injustice cannot therefore be disqualified as a valid ethical approach on the grounds of partiality. Second, the structure of impartiality in ethics cannot be taken for granted. The claimed perspectiveless objectivity could be a means to silence criticism about those claiming special insights into the world of the objective. Donna Haraway dubbed this the "god trick"; it strikes many feminists as both politically suspect and impossible to achieve (Lindemann 2004, 885).

My aim in this chapter is to detect possible transformations in the "mainstream" resulting from the impact of feminist bioethics. There is therefore a problem of defining "mainstream" in bioethics, because it would be inappropriate to exclude such a transformation even as we define the concept of "mainstream bioethics." Thus, I use the term "mainstream bioethics" here not in the sense of any substantial conceptual framework like liberal individualism but rather to indicate a range of methods, concepts, and approaches that have an accepted standing as well-reputed tools in the discourse.

In this discursive sociological sense of the term, the "mainstream" can be detected through symbols that are used in academic bioethical discourse to indicate that an approach is accepted, state-of-the-art, or well reputed. Such indicators include standard reference works, commonly used textbooks, or the selected keynote speakers at high-profile conferences. In this chapter I will use the *Encyclopedia of Bioethics* in a case study as just such an indicator of the mainstream in bioethics. It is possible to follow the selective and formative effect of this reference tool through its three editions (1978, 1995, and 2004), covering a period of more than 25 years. A disadvantage of this methodology is the arbitrariness of that choice, reinforced by the selection of only one theme: prenatal diagnosis. I use a simple hermeneutic methodology based on content analysis (Krippendorff 1980; Weber 1990). But relevant texts from encyclopedias can also be viewed as fragments of a discourse on how sexuality materializes within medically assisted reproduction (Maasen 1998; Roberts 2006). Discourses are powerful in at least three respects: (1) they are systems of inclusion and exclusion of words, issues, or narratives; (2) they define the limits and content of rationality; and (3) they shape the idea of truth (Foucault 1974). Discourses on the morality of prenatal diagnosis configure aspects of gender, moral selves, embodiment, and genetic identity and those technologically mediated sexual relationships (and social practices therein) that give genetics and reproductive medicine their specific meanings.

Prenatal Diagnosis in the *Encyclopedia,* 1978, 1995, and 2004

I chose prenatal diagnosis (PND) because it is a joint practice of science (genetics), medicine (obstetrics), procreation (mothering), and socially defined constraints (individualization of "preventive" responsibility, eugenics), in which women's experiences, moral agency, and ethical responsibility are crucial. The ethical issues in this complex arrangement of social practice can be constructed in different ways, highlighting the perspectives of one or other of the involved groups. PND is, moreover, a topic that has been thoroughly discussed from ethical perspectives by feminist scholars: "Reproduction," as Helen Bequaert Holmes and Laura Purdy (1992, xi) observe, is "the most obvious place where sex makes a difference." Hence, the need for feminist approaches was evident.

The Population and Community Perspective

The first edition of the *Encyclopedia of Bioethics*, edited by Warren T. Reich, appeared in 1978. It contained an article on clinical aspects of PND by geneticist Aubrey Milunsky and another on ethical issues by pioneer bioethicist John C. Fletcher. Milunsky's article was not restricted to purely medical topics but also covered societal and policy issues. It suggested, for instance, that PND should be applied to *all* pregnancies, a goal whose attainment was delayed in his view only by a shortage of trained personnel and facilities. Milunsky's article told how technological progress was leaving "in its wake a concerned society wrestling with the ethical and legal implications of such challenging progress" (1334). The geneticist's answer to this challenge was to explain the true "philosophy of prenatal genetic diagnosis": PND, as he puts it, does not aim to remove defective offspring but to provide "parents at risk with the option and assurance of selectively having unaffected offspring" (ibid.). This statement reinterprets a means to enable women to selectively abort affected fetuses as a means for "the provision of life for children who may never even have been born . . . The need to consider abortion after prenatal studies is . . . infrequent" (ibid.). The audience Milunsky is addressing with this reinterpretation is the "concerned society." It is obviously not the woman patient of PND, who would probably benefit little from this explanation, especially if she is one of the "infrequent" cases.

The intention to reassure concerned parts of society also manifests itself in the use of euphemisms like "therapeutic abortion" (1335) or the description of PND as disease "prevention" (ibid.). These words make sense only from the viewpoint of a population geneticist who excludes the perspective of individuals from consideration.

There is one single passage in Milunsky's article in which the word *woman* is used in relation to an ethical issue. It appears in a list of "issues concerning abortion": "should a woman with phenylketonuria (an inherited form of mental deficiency) herself be allowed to produce defective offspring in virtually every pregnancy?" (1334). These words reveal (1) a strong paternalistic attitude toward the mentally disabled woman in the example, who is treated as an irrational subject to be subjugated to a social order (should she "be allowed to?"); and (2) the maternal relationship, described in technological language as a relation of production (cf. Rothman 2000, 28). The offspring is the product, and is (3) subject to quality control: it can be "defective"—another term from the language of technology.

In other passages the pregnant woman is systematically made invisible. First linguistically: she rarely appears in the words used. The text mentions parents, fathers, fetuses, and pregnancies, but not often women or mothers. Even the option of abortion is provided not to the woman but to "parents who wish it" (1333). The invisibility of the woman *as an individual* is reinforced by iconography. An explanatory figure entitled "Major steps in establishing a prenatal diagnosis of a genetic disorder" shows no image of a woman, only an isolated uterus containing a fetus. The syringe aspiring amniotic fluid is shown entering the uterus directly through the uterine wall with no surrounding tissue, muscle, or skin. However, on the right side, there is a tiny picture of a whole male torso, donor of a blood specimen for carrier detection. The viewer sees a fetus in the uterus-vessel, a pregnancy without a woman, alongside the father in clothes.

Many of the ethical and policy issues the article discusses have a common feature: they all deal with limiting the rights and freedom of women:

- Should a woman with an inheritable disability be allowed to have children?
- Should fathers be excluded from decisions about abortion?
- Should amniocentesis be mandatory, because voluntary programs are evidently ineffective?
- Should those opposed to abortion on religious (or other) grounds be permitted to continue a pregnancy with a "defective" fetus?
- Should legislation consider tort in the case of "fetal damage"?
- Does a child have a right to be born normal and healthy?
- Who should define the criteria of "fetal quality" in borderline cases?
- Should a commitment to abort in the case of a diagnosed disorder be sought before the prenatal test?

In Milunsky's view, the answer to the last question is no. All parents have "a right to know as much information as is available on their fetus" (1335). But again, the parents, not the woman, have this right. Milunsky's defense of the autonomy to decide takes the parents as its subject: legislation for instance should not mandate the economic burdens on those parents who continue a pregnancy in spite of a diagnosis, because this would interfere with their "procreational privacy and constitutional rights" (1335).

John C. Fletcher's article that follows in the same volume has a different character. It is an extensive review of bioethical literature and obviously written for bioethicists. It covers five main topics in detail: (1) the risks of amniocentesis, (2) the issue of selective abortion, (3) the relation of PND to infanticide, (4) when to perform PND, and (5) social policy on genetic disease.

In his summary of the first topic, Fletcher adopts a population perspective: "Prenatal diagnosis serves to save life, in the sense that more normal fetuses are saved from abortions that would have been performed on the basis of unfounded genetic risk than there are at-risk fetuses aborted" (1337). Fletcher quotes two studies showing that amniocentesis does not affect the number of fetal deaths, birth difficulties, or malformations in any statistically significant way. "It is a safe procedure," in that it does not damage the pregnancy, Fletcher concludes; other ethical issues of PND may therefore be discussed independently. What is striking is not only the optimistic reading of the statistical evidence of his time, but also Fletcher's reliance on the population perspective. He does not discuss a potential *moral* difference between the death of a fetus caused by fetal anomaly and the (rare but still possible) death of a fetus caused by amniocentesis. Statistically they may be equivalent. But in terms of responsibility and guilt feelings they may appear fundamentally different, because the latter is a consequence of an action that could have been avoided. To discuss these differences would require the perspective of the individual. Second, Fletcher discusses a broad variety of ethical arguments for and against selective abortion. In conclusion, he takes a mediating position that "favors (1) acceptance of selective abortion in medically severe cases, along with a policy of financial assistance for families deliberately choosing to accept a defective infant and support for research (including fetal research) required to perfect genetic therapies; and (2) support for parents who conscientiously object to selective abortion, balanced with advocacy of malpractice on the part of genetic counselors who do not provide information about prenatal diagnosis because of their convictions on abortion" (1341). Here again, mediated by impersonal formulations, the reader sees society from an abstract moral point of view. "Acceptance," "assistance," "support," and "advocacy" are the terms delineating the favored ethical position. The disease, disability, and suffering of children are described as "medically severe," and a child with a disability is a "defective infant." The perspective of the woman who might take the decision and bear its consequences is again excluded from ethical debate.

This tendency is reinforced in Fletcher's discussion of the third topic, the moral equation of genetically indicated abortion with infanticide. Provocatively he raises the question of the change in moral status with birth: "What ought we to do about an infant born with Down's syndrome following a false negative diagnosis?" (1342). What strikes me here is that he opens this ethical dilemma from the position of an impersonal, all-encompassing "we" instead of the parents or, more precisely, the mother of the child. The dilemma is to be solved by an anonymous "we," symbolizing perhaps the moral community, the citizens of the state, or the hypothetical community of all rational subjects (*Gemeinschaft der Vernunftwesen*, in Kant's terms).

I will not pursue a detailed discussion of Fletcher's fourth and fifth concerns. They do not counteract the systematic exclusion of women from ethical discourse on PND. It is "the parents" who might wish for selective abortion in the case of sex selection or cosmetic abnormalities (like cleft palate). It is the "rights of individuals" (not the right of the pregnant woman) to decide against abortion in the case of a recognized diagnosis. Women are named openly only when Fletcher discusses the physical and psychological complications for women who undergo late second trimester abortions delayed by the need to confirm amniocentesis results. But even here the woman is not recognized as a moral subject but as a second passive patient experiencing serious complications.

Making invisible, of course, is a double-edged moral strategy. Women are excluded from the community of rational observers (or included only if they accept the role of a detached rational observer). The circle of persons concerned is generalized, and at the same time the moral and epistemological privileges of the participant perspectives are dissolved. The results of an evaluation on the level of all those generally concerned (as rational observers) are imposed on those directly and really concerned, and the moral imposition of rational observers "speak[ing] for others" (Crosthwaite 1998, 38) can no longer be detected.

The Provider Perspective

The second edition of the *Encyclopedia* in 1995 contains a much shorter article on PND by Mark I. Evans, Mordecai Hallak, and Mark P. Johnson. The paragraph on ethical implications fills only half a page (instead of 10 pages as in the 1978 edition). The part on "genetic testing and screening" ends with a separate article on "ethical issues," by Thomas H. Murray and Jeffrey R. Botkin, in which (on two-thirds of a page) some additional aspects of PND are discussed. The three subparagraphs of the genetic testing and screening article cover (1) the linkage of the two decisions to take a test and to abort, (2) screening technologies, and (3) possible mother-fetus interest conflicts.

The first discussion is intended to clarify the aim of PND "for couples who would not under any circumstances consider termination of pregnancy" (989). The way the question is introduced in the article makes it clear that for Evans, Hallak, and Johnson it is an ethical question from the perspective of the providers, the medical geneticists: "It has become a fundamental tenet of genetics that there is no linkage between the offering of prenatal diagnosis, the documentation of fetal abnormalities, and the decision of whether to have an abortion" (ibid.). The article demonstrates why knowledge gained in PND can be extremely valuable even when termination is rejected: for decreasing "levels of anxiety," to prepare for what is coming, and to optimize care of the newborn patient. The persons to whom genetic services are provided are now designated as "couples" instead of "parents." This signifies a step toward a clarified provider-client relationship, which at the time of PND is not yet the relationship to parents of a child.

Second, the article highlights the importance of technologies like ultrasound and maternal serum alpha-fetoprotein (MSAFP) screening from a public health viewpoint. Twenty percent of all chromosomal abnormalities would not be detected if PND were offered only to women age 35 or older. MSAFP screening was originally met with skepticism and anxiety "by women who previously were considered low risk and suddenly shifted to being high risk. *However, after several years of experience, patients have learned* to cope with the alteration in anxiety and, by and large, to undergo the further testing necessary to clarify their situations" (989, emphasis added). Pregnant women are perceived as a transient group of patients among whom a learning effect can be detected. This is the viewpoint of the providers of a service to the population. The individual woman participates in this group only for the duration of the pregnancy, so she cannot be the one who has learned to cope over the years.

The third issue is the change in perception of the mother-fetus relationship with the advent of ultrasound and fetal treatments. "The distinction between mother and fetus has become generally understood" (990), with the effect of elevating the ethical and legal standing of the fetus relative to the mother in conflicts of interest between the two. Obstetricians, however, "have long held the concept of having two patients—mother and fetus" (989). Thus, according to Evans, Hallak, and Johnson, the nonprofessional perception has changed, mediated by prenatal screening. Here, I do not want to challenge the truth of this statement or claim that the diagnostic technology led to a general perception of the fetus as an ethical and legal entity (for discussion, cf. Duden 1991). But again the authors' intention becomes clear: to defend prenatal screening and diagnosis against criticism from those who defend the ethical and legal status of the fetus against the mother.

The separate "Ethical Issues" article by Murray and Botkin covers genetic testing and screening together. I mention it here because it includes viewpoints that have been raised by feminist bioethicists, including first the disproportionate burden on women: "When decisions are made whether to continue a pregnancy, women must bear the direct consequences, whatever choice is made" (1006). It also notes the difficulty of autonomous choice: "The very availability of these services, in conjunction with the society's ambivalent attitude toward those with disabilities, may carry an implicit message to couples about appropriate or responsible behavior during pregnancy" (1008), or "unintended verbal cues that promote the counselor's values" may undermine nondirective counselling (ibid.).

While these points are mentioned, the authors' perspective remains external to women's experience. In coining their ethical questions they adopt, consciously or unconsciously, a provider's perspective. The health care *service* is discussed from an ethical point of view. This explains their selection of the eleven ethical issues related to PND:

1. Women typically bear a *disproportionate burden*.
2. There is a *gap* between diagnostic abilities and treatment abilities.
3. PND requires an *environment* ensuring informed decisions, emotional support, and available guidance.
4. Problems of *confidentiality* arise if, for example, nonpaternity is discovered.
5. *Access* to genetic testing and screening will become a matter of justice.
6. *"High risk"* is a value-laden concept.
7. There is a need to define *indications* for PND (risk level and severity of conditions).
8. Professionals must develop more explicit *standards* for the provision of PND services.
9. *Autonomous choice* may be difficult.
10. *Knowingly* giving birth to a seriously impaired child could be considered child abuse.
11. As therapeutic abilities improve, "a conflict will arise between responsibility to treat the fetus and respect for the autonomous refusal of the mother" (1008).

In particular, the formulation of item 11 reveals an objective perspective, in which different interests are seen to collide. The solution that Murray and Botkin offer is worth mentioning: "Fortunately, the typical desire of parents to promote the welfare of their children despite personal sacrifice should make such conflicts rare" (ibid.). For a woman (or a couple) in this situation, this solution is evidently inadequate, because the conflict will arise *because* (not in spite) of their desire to promote the welfare of their child in considering burden, risks, and side effects of an intrauterine treatment. The solution works only in an abstract universe of conflicting values and interests.

The working premises of liberal individualism that dominated contemporary philosophical approaches to bioethics fit with much less trouble into a provider's or health care system's perspective than the particular and individual perspectives of those involved. There is thus a perspectival bias inherent to liberal individualism that manifests itself in the selection of ethical issues.

Women at the Center

The third edition of the *Encyclopedia* was issued in 2004 under a new editor, Stephen G. Post. The article on prenatal diagnosis, included in a chapter on reproductive genetic testing that also covers preimplantation genetic diagnosis (PGD), differs from both its predecessors. The authors are both women: Nancy Press and Kiley Ariail. Whereas Evans, Hallak, and Johnson, comparing amniocentesis with chorionic villus sampling (CVS) in 1995, stated that the decision to terminate pregnancy is more easily made earlier in pregnancy (998), Press and Ariail additionally highlight the shorter waiting period for results following CVS than those from amniocentesis—three to eight rather than ten to fourteen days. This, they write, represents a significant advantage in the context of parental anxiety.

The chapter clearly differentiates between screening techniques and diagnostic tests, whereas in the 1995 version all methods were subsumed under "methods used for prenatal diagnosis" (see table 1 there). Amniocentesis and CVS are used for diagnosis in high-risk women, "but almost all pregnant women are offered a variety of other prenatal screening tests" (998). Basically, a screening test is "offered to a population of apparently healthy persons in order to find those few at increased risk" (ibid.). Even questions like "What is your age?" or "Is there any genetic disorder in your family?" or "What is your ethnic background?" can be classified as screening tests, because they are used to identify women at increased risk. The technological screening tests that are now standard, including MSAFP, the triple-marker screen, and ultrasound, are relatively cheap and free of risk, but they also have a high rate of false positive results. Therefore, "each additional screen raises the risk for any individual woman of getting an initial positive result at some time during pregnancy." The disturbing effects on the experience of pregnancy are reinforced because "these tests are not all done at the same time during pregnancy" (998).

A special paragraph on "prenatal screening and the experience of pregnancy" captures the dramatic transformation of the experience of pregnancy of the *low-risk* women by MSAFP "—that is, the great majority of pregnancies." Because there is no one-age screening protocol that includes all risks, "it is possible for a woman to go through a period of waiting for results of one test only to then begin all over again with testing for another condition... All of this could produce a healthy baby and a disastrously upsetting and expensive pregnancy" (1000). The authors critically discuss the argument that the tests serve in most cases to reassure anxious women: empirical data suggest that anxiety is generally relieved by a negative result. These data, however, also suggest that for some women "the anxiety persists, along with difficulty believing their fetus is healthy" (1001). Second, some feminist critics point to the "irony in which the reassurance provided by testing may be necessary, in great part, due to anxiety raised by the testing itself" (ibid.).

An important difference from the earlier editions can also be seen in the way the 2004 article introduces the issue of late abortions. Multiple-marker screening cannot be done until the fifteenth week of pregnancy, and most women are screened at 16 weeks or more: "This means that diagnostic work-up for a positive test is done toward the end of second-trimester, and a woman who wanted to terminate the pregnancy based on the results of a diagnostic test would be facing a late second trimester termination" (999).

In this account it is the woman who is the subject of prenatal care. She is also the subject of the decision about termination. But the issue is not presented as a difficult decision (as in the earlier versions) but as an issue of "facing a late second trimester termination" with all its implications. This wording provides room for the whole procedure of inducing the birth of a fetus of this size and age, actively lived through by the woman and experienced not just as an issue of contradictory values.

Apart from the general ethical issue of abortion that remains fundamental to PND (with its "bifurcated conversation in the United States"; 1001), Press and Ariail refer to three sets of ethical issues pertinent to the situations created for pregnant women. First, the meaning is often unclear for the woman concerned, because "there is a lack of clarity about the centrality of pregnancy termination to an offer of prenatal testing" (1000). Today, apart from rare cases, the only preventive measure remains termination of the pregnancy. Data suggest that the vast majority of women who receive positive results do terminate their pregnancies. And a hypothetical positive effect of PND for those unwilling to terminate lacks confirmation: "There are no empirical data demonstrating that advance preparation actually has an effect on adjustment to the birth of a child with disability" (1001). A change in terminology can be noticed in comparison with the earlier articles in the *Encyclopedia*. "Abortion" is often replaced by "termination of the pregnancy," a description that highlights what it means for the pregnant woman and avoids the terminology of criminal law.

The contestations "over the experience of these tests" refer to the question of whether PND provides reassurance as a net benefit of testing for women, or whether the reassurance provided by testing is necessitated, in great part, by anxiety raised by the offer of testing itself or by screening tests performed earlier in pregnancy. This issue was not mentioned in the earlier versions of the article.

The social implications of these tests, the third set of ethical issues, are related to the problematic relationship of individual reproductive choices to societal effects. This includes the disability critique that PND is simply a eugenic program for avoiding the birth of as many disabled humans as possible. But it also includes the limits of autonomy: "Are prenatal testing decisions truly autonomous?" (1001). Is there really an informed consent? And why do women say yes to the offer of a test? The question is not about the necessity of informed and free decisions on testing and pregnancy termination, but "about the possibility and actuality of such autonomy" (1002). There are concerns that women do not adequately understand the implications of an offer of testing despite attempts to improve the informed consent process: "Empirical data suggest that, especially *low risk* women who are offered prenatal testing in a context of routine prenatal care, are likely to conflate prenatal testing for fetal anomalies with tests which can directly benefit themselves and their fetus" (ibid.; Press and Browner 1997). It is possible "that some women would not have started down the prenatal testing path if they had truly understood the implications in terms of pregnancy termination" (ibid.). A second, broader concern is that the very existence of large-scale testing programs, together with the routinization of testing, "compromises the possibility of individual autonomous decision making" (Press and Ariail 2004, 1002).

Press and Ariail also question the argument of the previous articles that the individualization of choice is an efficient safeguard against eugenics. The question arises because there is a known aggregate effect of all free individual decisions: "the net effect might be considered eugenic" (ibid.). Is there a sound ethical difference between eugenics premised on individual, autonomous choices and other forms of eugenics? The authors do not present a final answer to this. There are bioethicists, they write, who do not consider the aggregate effect to be problematic. Press and Ariail argue that, to defend the position that eugenics resulting from the superposition of many individual free choices is not necessarily bad, a clear social consensus would be required on what prenatal tests should be available. Without "an orderly process from gene discovery to test development and then to making that test available to the public" (ibid.), decisions remain arbitrary. The authors speak for the United States, but could have spoken for many other countries as well, when they say that tests "stumble" into becoming standard care "due to medico-legal concerns," instead of a circumspect and patient-centered evaluation. Their suspicion of the ideology of autonomous choice as an overall legitimating strategy for the expansion of prenatal testing programs is thus coupled to a proposal for a transparent orderly process from genomic discoveries to the offer of tests.

In Press and Ariail's article, the perspective of the pregnant woman to whom prenatal tests are offered is significant. In the language they use, the "pregnant woman" is the explicit subject. She is offered screenings and tests; she might want to terminate a pregnancy; "women and/or couples" are supposed to make informed decisions. Some key points raised by feminist authors are made (for example, that PND has radically changed the experience of pregnancy so that it has become a round of risk detection, risk assessment, and decisions, with all the accompanying moral quandaries on the shoulders of women). This reflects the work done by Barbara Katz Rothman, Rayna Rapp, and others on amniocentesis and the "tentative pregnancy" (Rothman 1986; Rapp 1999). Women may anticipate (or experience) blame by society if they refuse testing or abortion in a case of diagnosed anomaly. The decision requiring justification to one's health care provider and one's peers is not the decision to be screened or tested or to abort, but the decision *not* to be screened or tested, or even, in the end, the decision *not* to abort.

Comparison: The Indications Issue

Tackling the same topic, the articles in the three editions of the *Encyclopedia* tell strikingly different stories about "the ethics" of PND. The greatest difference appears between the 2004 article and the previous two versions. Introducing an awareness of the genuine perspective of the women concerned, their interests and experiences (according to Sherwin, "the most obvious difference between feminist and non-feminist approaches" [1992, 100]) changes not only the list of issues addressed, but also the way they are conceptualized and resolved. I want to illustrate this by comparing directly one issue that is treated in all three versions: the "indications" for prenatal diagnosis.

Fletcher (1978) discusses the question of indications from the viewpoint of two borderline cases: parents who threaten abortion unless there is confirmation of "normality" of the fetus, and parents who request amniocentesis for sex selection. In both cases, the issue, in Fletcher's account, is whether parental anxiety or parental gender preference "is a sufficient cause for prenatal diagnosis" (1342). He singles out cases in which the life of a fetus will be saved by prenatal diagnosis, either by providing evidence for the desired normality ("since diagnosis is overwhelmingly negative" [1342]) or by showing the desired sex of the fetus ("if parents threaten abortion it would be right for the physician to comply" [1343]). Saving a life is a sufficient cause; therefore, the requests can be admitted. In this treatment, the issue of indications is understood as one of sufficient reasons for providing access to the diagnosis. Problems like this are treated within a vision of "the rationality and consistency of ethical positions" (ibid.).

The account by Murray and Botkin (1995) of the same issue is quite different. They divide the problem of indications into defining sufficient risk levels for serious conditions and defining conditions that are sufficiently severe to warrant prenatal testing. They also discuss sex selection as an extreme example that is, however, still comparable to the "host of genetic conditions" that have less-than-severe health implications or a later age of onset. They do not provide an answer but indicate the direction in which answers will be found: "Our answer as a society may depend on how much control we believe parents should have over the genetic composition of their children" (1008). I do not here have space to discuss the gene myth that manifests itself in the term "genetic composition of children" (cf. Neumann-Held and Rehmann-Sutter 2006). More important for our discussion is the confidence in a vision of ethics as dependent on the ideal of autonomy that is evident here. Ethics has the role of defending or limiting the liberty of individual (parental) decisions; the choices themselves are to be made and legitimized by the individuals (parents).

Press and Ariail (2004) do not discuss the "indications" issue as a separate topic. The problem of selecting which tests are offered to whom, however, appears as an issue of "decision-making." They observe (and complain about) "the lack of a mechanism for rational deliberative decision-making in the United States

TABLE 2.1
The indications issue of PND in the different editions of the Encyclopedia of Bioethics

Edition	Indications Issue Is a Problem of	Ethical Vision
1978 Fletcher	Sufficient ethical reasons for admission to PND	Rationality and consistency of ethical positions
1995 Murray and Botkin	How much control parents should have over the genetic composition of their children	Liberty of choice
2004 Press and Ariail	Women's agency	Open and fair procedures of decision making

about why and which prenatal tests are developed and offered" (1000). With this procedural approach to the question of indications, the authors are able to address issues of power in the decision-making processes: "Healthcare providers are the de facto gatekeepers, relying on recommendations from professional organizations, actions of insurance payers, patient demand, and their own consciences" (1002). They can introduce a critical perspective on societal contexts and effects ("Can the aggregate impact of autonomous choices be eugenic?" [ibid.]). In this framing it is possible to discuss better procedures ("an orderly process from gene discovery to ... making that test available to the public" [ibid.]) that take into account power distributions and the aggregate effects of screening and testing on the pregnancy of individual women and for society.

Table 2.1 summarizes the results of this comparison of how the indications issue is treated. An understanding of this issue as a problem of ethical reasons for admission to PND corresponds to a *rationalist* ethical vision of the soundness and consistency of ethical reasons. An understanding of the issue as a problem of how much control parents should have over the genetic composition of their children corresponds to a *liberal* ethical ideal of the freedom of choice. And the understanding of the issue as a problem of decision making corresponds to a *procedural* ethical vision of an open and fair decision-making processes. All three approaches are related to very different political philosophies. Rationalism is a political ideal in which the well-ordered society may be understood by any intelligent rational mind. Liberalism is a political ideal of a society in which the constraints that are imposed by collective bodies (like the state or society) on individuals are minimal in order to enhance autonomy. Proceduralism is a political ideal that values transparency, openness, and fairness of decision making and in which the execution of power in discourses is assessed critically. These three imply very different visions of living together in general and of implementing technology in society in particular.

The Pertinence of Feminist Bioethics

It would be an understatement to say that feminist bioethics frames the ethical issues differently. It is more than framing. Framing means three things: selection, prioritizing, and contextualizing. The "frame" selects certain things and excludes others from (literally) its "opening"; it prioritizes certain things by putting them in the middle and at the right angle; through its texture, it connects the framed vision with a background and surrounding objects and people. Feminist bioethics certainly has a strong impact on all of this. But when I compare how the indications issue in PND has been discussed in the series of three authoritative encyclopedia papers, I am inclined to say that the change was deeper than mere selection, priorities, and theoretical surroundings. The change in "the structure" of bioethics that Crosthwaite (1998) pleaded for, and that we could follow in the comparison, is in seeing the *kind* of problem. It is a change in moral perception itself.

By "moral perception," I mean the extraction and use of information about ethically relevant aspects of a situation that leads to the acknowledgment of moral or ethical issues (for perception in general, cf. Dretske 1995 and Rehmann-Sutter 1996, chap. 8). It is not that this information is lying around outside us and we just pick it up selectively. Information here is something a person *understands* (not just records as bits and bytes) and, therefore, moral perception is a practice of understanding as well, an interpretation of aspects of the situation concerned. The receptive and interpretative aspects of the practice of perception cannot be split. Both contribute to the relationship that each act of perception constitutes. With a different kind of moral perception, the subject relates itself differently to the situation. It is on this level that feminist ethics, and so feminist bioethics, starts.

Modern, pre-Gilligan ethics' preference for impersonal rules, objective principles, and universally justified duties and its corresponding ideal of moral rationality not only excluded women's perspectives from its apprehension of "ethical issues" but also tended to devalue perspectives in morality altogether. The essence of an "ethical issue" was considered to be abstract, general in form, and independent of unique circumstances, social contexts, or cultural backgrounds like gender, patriarchal social structure, or other unequal power distributions. Seeing a situation from a socially located standpoint has been classified by this approach to ethics as only secondarily important. Feminist bioethics brought women's perspectives back into ethical discourse. And at the same time, feminist scholars in bioethics defended the fundamental significance of perspective and relationships in ethical deliberations as indicators of the position from which someone is speaking.

In the defense of women's perspectives in bioethics, however, I see more than the correction of their former exclusion by mainstream discussions. The defense can make us realize that ethics is not an exchange of arguments with other minds in an abstract space of rationality. Even those philosophers who would describe what they do in such terms see and speak from somewhere: perspective cannot be eliminated. The whole strategy of elimination of perspective that underlies the fight for objectivity and universality is ethically questionable, because it tends to cover up *ethically relevant* aspects of the situations under analysis. The key aspect that is hidden in objectivist universalism is the fact that those who are doing ethics—the bioethicists—are real people participating in some way or other in the situations they speak about. The situation is created in a discourse. How ethical issues and possible solutions are conceptualized locates bioethicists within a communicative situation and relates them to others who participate or are practically affected. The method of bioethics realizes a relationship. To see and to reflect on this practice *of ethics*, bioethics needs sensitivity to the ethical relevance and normative construction of relationships.

An awareness of the unavoidable *perspective* of bioethics was in my view the first of three key contributions of feminist approaches to bioethical discourses. With it came an awareness that philosophers were and are real people doing things in real situations with other real people. Moral philosophy does not happen in a pure, rational superworld. "Good practice" in moral philosophy and bioethics means first of all being prepared to reflect and try to free oneself from prejudice and partiality. Even after recognizing the unavoidable perspectivity of ethics itself, it makes a difference whether somebody is seeing/thinking/speaking from a standpoint with or without being aware of this fact, and with or without including this fact in her or his reflections. Only an awareness of one's own perspective makes one open to recognizing others in one's concrete situations and perspectives (Benhabib 1987). The case study on PND shows that this change in attitude (or in perspective) manifests itself in a variety of concrete ethical issues that are either described differently or were not previously recognized by professional bioethicists. (The same can be shown in other fields of bioethics; see, for example, Tong 1997, part II.) But most important, the recognition of women's perspectives reveals the moral implications of neglecting them.

Barbara Katz Rothman, in her empirical work on pregnant women's perception of genetic testing, has provided concrete evidence for the existence of a whole range of ethical issues that can only be recognized by asking women how they feel and think about their experiences. I refer to just one of these. Women who had an abortion after PND reported their grief; the impossibility of that choice; the challenges to their concept of being "mature," to their morality, religion, to all of their basic values; and a deep upheaval in their moral identity, not to be confused with rejecting the technology of amniocentesis. One woman said: "You feel like you're a victim." Rothman offers an ethical analysis of this feeling of being victimized: "They are the victims of a social system that fails to take collective responsibility because we individualize the problem. We make it the woman's own. She 'chooses' and so we owe her nothing. Whatever the cost, she has chosen, and now it is her problem; not ours" (Rothman 1991, 384). The ideology of individual choice is thus more than the basic category of one of the "mainstreams" in bioethics. It is a strategy of legitimization (a biopolitical measure). Bioethics cannot claim impartiality without discussing it critically. Such discussion at an ethical level, however, is prevented by redefining women as emotional and suffering from "guilt feelings." Precluding women from the community of those who define how the ethics of biomedicine and biotechnology should be discussed avoids collective responsibility.

This move brings the social context back into the picture. A *radically contextual thinking* is a second key contribution of feminist bioethics. The criticism of individualization of ethical problems (not only as a way of thinking but as a strategy) is one consequence of contextual thinking, but there are many others. The insight that contexts are relevant for understanding an ethical issue properly, that at least some essential parts of the context are intrinsic to the issue, is old. Identification of an ethical issue is a totally different procedure than the isolation of a protein in biochemistry: it does not mean purifying it against the other components in a mixture "but rather identifying which contextual elements are *essential* for an understanding of the key moral aspects of the issue, and explaining how they establish its particular character" (Rehmann-Sutter, Düwell, and Mieth 2006, 1). Contexts can mean different things: (1) a list of conditions, the "concrete circumstances" that make up the special complexity and particularity of a case; or (2) the texture of relationships with others. There is a "relational" variant of contextualism that is different from what I call "conditional" contextualism (see Rehmann-Sutter 1999), because it implies a different account of moral commitment or obligation. An obligation, in moral relationships, is not created by reasoning but by the relationships themselves. The particularity of a situation (elucidated by contextual thinking) is not a threat to the validity of ethical obligations but rather a chance for their realization.

The special attention given by feminist bioethics to relationships gave contextual thinking in ethics a relational turn. The particular "feminist" point in relational contextualism, however, is the attention given to the gendered distribution of power in these networks of relationships. This, I think, is one of the key constituent features of the structure and contexts of practical issues in biomedicine. Without considering it we would have a false picture of the relationships that are essential for understanding the "moral character" of an issue. Without reflecting on the power components in the extended physician-patient relationship in prenatal diagnosis, to take our example, we would be unable to see what it means for individuals to decide about tests and termination. And the claim for an open and circumspect procedure of decision making about the introduction of new tests and screenings would not have ethical force.

But relationships need a critical eye. Relationships need not be good per se. An oppressive exploitative relationship is still an interconnection between human beings. To discriminate between "good" and "bad" relationships, or perhaps more realistically, to find the "better and "worse" parts in a relationship and develop the competence to transform relationships, an account is needed of their ethical structures and qualities. Which *kinds* of relationships are ethically better than others? How can participants see the differences between the strands of a relationship? Which vulnerabilities arise from the dependency that is implied by one way or the other?

Rosemarie Tong (1996) wrote about three key approaches in feminist bioethics: (1) liberal feminism, focusing on autonomous choice, reasoning largely within the liberal individualist philosophical framework but from an explicit gender perspective; (2) radical feminism, illuminating women's limited control over social institutions like health care, sexuality, or reproduction and rejecting "care" as a *prima facie* positive value because of its role as a specifically "feminine" value in patriarchal society; (3) cultural feminism that identifies itself with a feminine ethic of care. Caring relationships, in the third approach, became a critical benchmark for evaluating policies and practices: do they foster or dissolve caring relationships? (Dodds 2000, 221). However, the genitive in the title "ethics of care" can be meant in the sense of ethics drawing on the ideal of care, or of ethics taking care in a critical focus, thus leaving room for both perspectives on caring relationships that are so particularly important in understanding health care: the ethical ideal of sustaining relationships of empathy and mutual intersubjectivity (for example, Held 1993, 60), *and* the deconstructive-reconstructive approach to relationships as a field for the reformulation of ethical virtues, values, and ideals.

The third key element in feminist approaches to bioethics is their step beyond the doctrine of *autonomy as independence*. In the case study, we saw skepticism toward the possibility of autonomous choice in PND about testing or termination. On the other hand, autonomous choice was not used as an overarching legitimatory tool for the extension of PND regimes. This ambivalence toward autonomy as an impracticable ideal and yet insufficient for legitimacy, reflects the current fascinating and conceptually groundbreaking discussion that sees relational concepts of autonomy not as opposed to relatedness, but as a form of true authenticity or harmony with one's self (Meyers 1989; Kittay 1999; Mackenzie and Stoljar 2000). All of the three feminisms in Tong's terminology will have an impact here: liberal feminism probably more on the issues of coercive subtexts that are hidden under the slogans of "free and informed consent" in cultural or social contexts; radical feminism probably more in claiming control over the structure of health care systems or other institutions; cultural feminism probably most as a deepened understanding of the autonomy of the self not as a metaphysical prerequisite of "humanness" but as an accomplishment of mutual care. It is perhaps this strand of innovative thinking that changes the "structure" of bioethics most sustainably.

Conclusion

The old idea of ethics as a monochromatic ray of rationally reconstructed morality, capable of clarifying all moral problems, must be abandoned. Such a morality never existed except in imagination. Morality and ethics in their practices seem more like a multibranched river flowing around islands of established social practice and along banks of stabilized institutions, constantly changing the shape of the riverbed. The strength of ethics lies not in its capacity to reduce but in its capability to transform the conflicts and contradictions in society; the aim of moral philosophy in bioethics is not to find one set of principles but to work on a diversity of methods. Each of them is as good as the understanding it generates. A new mainstream, which includes the contribution of feminist bioethics, should be not another fortified canal but the strongest branch of an open river.

ACKNOWLEDGMENT

The author thanks Jackie Leach Scully and Suzanne Braga for helpful and clarifying comments on a draft version.

REFERENCES

Benhabib, S. 1987. The generalized and the concrete other: The Kohlberg-Gilligan controversy and moral theory. In *Women and moral theory*, ed. E. F. Kittay and D. T. Meyers, 154–77. Lanham, Md.: Rowman & Littlefield.

Crosthwaite, J. 1998. Gender and bioethics. In *A companion to bioethics*, ed. H. Kuhse and P. Singer, 32–40. Oxford: Blackwell, 1998.

Dodds, S. 2000. Choice and control in feminist bioethics. In *Relational autonomy: Feminist perspectives on autonomy, agency, and the social self*, ed. C. Mackenzie and N. Stoljar, 213–35. New York: Oxford University Press.

Dretske, F. 1995. Perception. In *The Cambridge dictionary of philosophy*, ed. R. Audi, 568–72. Cambridge: Cambridge University Press.

Duden, B. 1991. *Der Frauenleib als öffentlicher Ort: Vom Mißbrauch des Begriffs Leben.* Hamburg: Luchterhand.

Evans, M. I., M. Hallak, and M. P. Johnson. 1995. Genetic testing and screening. II. Prenatal diagnosis. In *Encyclopedia of bioethics*, rev. ed., ed. W. T. Reich, 985–91. New York: Simon & Schuster Macmillan.

Fletcher, J. C. 1978. Prenatal diagnosis. II. Ethical issues. In *Encyclopedia of bioethics*, ed. W. T. Reich, 1336–46. New York: Free Press.

Foucault, M. 1974. *Die Ordnung des Diskurses.* München: Hanser.

Gilligan, C. 1982. *In a different voice: Psychological theory and woman's development.* Cambridge, Mass.: Harvard University Press.

Held, V. 1993. *Feminist morality.* Chicago: University of Chicago Press.

Holmes, H. B., and L. M. Purdy, eds. 1992. *Feminist perspectives in medical ethics.* Bloomington: Indiana University Press.

Jonsen, A. R. 1998. *The birth of bioethics.* New York: Oxford University Press.

Kittay, E. F. 1999. *Love's labor: Essays on women, equality, and dependency.* New York: Routledge.

———. 2006. The concept of care ethics in biomedicine: The case of disability. In *Bioethics in cultural contexts: Reflections on method and finitude*, ed. C. Rehmann-Sutter, M. Düwell, and D. Mieth, 319–39. Dordrecht: Springer.

Krippendorff, K. 1980. *Content analysis: An introduction to its methodology.* Beverly Hills, Calif.: Sage.

Lindemann Nelson, H. 2004. Feminism. In *Encyclopedia of bioethics*, 3rd ed., ed. S. G. Post, 884–91. New York: Macmillan.

Maasen, S. 1998. *Genealogie der Unmoral: Zur Therapeutisierung sexueller Subjekte.* Frankfurt: Suhrkamp.

Meyers, D. T. 1989. *Self, society, and personal choice.* New York: Columbia University Press.

Milunsky, A. 1978. Prenatal diagnosis. I. Clinical aspects. In *Encyclopedia of bioethics*, ed. W. T. Reich, 1332–36. New York: Free Press.

Murray, T. H., and J. R. Botkin. 1995. Genetic testing and screening. VII. Ethical issues. In *Encyclopedia of Bioethics*, rev. ed., ed. W. T. Reich, 1005–11. New York: Simon & Schuster Macmillan.

Neumann-Held, E. M., and C. Rehmann-Sutter, eds. 2006. *Genes in development: Rereading the molecular paradigm*. Durham, N.C.: Duke University Press.

Press, N., and K. Ariail. 2004. Genetic testing and screening. I. Reproductive genetic testing. In *Encyclopedia of bioethics*, 3rd ed., ed. S. G. Post, 996–1004. New York: Macmillan.

Press, N., and C. H. Browner. 1997. Why women say yes to prenatal diagnosis. *Social Science and Medicine* 45:979–89.

Rapp, R. 1999. *Testing women, testing the fetus: The social impact of amniocentesis in America*. New York: Routledge.

Rehmann-Sutter, C. 1996. *Leben beschreiben: Über Handlungszusammenhänge in der Biologie*. Würzburg: Königshausen & Neumann.

———. 1999. Contextual bioethics. *Perspektiven der Philosophie* 25:315–38.

Rehmann-Sutter, C., M. Düwell, and D. Mieth, eds. 2006. *Bioethics in cultural contexts: Reflections on method and finitude*. Dordrecht: Springer.

Roberts, C. 2006. Enacting gender in reproductive medicine. In *Prenatal testing: Individual decision or distributed action?* ed. B. Wieser, S. Karner, and W. Berger, 87–100. Vienna: Profil.

Rothman, B. K. 1986. *The tentative pregnancy: How amniocentesis changed the experience of motherhood*. New York: Viking.

———. 1991. Prenatal diagnosis. In *Bioethics and the fetus*, ed. J. Humber and R. Almeder, 171–86. Series: Biomedical Ethics Review. Totowa, N.J.: Humana Press. Reprinted in *Ethical issues in modern medicine*, 5th ed, ed. J. D. Arras and B. Steinbock, 378–84. Mountain View, Calif.: Mayfield, 1999 (quoted therefrom).

———. 2000. *Recreating motherhood*, 2nd ed. New Brunswick, N.J.: Rutgers University Press.

Sherwin, S. 1992. *No longer patient: Feminist ethics and health care*. Philadelphia: Temple University Press.

Tong, R. 1996. Feminine and feminist approaches to bioethics. In *Feminist bioethics: Beyond reproduction*, ed. S. Wolf, 67–94. New York: Oxford University Press.

———. 1997. *Feminist approaches to bioethics: Theoretical reflections and practical applications*. Boulder, Colo.: Westview Press.

Weber, R. P. 1990. *Basic content analysis*, 2nd ed. Thousand Oaks, Calif.: Sage.

Wolf, S. M., ed. 1996. *Feminism and bioethics: Beyond reproduction*. New York: Oxford University Press.

CHAPTER THREE

Broadening the Feminism in Feminist Bioethics

RICHARD TWINE, PH.D.

This chapter was prompted by the disparity between forms of feminism practiced in feminist bioethics[1] and generally similar fields, for example, feminist science studies. The latter can be seen to adopt postmodern feminist arguments to a much greater degree. Both fields face challenges to move from the "margins to the center," yet in that very process, and due in part to the politics of that process, each field can perform its own exclusions.

Does the desire to be accepted by "mainstream bioethics" set up a dynamic as to what type of feminism is put forward? Does this lead to an exclusion of some feminist perspectives that might be less palatable to "mainstream bioethics"? Although feminist bioethics and feminist science studies are not directly comparable,[2] their degree of common subject matter renders their lack of communication in need of explanation. Some of the postmodern tools that have proved of benefit to feminism, such as the critique of the partiality of "reason" and a suspicion of "truth" and "progress," are of similar relevance to feminist bioethics. Moreover, this chapter will explore the commonalities between feminist bioethics and other critical bioethical discourses, for it would be a mistake to separate the feminist critique from other challenges to bioethics. Finally, the broadening of the feminism in feminist bioethics can have the added benefit of addressing the wider academic divide between bioethics and science studies.

Bioethics, it should be noted from the outset, is a contested field. Indeed, it may not even be a useful metaphor to conceptualize a "center of bioethical discourse" within which critical voices strive to have a presence. If, as one assumes, this proposed "center" is populated by a hegemony of abstract philosophical bioethicists who conceive of ethical theory, ethical agents, and bioethical subject matter in a particularly narrow way, it is not clear that they constitute either a center or a majority. One's impression of bioethics can change markedly, depending on which meeting or conference one might happen to attend or which journal one happens to read. Anecdotally, there was a notable difference between my experience of attending the International Network for Feminist Approaches to Bioethics (FAB) / International Association of Bioethics (IAB) World Congress[3] (Sydney, November 2004) and attending general bioethics events in the United Kingdom. Generally, there was a greater expression of interdisciplinarity and attention to issues of power in the former.

In exploring these questions, I will focus on two main strands. First, I will outline the sort of feminism deployed by feminist bioethics and think through both omissions and areas of de-emphasis, to briefly compare this to similar areas of feminist inquiry, namely, ecofeminism and feminist science studies. Second, I will locate this analysis within the wider debate taking place about the partiality of bioethics and focus especially on a new discourse of "critical bioethics." In conclusion, I will consider some of the advantages of a more pluralistic, coalitionary feminism, both to feminist bioethics and to bioethics generally.

Reflecting on Feminist Bioethics

There are concerns that in the process of striving to move to the center of bioethical discourse, feminist bioethics may be liable to compromise, or "management." This concern is important precisely because the aim should be to reconceptualize that center space rather than to be a quaint sideshow. Yet in the formation of an entity known as "feminist bioethics," there is clearly a need for nuanced reflection on which "feminism" and what "bioethics" are being deployed, given how contested each term is. I do not want to suggest that a given branch of feminist discourse is somehow better but to delve a little into the reasons for their differences. What I do want to suggest is that the best way forward for a feminist reconceptualization of bioethical discourse is to deploy a plurality of feminisms while insisting on a critical bioethics.

The sociologist David Morgan once wrote, "Sociology that ignores the question of gender is simply bad sociology" (1992, 172). Similarly, when reviewing the state of feminist bioethics in the 2001 special issue of the *Journal of Medicine and Philosophy*, Rawlinson wrote, "To ignore the results of this collection of research at this point in the history of the discussion is just not to do ethics very well... Given the body of research that goes under the name of 'feminist bioethics,' it is impossible to ignore the gender marking of the supposedly generic subject of philosophy and bioethics" (340). Both writers have been keen to emphasize the misconception that the signifier "feminist" somehow refers only to "women's issues," instead emphasizing that gender savviness is an important corrective to the assumptions of masculine universality and a way toward a more nuanced analysis of social and ethical action.

Clearly, there is a tension between the implied interdisciplinarity of the IAB definition of bioethics as the "study of the ethical, social, legal, philosophical and other related issues arising in health care and in the biological sciences"[4] and those who hold a much narrower vision of bioethics. In common with the social science critique of bioethics (see De Vries and Conrad 1998; Gervais 1998; Light and McGee 1998; Spallone et al. 2000; Haimes 2002; Levitt 2003; Hedgecoe 2004; Twine 2005), much labor has gone into reconceptualization work by feminist bioethicists, notably on alternative understandings of moral agency. Yet there is not a neat overlay between feminist bioethics and the social science critique. Consequently, it would misrepresent the diversity within feminist bioethics to portray it as simply involved in a concerted attack, in alliance with social scientists and other critical bioethicists, against some notion of a centered and hegemonic mainstream bioethical discourse. One important question to consider is where feminist bioethics positions itself on the issue of interdisciplinarity and the role of empirical research in bioethics. Although one might have said previously that feminist bioethics was as dominated by philosophers as the rest of bioethics, this is increasingly not the case.

When I first encountered feminist bioethics, my initial impression was that the feminism being discussed sat a little oddly with that being practiced elsewhere. As someone who was more familiar with feminist theories of the body, ecofeminism, and feminist science studies, I thought feminist bioethics seemed out of touch with some of the debates inspired for the most part by feminism's encounter with postmodernism. Although that impression has not totally vanished, it has become clear to me that, as feminist bioethics has developed, it has shown a pluralism that now covers a wider range of feminism.

Although wrongly stereotyped for a long time as essentialist, ecofeminism and the constellation of feminisms that theorize gender and the environment provide a good source of coalition (see Twine 2001, 50) for feminist bioethics.[5] There can be a mutual concern to widen the meaning of the "bio" in bioethics (see Twine 2005) and a related need to think widely when conceptualizing "health" so that we include what humans do to the environment as bioethical issues. An obvious anthropocentric concern here is that the mastery of nature has had deleterious effects on human health, sometimes disproportionately experienced by women, although ecofeminist ethics go further than this, giving value to the life of animals and ecosystems. If we took ecofeminist ethics seriously within bioethics, we could no longer simply gloss over the impact on human/animal relations when discussing the social and ethical aspects of biotechnology, as this would also be "bad ethics" and tend to echo the glossing over of women's experience by *andro*centric bioethics. There is also scope for shared theorizing between ecofeminist and feminist bioethics on the area of contextual ethics (see, for example, Cuomo 1998; Plumwood 2000). In spite of these points of commonality, no cross-conversations are taking place.

Turning to the relationship between feminist bioethics and feminist science studies, the situation is almost as bad. If one were to falsely reduce the reason for this to one factor, then it would almost certainly revolve around the different response to postmodernism found within these two areas of feminism. Although by no means synonymous with postmodernist theory, feminist science studies has been one area that has significantly embraced its insights,[6] while feminist bioethics has on the whole been more skeptical. It is difficult to account for this satisfactorily; however, there are different traditions of influence at play. For example, feminist science studies has been influenced by cultural studies in a way that feminist bioethics has not, while the latter has undoubtedly been influenced by more foundational philosophical traditions that have run counter to certain postmodern theoretical assertions. In saying this, I would claim that we are in a productive transitional period that provides fertile opportunities for feminist bioethics to explore coalitions and relations with other feminisms. I base this on the observation that since the late 1990s feminist bioethics has indeed become more pluralistic and more open to postmodern feminism.

Postmodern Thought in Feminist Bioethics

It has been argued that, at the outset, feminist bioethics split into two main groups—a liberal feminist perspective that centered on issues of choice and a radical feminist perspective that focused on issues of control—but that now it has begun to engage with a "third wave" feminism that is clearly inflected with postmodernist thought (Tong 2003, 92–93). Clearly such an engagement poses potentially radical change for feminist bioethics; it may have emerged partly due to a dissatisfaction with the underlying understandings of power posed by liberal and radical feminism. Postmodern theory has been evoked to produce a more nuanced theory of power that—taking Foucauldian cues—abandons the view that power is an extrinsic top-down repressive force. Feminists and others have used this to try to move beyond free will/determinism polarity to an understanding of power that is also better suited to thinking through the intersections between gender and other relations of power. Sometimes it may be felt that this can translate into a de-emphasis of power issues—it is quite striking how terms such as "oppression" and "domination" are used less in the feminist academy than they used to be, presumably as they might imply a commitment to top-down theories of power.[7]

There are also other issues at play in the skepticism some feminist bioethicists have toward postmodernism that partially feeds into the lack of conversation with other contemporary feminisms. Postmodernist thought is generally guarded toward ethics, considering it a field that may veer toward false universalisms, eternal truths, and normalizing pronouncements on identity and behavior. Applied ethics, on the other hand, is likely to be wary of the possibilities of relativism and idealism in postmodern thought and to ask questions of the usefulness of its insights when at least one goal is to have a voice in public policy.

One move in feminist bioethics of relevance to this discussion has been the argument for a core feminism, a unity call around basic feminist concerns (Sherwin 1992a; Donchin and Purdy 1999). Although some might be skeptical of the move to elide differences between feminisms, Sherwin (1992a) intended to outline for practical purposes core views consisting of "a recognition that women are in a subordinate position in society, that oppression is a form of injustice and hence is intolerable, that there are further forms of oppression in addition to gender oppression... , that it is possible to change society in ways that could eliminate oppression, and that it is a goal of feminism to pursue the changes necessary to accomplish this" (29). Although now written some time ago, this might strike one as slightly simplifying. For example, the third statement arguably contradicts the first, given that it underlines significant differentials of power *between* women, and "gender oppression" is also bound up in the power of some men over others in competing notions of hegemonic masculinities (see, for example, Connell 1995). As Donchin and Purdy (1999) later pointed out when they came to build on Sherwin's notion of a core feminism, this approach would not be palatable to all feminists. They wrote: "Postmodernists, for example, doubt the usefulness both of reason and of the category 'woman.' At this point, however, neither doubt seems compelling. Showing that some version of reason is flawed does not justify rejecting such a crucial concept altogether. 'Woman' too, may need some work to ensure that it recognizes morally relevant differences among us, but given its importance as a moral category, it remains to be shown that eradication rather than redefinition is the best approach" (2).

It's not clear that taking the constructedness of categories such as "woman," "reason," or "nature" into account, as postmodern feminists do, implies their ontological dissolution, as Donchin and Purdy seem to suggest. Therefore, there might be less disagreement than at first thought. In the context of ecofeminist ethics, there has been a process of acknowledging and explicating the constructedness of "natures" and of "reason," yet it is not clear that this process then removes the possibility of deploying some version of a realist sense of nature (although now no longer understood as exclusionary or purified of the human) as an important moral category, or of giving up on reason. In fact, the ecofeminist philosopher Val Plumwood (1993) is explicit that her rationale is to redefine these terms. Similarly, I read the postmodern turn as implying a reconceptualization (not eradication) of such categories which grants them a history and social context. There is also good reason for postmodern feminists not to allow their deployment of social constructionism to veer into idealism. For to do so would actually be to collude with the denigration of materialities so often identified with andro- and anthropocentric power relations, the denial and mastery of embodiment and so on. The need for feminist bioethics to (carefully) retain the category of "woman" is brought home in its goal to influence and operate as an effective feminist discourse in policy-making contexts (Tong 2003, 93). It is fair to say that this marks a significant difference from feminist science studies that has become, for better or worse, very theoretical[8] (for example, Lykke and Braidotti 1996; Haraway 1997; Mayberry, Subramaniam, and Weasel, 2001). Yet it ought not to mean that to operate in policy circles feminism has to somehow revert to a less nuanced use of conceptual frameworks. A significant challenge for feminist bioethics and feminist science studies must then be to translate complexity into policy and to take great care when drawing on what is sometimes referred to as strategic essentialism.

If idealism has been one concern. another has been relativism. The antifoundational perspective of postmodernist theory has been used within feminist science studies to point to the partiality, the constructedness, of scientific knowledges and "truths." Inasmuch as *ethics* has unreflectively been positivist and so mimetic of such grand narratives of truth, progress and universalism, such an antifoundationalism has significant import for its own feasibility. Ethics may be thought of as positivist in at least two ways. The first refers to the codifiability pretensions (the idea that they may be applied universally) of a substantial part of normative theory that remains faithful to a decidedly non-leaky ethical framework which tends to exclude social complexity. It is this sort of inattention to social context that has concerned virtue ethicists. The idea of principlism, although useful, is a good example of a catchall framework that has been widely applied in bioethics. Second, some accounts of *bio*ethics share a conception of rationality—one that valorizes both dispassionate analysis and a rationalist ontology of the self—broadly similar to that at play in contemporary paradigms of science and so quite antithetical to movements such as postmodernist theory, feminist science studies, and ecofeminism that have put considerable labor into critique and reformulation of dualistic ontology. At this point we can glimpse the at times wide schism between bioethics and science studies,[9] of which that between feminist bioethics and feminist science studies may be a similar, yet perhaps not as polarized, "family conflict."

In contrast to much of bioethics, feminist science studies now has a significant history of employing postmodern insights into the study of science that put into cultural, political, and historical context what might be assumed to be neutral scientific knowledge. Yet it is not clear that such a line of argument, one that renders problematic scientific truth claims, one that exposes science as value-laden, necessarily implies the moral equivalence of all truth claims and so a turning of the back on the ethical. What it does do, as Bauman argued, is render ethics more self-reflexive to its prior modernist assumptions over, for example, absolutes and universalisms (1993, 4). So as with the case of the category "woman" above, we might be being challenged to recognize complexity when doing critically minded bioethics, rather than being presented with a body of thought that is necessarily politically or ethically paralyzing.

The pivotal figure at this point of the discussion is Margrit Shildrick. Having written extensively on feminist theories of embodiment (for example, 1997, 2002; Shildrick and Price 1998), Shildrick is one of the few scholars to have then moved into feminist bioethics (2001) and comment on the relationship between feminist bioethics and feminist science studies (2004).[10] Moreover, she has spoken most overtly about the failure to date of feminist bioethics to engage with postmodernist theory. In reviewing the successes of feminist bioethics, she writes of the challenge to the "assumption of a given sovereign subject whose agency precedes and acts on particular contexts, rather than emerging from and being immersed in them... The emphasis has been redirected to the specificity of the needs and desires of each person, to the mutuality of the biomedical encounter, and to an ethics of interconnection and care which deliberatively extends the focus of bioethics to encompass everyday issues of bodily well-being as well as the more dramatic scenarios of life and death" (2004, 150). Thus, she applauds the feminist interruption that has worked to embody bioethics (for example, Donchin and Purdy 1999) but is less enamored by what she sees as persistent "investments in humanist and modernist discourse that leave it stretched , both in the face of the problematisation of the body offered by postmodernist theory, and by the bioscientific developments of postmodernity" (Shildrick 2004, 150).

Here Shildrick has a point. She concentrates on genetics and genomics,[11] and these areas of contemporary science are starkly postmodern in their intermixing of the old and new. Areas of technoscience such as cosmetic surgery and some of the new genetics unambiguously deploy modernist normalization and optimization discourses directed at bodies. The understanding of the body is classically abstracted, dualistic, but newly malleable and open to therapeutic applications. On one hand the body is seen simplistically as the shadow of its dualistic reference "nature" and so, given our humanist heritage, as a resource to be worked on and "enhanced." But simultaneously the new malleability of the body in contemporary technoscience, as Shildrick argues, encourages a postmodern challenge to binary oppositions such as culture/nature, individual/society, self/other, human/animal and natural/artefactual. I have argued elsewhere (Twine 2005) both that science is ambiguous in this way and that bioethics has been uncritical to its own use of dualistic thinking. I would want to echo Shildrick's questioning of the suitability of the tools of (feminist) bioethics for asking the right questions about such complexity. At the least, reconstituting the field of bioethics as more interdisciplinary in its breadth is vital to imagining the ethical implications of contemporary changes to health, the body, and the biosphere.

Perhaps the strangest complexity is that contemporary technoscience supersedes the *conceptual* deconstructions of critical postmodern theory with material deconstruction and transgression. The figure of the animal serves as a good example. The human/animal hierarchical dualism has been criticized on both grounds of human rights and animal ethics. It has facilitated the application of discourses of animalization to various human groups seen as less rational and closer to nature, but has only had that discursive power due to the very naturalization of human domination over other animals that it perpetuates. Consequently, it has been challenged in a shallow sense any time that a constructed group has resented being compared to animals, and more deeply by those who have been just as interested in animal ethics. However, proponents of this critical deconstruction would no doubt be surprised now to see the material deconstruction of this boundary as represented most clearly in transgenic technologies. There is, of course, no sudden cutoff point to our constructed epochs, so it is not surprising that we see older understandings of the body conjoined to persistent hierarchies of, for example, gender and species in the new materializations of technoscience. But the main point here is that we must equip our bioethics to understand such changes and to make ethical sense of ambiguous social and technological change.

Feminist Bioethics and Critical Bioethics

In addition to the emerging question of the use of postmodernist theory, further critical strands within bioethics are of use to the goals of feminist bioethics. We have already seen prominent attacks from within bioethics that herald a reflexivity to the types and uses of rationality employed by bioethicists. For example, Campbell (1999) spoke of the partiality of our Western mode of reasoning, and Gillett (2003), in more detail, has examined the types of reasoning in bioethics, arguing that in some cases they might be better seen as irrational. When bioethics is so abstracted from the sociopolitical realities of everyday life, it can seem not only irrational but also naïve or even disturbing. One can detect the positivism at work here in the valorization of a distinctly dispassionate reason. We see examples of this in the debate around the enhancement of nondisease traits (Savulescu 2001) and other techno-fix bioethics that can consider the compulsory sterilization of materially deprived couples (Archard 2004) over the injustice of poverty.

More recently, we have seen the emergence of "critical bioethics" (Hedgecoe 2004; Twine 2005). These two works arose independently but have in common a call for greater reflexivity and a discussion of the relationship between the social sciences and philosophy in the context of bioethics. Moreover both approaches take care to avoid an oversimplified denunciation of philosophical bioethics.[12] While Hedgecoe's concept focuses more on methodological issues, my version asks questions of the breadth and scope of bioethics.[13] Although we are both interested in the relationship between the social sciences and bioethics, Hedgecoe concentrates on the issue of empirical research, and I devote more time to sociopolitical dimensions. Furthermore, while we both flag reflexivity as a central element of critical bioethics, we take this in different directions with, for example, my call for a closer relationship between bioethics and environmental ethics.

Specifically, I conceptualized critical bioethics as consisting of three elements—interdisciplinarity, self-reflexivity, and the avoidance of uncritical complicity—which I explored through a general strategy of critiquing the presence of dualisms in bioethics (Twine 2005). Interdisciplinarity is important because restricting bioethics to the narrow preserve of a branch of philosophy stakes a certain claim over the ethical and discounts the important contribution of other disciplines or other philosophical perspectives. The narrowing of bioethics to medical ethics,[14] or sometimes "biomedical" ethics, represents an *unreflexive* anthropocentric conception of the "bio" in bioethics that brackets out environmental and animal ethics and tends to downplay sociopolitical, socioeconomic, and ecological inputs into human health. A greater degree of self-reflexivity, as Hedgecoe (2004) concurs, positions us to be attentive to the way in which what counts as a bioethical problem is in part a social process (126). With the third element, I underlined the danger of employing a philosophical perspective that espouses a similar rationalist worldview as the science it claims to ethically watch over. Here the intention is to position bioethics critically, to respond to the oft-heard claim of complicity.

Hedgecoe's concept of critical bioethics is a deeper exploration of the relationship between the social sciences and "philosophical bioethics," requiring "bioethicists to root their enquiries in empirical research, to challenge theories using evidence, to be reflexive and to be sceptical about the claims of other bioethicists, scientists and clinicians" (2004, 120). His concept can be seen as an expression of concern over both the dislocation from social realities of some bioethics and the conservative paradigmatic nature of some of its ethical-theoretical tools. In addition the account of reflexivity is explored on a few levels, but particularly in the sense of the self-awareness of bioethicists, so that "in critical bioethics reflexivity is about acknowledging one's personal context, but not accepting that this undermines the legitimacy of one's claims" (ibid., 138–39). By positing the importance of reflecting on one's social position, one's experiences, and one's place within multiple relations of power, Hedgecoe favors the model of the honest, engaged bioethicist over a detached, god's-eye view that would deem such reflections largely irrelevant.

It is clear, I hope, how these concepts of critical bioethics may be complementary to feminist bioethics. My definition of critical bioethics was conceptualized with the assumption that feminist bioethics was very much part of the same project. Feminism is an interdisciplinary field, it is closely concerned with reconceptualization, it cannot fail to be concerned with the sociopolitical and socioeconomic domain, and it is historically well positioned to be attentive to the partiality of particular ideas of reason. Given the feminist experience of exclusion, decontextualized understandings of health and dualistic thinking, I would hope that feminist bioethics would also be sympathetic to my broadening of bioethics to encompass stronger links with environmental contexts and the inclusion of animal ethics. From Hedgecoe's concept we can also note a relevant complementarity, especially in his call for critical bioethics to be empirically rooted and his discussion on reflexivity. The former dovetails with the phenomenological and experiential foci of feminist bioethics. Although feminist bioethicists have commented little on the recent debate about the role of empirical research in bioethics, it has been from the outset critical of bioethical abstraction (Sherwin 1992a, 17) and it would be difficult to conceive of a sustainable feminist bioethics that was not thoroughly complemented by empirical research. Hedgecoe's discussion of reflexivity essentially corresponds to a methodological self-awareness that has now been practiced by feminist writers for many years, as they have sought an alternative model to the idea of disengaged, value-free objectivity (for example, Sherwin 1992b, 173). Given the diversity within feminist bioethics, there may be differing responses to social science ventures into bioethics, but generally there is both much to discuss and to complement.

Conclusion

I have sought to briefly outline the importance for feminist bioethics of reflecting on the types of feminism on which it draws, and I have noted that this reflection is already under way. To intensify this process, productive coalitions could form that not only would imply changes for feminist bioethics but also could further enrich contemporary debates within bioethics and bring out into the open the wider schism between bioethics and science studies. Specifically, I have argued for a closer engagement between feminist bioethics and other feminisms, notably ecofeminisms, postmodern feminisms, and feminist science studies. If these four areas could in various research contexts be occasionally but coherently brought together, much could arguably be achieved in terms of thinking through concepts of gender, power, health, and the biosphere. Such an exercise would also have a bearing on the three foci of critical bioethics mentioned above: interdisciplinarity, reflexivity to bioethical subject matter, and complicity. For example, bioethics generally will have to become more overtly a movement also for *environmental* justice.

There is much scope for commonality in a potential engagement between feminist bioethics and social science approaches and with critical bioethics perspectives. Feminist bioethics ought to be a strong advocate of empirical research in bioethics understood not as a public opinion exercise but as nuanced examinations of the contextual everyday processes of ethical reflection, discourse, and decision making, as well as the experiential knowledge given by both lay and professional actors in bioethically relevant domains. Furthermore, coalitionary endeavors would continually contest which domains were deemed "bioethically relevant," for example, to counter the sequestration of the body and emotionality from bioethics as well as other dangers such as capture, complicity, or technologization.

Bioethics is a contested field that offers up varying contexts, some in which feminism is still marginalized, but also others in which it very much has a voice. The idea of a feminist bioethics remains likely to contradict the understanding of those committed to a notion of bioethics in terms of value-free dispassionate reason. Moreover, feminist bioethics remains marginalized in those areas and committees where bioethicists are sought out to give expert advice. Ethical deliberation over stem cell research provides a good example. In many cultures, this debate has been reduced somewhat to a discussion over the moral status of the embryo. The feminist bioethical riposte to this framing queries the vanishing of female embodiment at play here as well as the voices of women who may be asked to donate "spare" embryos from either IVF or preimplantation genetic diagnosis (PGD) (see Franklin and Roberts 2006). In spite of the value of such feminist research, it has not yet successfully been outlined in those prized expert spaces within which bioethicists are increasingly being welcomed. Engaging in the kind of practical and theoretical coalitions argued for here can assist in producing a more strongly joined up feminist voice. This fate is not one of academic compartmentalism but of changing more fundamentally the study of the ethical, social, legal, philosophical and other aspects of health care and the biosciences.

ACKNOWLEDGMENT

I gratefully acknowledge the support of the Economic and Social Research Council (ESRC). This work was part of the program of the ESRC Centre for Economic and Social Aspects of Genomics (Cesagen).

NOTES

1. I would see the concern of feminist bioethics not only as the analysis of how bioethical issues affect diversely positioned women, but also as the attempt to question what counts as a bioethical issue and what role gendered relations of power play within these. Like feminism generally, then, feminist bioethics is interested in the social construction of both femininities *and* masculinities.

2. Feminist bioethics is far broader in coverage, and feminist science studies is arguably more concerned with power than ethics.

3. The 2004 conference was significant in that on the middle day there were joint FAB/IAB themes and panels, and so bioethicists not usually inclined to feminism were given a new opportunity to learn.

4. www.bioethics-international.org.

5. It is worth noting that two recent papers on feminist bioethics make nods in the direction of including environmental concerns within the feminist and bioethical project (see Sherwin 2008; Shildrick 2008). However, neither makes reference to the myriad fields combining feminism and environmentalism, such as ecofeminist ethics or feminist political ecology.

6. I am thinking most obviously of the work of people like Donna Haraway and Sarah Franklin.

7. It is a mistake to let go of these terms, even if they do imply a commitment to overly top-down understandings of power. It was thus refreshing to hear them again at the FAB conference in Sydney, November 2004.

8. Feminist science studies is a theoretically rich and sophisticated field. I do not think there is anything specific to FSS at play here, but the divide between theory and activism is found increasingly throughout all feminist academic discourse. It is a challenge for FSS to think more about a policy voice, something that would no doubt be helped by the creative coalition with feminist bioethics that I advocate in this chapter. It should be noted that FSS is currently relevant to policy in *certain* areas, for example, redefining science disciplines and female access to them.

9. Regrettably, although not surprisingly, feminist science studies faces its own battles for legitimacy within the wider field of science studies.

10. Shildrick was also a keynote speaker at the FAB conference in Sydney, November 2004.

11. As Shildrick would no doubt agree, we have to be constantly reflective to the technologization of bioethics and think widely about what is (feminist) bioethical subject matter.

12. The phrase "philosophical bioethics" is used by Hedgecoe. I would prefer to avoid it because it carries a risk of collapsing all varieties of bioethics that might see themselves as philosophical.

13. Thank you to Adam Hedgecoe for his framing of the difference between our two concepts of "critical bioethics" (personal communication, March 2005).

14. As I argue (2005), such a narrowing is in contradistinction to the wider view of bioethics, as envisaged by V. R. Potter, who originally coined the term "bioethics" in the early 1970s.

REFERENCES

Archard, D. 2004. Wrongful life. *Philosophy* 79:403–20.
Bauman, Z. 1993. *Postmodern ethics*. Oxford: Blackwell.
Campbell, A. 1999. Presidential address: Global bioethics—dream or nightmare. *Bioethics* 13 (3/4): 183–90.
Connell, B. 1995. *Masculinities*. Cambridge: Polity Press.

Cuomo, C. 1998. *Feminism and ecological communities: An ethic of flourishing.* London: Routledge.

De Vries, R., and P. Conrad. 1998. Why bioethics needs sociology. In *Bioethics and society: Constructing the ethical enterprise,* ed. R. De Vries, and J. Subedi, 233–57. Upper Saddle River, N.J.: Prentice Hall.

De Vries, R., and J. Subedi, eds. 1998. *Bioethics and society: Constructing the ethical enterprise.* Upper Saddle River, N.J.: Prentice Hall.

Donchin, A., and L. Purdy, eds. 1999. *Embodying bioethics: Recent feminist advances.* Oxford: Rowman & Littlefield.

Eldridge, J., J. MacInnes, S. Scott, C. Warhurst, and A. Witz., eds. 2000. *For sociology: Legacies and prospects.* Durham, U.K.: Sociology Press.

Gervais, 1998. Changing society, changing medicine, changing bioethics. In *Bioethics and society: Constructing the ethical enterprise,* ed. R. De Vries and J. Subedi, 216–32. Upper Saddle River, N.J.: Prentice Hall.

Franklin, S., and C. Roberts. 2006. *Born and made: An ethnography of pre-implantation genetic diagnosis.* Princeton, N.J.: Princeton University Press.

Gillett, G. 2003. Reasoning in bioethics. *Bioethics* 17 (3): 243–60.

Haimes, E. 2002. What can the social sciences contribute to the study of ethics? Theoretical, empirical and substantive considerations. *Bioethics* 16 (2): 89–113.

Haraway, D. 1997. *Modest_Witness@Second_Millenium.FemaleMan©_Meets_Onco Mouse™: Feminism and technoscience.* London: Routledge.

Hayry, M., and T. Takala, eds. 2003. *Scratching the surface in bioethics.* Amsterdam: Rodopi.

Hedgecoe, A. M. 2004. Critical bioethics: Beyond the social science critique of applied ethics. *Bioethics* 18 (2): 120–43.

Levitt, M. 2003. Better together? Sociological and philosophical perspectives on bioethics. In *Scratching the surface in bioethics,* ed. M. Hayry, and T. Takala, 19–27. Amsterdam: Rodopi.

Light, D., and G. McGee. 1998. On the social embeddedness of bioethics. In *Bioethics and society: Constructing the ethical enterprise,* ed. R. De Vries and J. Subedi, 1–15. Upper Saddle River, N.J.: Prentice Hall.

Lykke, N. and R. Braidotti, eds. 1996. *Between monsters, goddesses and cyborgs: Feminist confrontations with science, medicine and cyberspace.* London: Zed Books.

Mayberry, M., B. Subramaniam, and L. Weasel, eds. 2001. *Feminist science studies: A new generation.* London: Routledge.

Morgan, D. 1992. *Discovering men.* London: Routledge.

Plumwood, V. 1993. *Feminism and the mastery of nature.* London: Routledge.

———. 2000. Integrating ethical frameworks for animals, humans and nature: A critical feminist eco-socialist analysis. *Ethics and the Environment* 5 (2): 285–322.

Rawlinson, M. 2001. Introduction. *Journal of Medicine and Philosophy* 26 (4): 339–41.

Savulescu, J. 2001. Procreative beneficence: Why we should select the best children. *Bioethics* 15 (5/6): 413–26.

Sherwin, S. 1992a. Feminist and medical ethics: Two different approaches to contextual ethics. In *Feminist perspectives in medical ethics*, ed. H. B. Holmes, and L. Purdy, 17–31. Indianapolis: Indiana University Press.

———. 1992b. *No longer patient: Feminist ethics and health care.* Philadelphia: Temple University Press.

———. 2008. Whither bioethics? How feminism can help reorient bioethics. *International Journal of Feminist Approaches to Bioethics* 1 (1): 7–27.

Shildrick, M. 1997. *Leaky bodies and boundaries: Feminism, postmodernism and (bio)ethics.* London: Routledge.

———. 2001. Some speculations on matters of touch. *Journal of Medicine and Philosophy* 26 (4): 387–404.

———. 2002. *Embodying the monster: Encounters with the vulnerable self.* London: Sage.

———. 2004. Genetics, normativity, and ethics: Some bioethical concerns. *Feminist Theory* 5 (2): 149–65.

———. 2008. The critical turn in feminist bioethics: The case of heart transplantation. *International Journal of Feminist Approaches to Bioethics* 1 (1): 28–47.

Shildrick, M., and J. Price, eds. 1998. *Vital signs: Feminist reconfigurations of the bio/logical body.* Edinburgh: Edinburgh University Press.

Spallone, P., T. Wilkie, E. Ettore, E. Haimes, T. Shakespeare, and M. Stacey. 2000. Putting sociology on the bioethics map. In *For sociology: Legacies and prospects,* ed. J. Eldridge, J. MacInnes, S. Scott, C. Warhurst, and A. Witz, 191–206. Durham, U.K.: Sociology Press.

Tong, R. 2003. Feminism and feminist bioethics: The search for a measure of unity in a field with rich diversity. *New Review of Bioethics* 1 (1): 85–100.

Twine, R. 2001. Ma(r)king essence: Ecofeminism and embodiment. *Ethics and the environment* 6 (2): 31–58.

———. 2005. Constructing a critical bioethics by deconstructing culture/nature dualism. *Medicine, Health Care and Philosophy* 8 (3): 285–95.

PART TWO

Theory in Feminist Bioethics

PETYA FITZPATRICK, M.A., AND
JACKIE LEACH SCULLY, PH.D.

Bioethical Theory

Bioethics, as a form of applied ethics, has always had a distinctive approach to the relationship of bioethical theory to practice. In its formative years, the majority of academics involved in constructing theory were philosophers, and today much of mainstream bioethics rests on concepts and approaches familiar to moral philosophy. Over time, and as it has become recognized as an area of inquiry in its own right, bioethics has begun to draw on theoretical approaches that are more reflective of its contemporary character. And because one distinctive feature of today's bioethics is its interdisciplinarity, theoretical development is being shaped not just by the obvious fields of medicine, law, theology, and public health but also by growing input from feminism, sociology, cultural theory, ancient philosophy, and literary theory (London 2001). Still, mainstream bioethics remains dominated by the use of foundational concepts derived from moral philosophy and ethics.

A second feature of bioethics is its practical orientation, and this has had an immense impact on the kind of theory it finds helpful and how that theory is used. Bioethics has long been criticized for its thoroughgoing instrumentalism: in line with its task of regulating biomedicine, and against a cultural background of growing disenchantment with the possibility of creating all-encompassing ethical frameworks, there is a sense in which bioethics remains focused on concrete goals and midlevel theories rather than metatheorization. This practical turn has been accompanied by speculation as to whether bioethics' *theorizing* will eventually become entirely redundant to or uselessly divorced from the (putatively more important) work of bioethics' *practice* (London 2001, 65). So the question is not just whether feminist theorizing has had any effect on the kind of theory used in bioethics, but also if it has made any difference, overall, to the way that bioethics uses theory.

Feminist Bioethical Theory

The central contribution of feminism to moral theory in general has been its capacity to identify "gender bias in the preoccupations, assumptions and perspectives of the dominant theories" (Nelson 2000, 494). This means that for a quarter of a century or more feminist bioethicists have targeted such preoccupations, assumptions, and perspectives in bioethics as neglectful of women's interests and the interests of other marginalized groups and thus ultimately oppressive. If the foundational assumptions of bioethics' theory remain unexamined, it is argued, the price paid will be a continuation of exclusionary and oppressive bioethical practice.

Having said that, the heterogeneity of feminist thought makes it especially difficult to meaningfully define what makes bioethics theory *feminist*, without excluding some of the range of approaches to theory that feminist bioethics clearly contains. Nevertheless, there are certain critiques of standard bioethics theories that are common to any approach calling itself feminist. These critiques have revealed a bioethics that is irreducibly gendered, with male identity and moral experiences posited as the norm. In this framework, feminists claim, the perspectives of women have been ignored, pathologized, and otherwise rendered invisible (Lloyd 1984; Brennan 1999; Donchin 2004). As well as neglecting and marginalizing the sort of moral experiences women undergo, bioethics' reliance on the theoretical structures of traditional philosophy means that it may draw unreflexively on particular models of moral identity, autonomy, and universalism, and on particular epistemic claims, that feminist ethical theory has already diagnosed as contaminated by the gendered social and political orders that devised them. Feminist bioethical theories adopt distinctive ontological and epistemological positions that challenge traditional assumptions about selfhood and the moral agent, and about the sorts of knowledge and ways of knowing that can reliably be addressed to moral problems.

Relational Autonomy

A prominent feature of recent feminist thinking on the self is an attempt to replace the atomized, unattached self central to the liberal theory of selfhood and agency with a model of the individual defined through her social roles, relationships, and history (Sherwin 1992; Tong 1993; Walker 1998; Mackenzie and Stoljar 2000; Donchin 2004). Revising the concept of selfhood stimulates a revision of the process of moral deliberation, because detachment and impartiality in moral reasoning are not always as possible—or not possible in the same ways—for a socially constituted self as they can seem to be for the self of liberal theory. Feminist argument attempts to frame moral problems in a form that pays greater attention to the aspects of social circumstances, history, emotions, and values (Nelson 2000). Finally, while traditional bioethics theory has claimed to be apolitical, feminist theories are avowedly political—not merely in their goals but in the recognition of the construction of the self through power relations that is pivotal to feminist theories of the moral agent and moral autonomy. Taken together, these differences constitute significant challenges to theories that have hitherto dominated bioethical thinking.

The feminist relational view of the self has major implications for the reconceptualization of standard bioethical principles such as autonomy. The *principle* of respect for (patient) autonomy has preeminent status in modern Western bioethical theorizing, and it is important to stress that the use of this theoretical principle as a tool to promote and protect personal freedom has been central to much overtly feminist ethical work. Nevertheless, the prevailing *concept* of autonomy in bioethics literature is still criticized by feminists for being grounded in a picture in which the self operates "outside of time, space and bodily circumstances" (Ruhl 2002), paying insufficient attention to the social context in which decisions are made (Nedelsky 1989; Donchin 1995; Keller 1997; Sherwin 1998; Mackenzie and Stoljar 2000). Such a configuration of autonomy can have little relevance to an ethical account of the lives of marginalized groups, whose capacity for self-determination is radically limited by structural power relationships. By taking note of material and economic circumstances, educational and social resources, and social institutions and social norms, relational theory examines the genuine availability of options that facilitate the making of self-determining choices. Additionally, by problematizing the neoliberal view that autonomy is constituted in the maximization of unfettered choice, and paying attention to the constitutive effect of discursive relations (especially relations of power), a relational model of autonomy raises the level of skepticism about the general notion of "autonomous choice" in bioethics and elsewhere. Already highly influential in feminist bioethical literature, the concept of relational autonomy has recently begun to draw the attention of nonfeminist bioethicists (Russell and Tokatilan 2003; Christman 2004).

Catriona Mackenzie's chapter makes a strong argument for the application of a relational view of autonomy, leading the reader through several problems of contemporary bioethics literature: the establishment of a regulated market in human body parts, sperm, and oocytes; cosmetic surgery and demand self-amputation; assisted reproductive technologies and genetic technologies. In the process, she demonstrates the shortcomings of the prevailing conception of autonomy—which she identifies as a "maximal choice" view of autonomy—and the assumptions that underlie it. She concludes with a concise but thoroughgoing overview of relational theories in bioethics literature to date, demonstrating what a relational view of autonomy brings to familiar bioethical debates.

Epistemology

A further theoretical challenge from feminism has been a reworking of the standard epistemological frameworks of bioethics. Feminists argue that distancing of the moral agent from the situated dilemma through an emphasis on universalizability, impartiality, abstraction, and rationality necessarily obscures the genderedness of dominant bioethical analyses. As a result, the specificities of women and women's interests—and indeed, the interests of other socially marginalized groups—are rendered invisible. Feminist bioethics has extended its concern to the "moral understandings" (Walker 1998) of activities taking place outside the spaces traditionally allocated to biomedical, and hence bioethical, encounter. Bioethics has been inclined to focus on theorizing around attention-catching "crisis" issues—stem cell research, euthanasia, cloning, abortion—while neglecting the more mundane "housekeeping issues" (Warren 1989), and especially the experiential aspect of ethics, for example, the communication between doctor and patient during counseling for genetic testing or the effects on a spouse of providing care for a person with dementia. Under feminist scrutiny, moral epistemology is thus revealed as a politically skewed activity, whereby matters associated with low-status activities, traditionally done by women, are neglected.

In examining women's "moral understandings," feminists have attempted to undermine the privileging of epistemic resources traditionally associated with socially dominant groups over other, marginalized ways of knowing things, and to formulate a complementary bioethics built on "the actual situations people find themselves in" (Held 1995). Such a formulation has wide implications for both the kinds of theory and the epistemic resources that bioethics relies on.

In her overview of feminist bioethical theory as a prelude to her exploration of the virtue of trust, Jessica Prata Miller refers back to the fact that both mainstream and feminist bioethics share an "urgent practical impulse" that has led them "to reject the search for an overarching theory of the good and the right, favoring instead a more piecemeal, contextual approach." For feminists, this emphasis has the advantage of avoiding and potentially undermining gendered theoretical frameworks through elucidation of empirical detail. Trust, for example, is not an abstraction: the main reason it holds interest for bioethicists is because it is a social relationship, with concrete consequences when trust is breached or misplaced. Miller takes a recognizably feminist approach in her argument that trust is emotional and affective, and that understanding trust requires attention to relationality, "particular details of concrete relations among the parties."

Care Ethics

Feminist work on relationality in trust is linked to what is perhaps the best-known theoretical work done in feminist ethics and bioethics—care ethics. Pioneered by feminist theorists in psychology and ethics such as Nell Noddings, Sara Ruddick, Carol Gilligan, and Virginia Held, this is a normative theory claiming that moral deliberation is done through an orientation of care for others. Gilligan's early suggestion that there is an observable gender difference in the ways that women and men approach morally troubling situations has been contested both within and outside feminism, but the idea of a contextualized morality continues to hold the interest of feminists and nonfeminists alike.

Care ethics—at least in the form of attention to asymmetric relationships as the basis for ethical concern—is gradually making its way into mainstream bioethics as a legitimate approach to moral problems, although not universally accepted as feminist. In fact, feminists have sometimes been its most vociferous critics, for example, rejecting Noddings's "feminine" approach to morality (Tong 1993), or the "maternal thinking" of Ruddick (1984, 1989) and Held (1987) on the grounds that it promotes an essentialist view of women by attributing to them particular characteristics (nurturing, emotionally giving, caring). Not all women may identify with these attributes or experience them as defining, valuable, or desirable. Traits universally attributed to women may be a product of their socialization within an oppressive society, in which case any theory based on supposedly intrinsic traits risks doing little more than reproducing women's oppression. Similarly, care theories have tended to assume a universal and benign experience of caring relations. Yet caregiving can be intimately bound up with women's social and political subordination (Kittay and Feder 2002). Caregivers, whether paid or unpaid, are most often women, and women who are in caring roles are often socially and financially disadvantaged. Moreover, a relationship of care, like any relationship, has potential for either carer or cared-for to be exploited, coerced, or abused, issues that are particularly fraught in situations where capabilities and power are inherently asymmetrically distributed.

In the past decade or so, some feminist bioethicists have attempted to reformulate a theory of care that addresses these concerns. Eva Feder Kittay, for example, developed a theory of dependency to articulate the ethical obligations incumbent on both the dependency worker and the dependent in the relationship (Kittay 1999; Kittay and Feder 2002; Kittay, Jennings, and Wasunna 2005). Like in other theories of care, obligations stem from the relationship that exists between carer and cared-for. However, Kittay strengthens the theory by also providing an account of society's obligations to dependency workers and defining circumstances (such as exploitation or abuse by the dependent) in which the obligation to the dependent no longer exists. According to Virginia Held (1995), society's obligations to carers should be defined by the general requirements of a just society. She suggests a reconciliation of care and justice whereby each is allowed influence in both the domestic *and* public spheres, for example by drawing on justice to prescribe minimal moral standards and on care to negotiate within that framework "questions of the good life or of human value over and above the obligatory minimums of justice" (Held 1995).

In part IV of this volume, two chapters consider the usefulness of an ethics-of-care perspective on research in vulnerable and minority populations: Ruth Groenhout discusses the inclusion of minority racial and ethnic groups in research, while Jennifer Baker, Terry Dunbar, and Margaret Scrimgeour consider whether care ethics can facilitate dialogue between indigenous communities and researchers.

Universalism and Particularity

Feminist bioethics' aim, exemplified in FAB's charter, is to formulate a bioethics, including theoretical positions, for women *and other marginalized groups*. This entails that feminist bioethics must be able to accommodate theoretical diversity in race, ethnicity, religion, sexual orientation, ability, and ideology. By being theoretically attentive to difference through focusing on the local and particular in moral life, feminists make explicit the social processes through which gender and other differences are turned into inequalities. This can be easier said than done: the crafting of feminist theory is itself complicated by the need to respond to the critiques of women who do not see themselves or their interests as being represented by feminism as it is practiced. Laurel Baldwin-Ragaven has more to say about this in the introduction to part IV. Beyond this, feminist bioethics, like bioethics as a whole, is faced with an ongoing tension between particularity and universalism. It should be clear from the account of feminist approaches given here that a globally relevant, universal bioethics is not a priority of feminist bioethics. However, as the scope and focus of global bioethics extend, accompanied by the demand for global or at least regional harmonization of biomedical regulation, feminists have been worried by the risk that relativized or standpoint epistemologies may be unequal to the task of challenging transgressions of human rights. The desire to respect the multiple cultures and traditions of the world has warred with the need to give coherent counterarguments to oppression and to articulate calls to action.

Acknowledging this difficulty, feminist bioethics remains committed to troubling the theoretical assumptions of the mainstream. In Mary C. Rawlinson's chapter, then, we see a critique from a historical and feminist perspective of the supposed universalism on which rights theory, and much of mainstream bioethical theory, is based. Feminist suspicion enables Rawlinson to locate the generic "person" of human rights and bioethics within highly specific conceptual traditions. Her example is the drafting of the 2005 United Nations Educational, Scientific and Cultural Organization's (UNESCO) *Universal Draft Declaration on Bioethics and Human Rights* (UDDBHR), whose creation involved identifying common, substantial goals, rather than seeking justification in all-inclusive grand theory (Rawlinson and Donchin 2005). There is much to be said in favor of an approach to bioethical problems that avowedly takes to the contextual and the concrete. However, on closer examination it is evident that certain problematic metaethical assumptions underlie the creation of this document. Rawlinson is not attacking the fundamental aims of universal declarations like this but uses feminist tools to trouble universalist rights theory by highlighting its historical origins and their consequences for how we understand the meaning of human rights today. In an original analysis that remains thoroughly within feminist theoretical tradition, she aims not to invalidate the progressive goals of such declarations but to uncover the need to revise a theory in which ongoing relations of subjection and the differences of power and wealth are rendered so problematically invisible.

REFERENCES

Brennan, S. 1999. Recent work in feminist ethics. *Ethics* 109 (4): 858–93.

Christman, J. 2004. Relational autonomy, liberal individualism, and the social constitution of selves. *Humanities, Social Sciences and the Law* 117 (1–2): 143–64.

Donchin, A. 1995. Reworking autonomy: Toward a feminist perspective. *Cambridge Quarterly of Healthcare Ethics* 4 (1): 44–55.

———. 2004. Feminist bioethics. *Stanford Encyclopedia of Philosophy*, www.seop.leeds.ac.uk/entries/feminist-bioethics/.

Held, V. 1987. Feminism and moral theory. In *Women and moral theory*, ed. E. F. Kittay and D. T. Meyers, 111–28. Totowa, N.J.: Rowman & Littlefield.

———. 1995. *Justice and care: Essential readings in feminist ethics*. Boulder, Colo.: Westview Press.

Keller, J. 1997. Autonomy, relationality and feminist ethics. *Hypatia* 12 (2): 152–64.

Kittay, E. 1999. *Love's labor: Essays on women, equality, and dependency*. New York: Routledge.

Kittay, E., and E. Feder. 2002. *Theoretical perspectives on dependency and women*. Lanham, Md.: Rowman & Littlefield.

Kittay, E. F., B. Jennings, and A. A. Wasunna. 2005. Dependency, difference and the global ethic of longterm care. *Journal of Political Philosophy* 13 (4): 443–69.

Lloyd, G. 1984. *The man of reason*. London: Routledge.

London, A. J. 2001. Theory and engagement in bioethics. *Theoretical Medicine* 22: 65–68.

Mackenzie, C., and N. Stoljar, eds. 2000. *Relational autonomy: Feminist perspectives on autonomy, agency and the social self*. Oxford: Oxford University Press.

Nedelsky, J. 1989. Reconceiving autonomy: Sources, thoughts, and possibilities. *Yale Journal of Law and Feminism* 1 (1): 7–16.

Nelson, H. L. 2000. Feminist bioethics: Where we've been and where we're going. *Metaphilosophy* 31 (5): 492–508.

Rawlinson, M. C., and A. Donchin. 2005. The quest for universality: Reflections on UNESCO's Preliminary Draft Declaration on Universal Norms in Bioethics. *Developing World Bioethics* 5 (3): 258–66.

Ruddick, S. 1983. Maternal thinking. In *Mothering: Essays in feminist theory*, ed. J. Trebilcot, 213–30. Lanham, Md.: Rowman & Littlefield.

———. 1989. *Maternal thinking: Toward a politics of peace*. Boston: Beacon Press.

Ruhl, L. 2002. Dilemmas of the will: Uncertainty, reproduction, and the rhetoric of control. *Signs* 27 (3): 645.

Russell, R., and J. G. Tokatilan 2003. From antagonistic autonomy to relational autonomy: A theoretical reflection from the southern cone. *Latin American Politics and Society* 45 (1): 1–25.

Sherwin, S. 1992. *No longer patient: Feminist ethics and health care*. Philadelphia: Temple University Press.

———. 1998. A relational approach to autonomy in health care. In *The politics of wom-*

en's health: Exploring agency and autonomy, by Feminist Healthcare Ethics Research Network, 19–47. Philadelphia: Temple University Press.

Tong, R. 1993. *Feminine and feminist ethics.* Belmont, Calif.: Wadsworth.

Walker, M. U. 1998. *Moral understandings: A feminist study in ethics.* New York: Routledge.

Warren, V. L. 1989. Feminist directions in medical ethics. *Hypatia* 4 (2): 32–45.

CHAPTER FOUR

Conceptions of Autonomy
and Conceptions of the Body in Bioethics

CATRIONA MACKENZIE, PH.D.

The principle of respect for autonomy dominates debates in many areas of bioethics. The central idea underpinning the principle is the simple but morally compelling idea that as moral agents we have the right to make important decisions about our lives and to determine what happens in and to our bodies. Few are likely to disagree with this idea, at least in principle. In practice, however, determining just what the right to self-determination means, how far it extends, and what it entails is complex and contested. For example, what kinds of claims against society or other people does my right to bodily self-determination entitle me to make? If I am in the terminal stages of cancer, does my right to bodily self-determination entitle me to seek the assistance of my physician to hasten my death? If I am infertile, does it entitle me to whatever assisted reproductive technologies I may need to enable me have a child who is genetically related to me? If I have body dysmorphic disorder and am convinced that one of my limbs is not part of my body, do I have a right to seek the assistance of a surgeon to amputate the offending limb? And does my right to bodily self-determination extend just to my own body, or does it extend to the bodies of my offspring, including, for example, a right to determine their sex or genetic characteristics?

The intention of this chapter is not to address these specific first-order questions. Rather, my aim is to diagnose some of the problematic assumptions about autonomy and about the moral relationship between persons and their bodies that underpin an influential conception of autonomy within bioethics, particularly in the English-speaking world, where bioethics has been dominated by utilitarian and libertarian liberal views. This conception, which I call the "maximal choice" conception of autonomy, involves two main assumptions. First, that the fundamental value on which health care decisions ought to be based is individual autonomy, and second, that individual autonomy is best promoted by maximizing the range of options available to individuals for exercising or increasing control over their bodies.

The maximal choice approach to health care decision making is ethically flawed and fails to place sufficient moral weight on considerations of social justice and equality. I will not attempt to provide a detailed argument for this claim here. Rather, the main focus of this chapter is to criticize the way maximal choice views understand autonomy. My charge, in brief, is that these views presuppose an excessively individualistic conception of autonomy and reduce autonomy to the expression of subjective preferences. I also want to question the way maximal choice conceptions understand persons' moral relationship to their bodies. According to these views, individual freedom involves extensive moral rights to dispose of one's body as one chooses, and these moral rights are grounded in ownership of one's body and body parts.

In the first section of the chapter, I characterize the maximal choice approach to autonomy and outline its main justificatory sources. I also provide some illustrations of the way this approach is deployed in four broad areas of debate within bioethics. In the second section, I state my main objections to the way autonomy and the moral relationship between persons and their bodies are understood by maximal choice conceptions. In the final section, I outline an alternative, feminist relational understanding of autonomy and explain why this approach to autonomy is more consistent with broader ethical concerns about social justice and equality.

Maximal Choice Conceptions of Autonomy

Maximal choice conceptions regard individual autonomy as a trumping value in health care decision making and assume that individual autonomy is best promoted by maximizing the range of options available to individuals. There are four overlapping justificatory sources for this conception of autonomy.

One is the familiar liberal view that we live in a pluralist society, characterized by significant diversity, indeed contestation, in views about the good. Given this diversity, there are no uncontentious criteria for making qualitative or normative distinctions among the different choices people might make about how best to live their lives or what values ought to guide their choices. A liberal society, therefore, should be neutral with respect to competing views of the good, but ought to provide maximum scope for individual liberty and make available to its citizens as many options and opportunities as possible, to best enable them to live according to their conception of the good.

Second, maximal choice conceptions typically adopt libertarian views of liberty, choice, and equality of opportunity. The maximal choice view of liberty is that as long as a person's choices do not cause undue harm to others, where harm is usually construed narrowly to include physical and some psychological harms but to exclude social harms, and as long as these choices are free from coercion and at least minimally informed, any restriction of liberty constitutes unjustifiable paternalism. Choice, on these views, is equated with the expression of individual subjective preferences. No matter how arbitrary, prejudiced, or manipulated a person's preferences might be, her ability to express her preferences through her choices is regarded as a good to be promoted. Combined with this approach to liberty and choice, maximal choice views tend to understand equality of opportunity as formal equality, or absence of legal or informal social constraints preventing certain individuals from having access to opportunities on the basis of race or ethnicity, sex, sexual preference, class, or religion.[1] Such views systematically overlook the effects of entrenched inequalities and injustices arising from social oppression or natural disadvantage. The rhetoric of maximizing choice thus pays little heed to whether a choice is in fact a significant option for particular people or groups in society, or to how options are socially distributed.[2]

Third, maximal choice conceptions construe bodily autonomy or bodily self-determination as maximizing control over one's body and having the freedom to dispose of one's body or body parts as one chooses. This view finds its colloquial expression in such slogans as "Whose body is it, anyway?" or "My body, my property." Although most jurisdictions do not recognize *legal* property rights in the body or body parts, proponents of maximal choice views regard this freedom as grounded in persons' *moral* ownership of their bodies. Maximal choice accounts that do not explicitly appeal to bodily ownership nevertheless construe the body instrumentally as a biological resource at the person's disposal, or at the disposal of another if she alienates the use of her body, or body parts, to them. Despite the fact that, at least within the English common-law tradition, the law does not recognize property relations in the body, the increasing pressure to commodify body parts, tissue, gametes, and so on justifies looking closely at this conception of the body.[3]

Finally, maximal choice views tend to regard state regulation and intervention as the main bogey to the exercise of individual autonomy, while looking to the market to maximize the range of choices available to individuals. While there are good reasons for wanting to limit the power of the state to intervene in people's choices, especially their reproductive choices, the role played by market forces in shaping both individual preferences and social opportunities is not always benign. In a context in which health care is increasingly controlled by powerful corporate interests such as pharmaceutical companies, and when biotechnology corporations can own patents in human life forms such as stem cell lines, this uncritical attitude toward the market is troubling.

Maximal choice conceptions figure in a range of different debates. These include, among others, debates concerning regulated markets in body parts, such as kidneys, corneas, blood products, sperm, and human eggs; and debates about contested surgeries, such as cosmetic surgery or demand self-amputation. They also include debates in the areas of assisted reproductive technology and genetic technology, such as those concerning commercial surrogate motherhood, prenatal testing and preimplantation genetic diagnosis, sex selection, genetic enhancement, and cloning. In all these areas, maximal choice conceptions are deployed to defend contested practices or technologies in the name of respect for individual autonomy.

The similarity in the structure of maximal choice arguments across these different areas is noteworthy. Their framing assumptions are that individual autonomy is a trumping value and that maximizing the options for bodily control, even extending to the bodies of one's offspring, is justified on the grounds of autonomy. They then proceed to discuss the benefits to individuals of legalizing the contested practice or making the specific technology available. Various harms that might outweigh these benefits, including social harms, are usually considered and then discounted, although in concession to such harms, limited restrictions on the exercise of individual autonomy, through some form of regulation for example, may be accepted. Finally, the conclusion is reached that any further restrictions would constitute unjustifiable paternalism. To illustrate, I want to consider arguments from four broad areas of debate: markets in organs, markets in oocytes, sex selection, and genetic enhancement.

The debate concerning morally permissible ways to increase the availability of organs, tissues, and blood products signals a site of tension in medical ethics and social policy between, on one hand, the injunction to respect the individual autonomy of potential donors and, on the other, the pressure on health systems created by increasing demand for body parts and shortages in supply. One proposed solution to this tension is to establish a current market in nonessential or renewable body parts, such as single kidneys, liver lobes, blood, bone marrow, or corneas. Two main arguments are adduced in support of such a market. One is the claim that persons have a right to determine what happens in and to their bodies, and this includes the right to use their bodies however they choose, including selling body parts and organs for material gain. Any attempt to limit this right, even on the grounds of protecting the interests of prospective donors/ sellers, is thought to constitute unjustifiable paternalism. The other is the claim that such markets simply provide prospective donors/sellers with extra options. Because nobody is under any obligation to choose these extra options if they do not wish to do so, then their availability can only enhance donors' range of choices and hence their autonomy. I will question both these arguments in the next section.

Defenders of markets in body parts acknowledge their potential risks and harms. In the case of a current market in organs, these include exploitation of the most desperate and disadvantaged members of society, inequities in the alloca- tion of health care resources that may attend their implementation, potential social harms arising from the commodification of human body parts, and under- mining the gift relationship—the altruistic donation of blood, organs, or gam- etes.[4] However, the interest in individual autonomy is claimed to trump these concerns. Thus, even if it is conceded that the option of selling a single kidney or cornea is likely to seem desirable only to the desperately poor, prohibiting the poor from pursuing this option or from pursuing other high-risk opportunities for earning income is considered unjustifiably paternalistic.[5] Nevertheless, in concession to such risks, defenders of current markets in organs usually argue for some form of government-regulated market.

Payment for egg or oocyte donation is currently permitted in some jurisdictions but prohibited in others. Arguments defending a regulated market in oocytes on grounds of individual autonomy employ argumentative strategies similar to those used by defenders of a regulated market in organs. For example, David Resnik argues that a market in oocytes promotes the liberty interests, or autonomy, of recipients and donors, as well as providing these parties with important benefits (Resnik 2001). Recipients benefit from such a market because it enables childless couples to have a child who is genetically related to the father and who has been gestated in the woman's uterus. A market in human oocytes also secures the right of such couples to procreative liberty, because reproduction is one of the most important ways in which people express their choices, values, and life plans. For the donor, the benefits are principally economic; for example, the money earned by a female university student may enable her to pay her fees or other educa- tional expenses. But a market in human oocytes also promotes the liberty rights of donors because it respects people's right to control what happens in and to their bodies.

Resnik does agree that the interest in liberty is not absolute. It may be justifi- ably constrained if it can be shown that the exercise of that liberty causes harm to others or to the person herself. Among the potential harms he considers are the risk of exploitation of donors who are poor or vulnerable and psychosocial harms to the children who are born through such market transactions. The broader social harms he considers include the risk that the commodification of human eggs may transform social and cultural attitudes toward the human body and so undermine respect for human life, and the risk that commodification will threaten the gift relationship. Resnik argues, however, that these potential harms are speculative and are outweighed by the risks to all parties that are likely to arise from an unregulated black market in human oocytes. A more prudential course of action is thus to establish a regulated market that would "pose a minimal infringement on the relevant liberty interests while protecting and promoting health, safety, human rights, and other values" (Resnik 2001, 24).

The extensive notion of reproductive liberty to which Resnik appeals also features prominently in debates concerning reproductive and/or genetic technologies, such as sex selection, postmenopausal pregnancy, using cadaveric or fetal eggs, genetic enhancement, and cloning. For the sake of brevity, I will focus on this appeal just in relation to sex selection and genetic enhancement.

As is well known, ultrasound and amniocentesis are widely used in some parts of the world to determine fetal sex in order to selectively abort unwanted female fetuses. In some contexts it is clear that the practice is coercively enforced and that it entrenches gender-based injustice, discrimination, and inequality. In India, where the widespread practice of sex selection has had a marked effect on sex ratios, sex selection is an ongoing concern for feminists, despite legislation banning the use of prenatal testing technologies for sex selection purposes.[6] In Western countries, although many medical professionals believe the use of these and other technologies for sex-selection purposes is a misuse, some appear to feel obliged to make them available to parents for "family-balancing" purposes or on the grounds of reproductive choice.

Defenders of sex selection, including some feminists, concede that there may be grounds for a ban on sex selection in countries in which there are powerful cultural preferences for sons. In such contexts, it is argued, the use of prenatal testing for sex-selection purposes seems to express similar misogynist cultural preferences as other practices like female infanticide, allowing unwanted girls to die of malnutrition and neglect, and subjecting women who do not bear sons to harsh punitive measures. However, it is argued that it is a mistake to assume that sex-selective preferences are universally harmful to women or always arise from coercive social pressures. In a Western context, where there is not a marked preference for male children, the sex-selective preferences of a woman or couple may well be an expression of voluntary choice, arising for example from a desire for gender balancing within a family, or from gender identification rather than gender stereotyping. Thus it is argued that in contexts where women enjoy significant economic and political autonomy, and where sex selection is unlikely to have a marked impact on sex ratios, the interest in reproductive liberty and in increasing the reproductive options available to parents should be protected.[7]

The appeal to parental reproductive liberty also figures significantly in arguments defending genetic enhancement. A number of bioethicists have argued that should the technology become available to allow genetic enhancement of the characteristics of one's offspring, it would be at least morally permissible for parents to seek to use to this technology on grounds of reproductive autonomy (Agar 1995, 1998; Harris 1998).[8] Two connected arguments are usually marshalled to support the appeal to parental reproductive autonomy. First, it is argued that concerns about enhancement are often based on a false genetic determinism and fail to appreciate the complex interaction of genes and environment in the development of phenotypic characteristics. Second, it is argued that given the role of the environment in the development of an individual's characteristics, the appeal to a distinction between therapeutic interventions designed to prevent harmful genetic conditions versus enhancements designed to benefit individuals by enhancing normal characteristics is questionable. When it comes to environmental input, parents do more than simply avoid exposing their children to harmful environments; they positively attempt to benefit them (for example, through choice of schools, music lessons, sports coaching). Is there any ground for distinguishing benefits deriving from environmental input and benefits deriving from genetic manipulation? If parents can send their children to expensive schools to promote the development of their capacities and better their life prospects, why not manipulate their genetic makeup to enhance their intelligence? Advocates of this "liberal eugenics" concede that enhancement should be limited to general-purpose capacities, such as intelligence or physical strength, with the aim of expanding the range of possibilities and goals open to the person (Agar 1995, 1998). Enhancements that aim to tailor individuals with capacities specified for particular goals (such as being a top-ranked tennis player) should be ruled out, however, on the grounds that they are likely to harm individuals by mismatching a person's capacities and goals. Similarly, any kind of genetic engineering that aims to restrict a person's goals by diminishing general-purpose capacities (for example, producing a slave class or a class of drones) should be ruled out.

Autonomy and the Body

Why are maximal choice approaches to autonomy problematic? After all, isn't it true, as feminists have been the first to point out, that the ability to exercise control over one's body is crucial for autonomy? And hasn't the defense of this right been important not only in protecting women from unwanted bodily violations but also in enabling us to exercise greater control over our fertility, and hence our lives, through access to contraception and abortion? To respond to this concern, my argument is not that control is unimportant for autonomy. Nor am I questioning that sometimes expanding the range of bodily options available to a person can be important for enhancing her autonomy. However, I will argue that maximal choice views conflate two distinct notions of bodily control, misconstrue the moral significance of embodiment, and assume a questionable conception of autonomy.

When we say that there is a moral requirement to respect the bodily autonomy of others, we usually mean two things. First, we mean that we may not physically interfere with another person's body or intrude upon her personal space unless, in some direct or indirect way, she has consented for us to do so. Let us call this the right to noninterference. Second, and connected with this, we usually mean that it is up to that person to decide what happens in and to her body, and that no one else may make such decisions for her. Let us call this the right to bodily self-determination. What is the relationship between the right to noninterference and the right to bodily self-determination, and how far does the latter extend? The right to bodily noninterference is essentially a negative right, a right to be free of trespass to the person. The control over one's body that it secures is control over one's bodily integrity. It enjoins others to respect the inviolability of one's person. I would argue that the right to bodily noninterference is an uncontroversial human right, although one that is routinely violated. The right to bodily self-determination, however, extends beyond this negative right and may involve claim rights to the provision of positive forms of assistance. The right to noninterference is necessary but not sufficient for bodily autonomy. For example, while freedom from bodily violations, such as rape or sexual harassment, is necessary, it is not sufficient for women's bodily autonomy, which requires more extensive forms of bodily self-determination, such as access to contraception, abortion, and arguably, some forms of assisted reproductive technologies. However, rights to extensive forms of bodily self-determination cannot simply be taken to follow from the right to noninterference, nor does a right to bodily autonomy automatically entail extensive claim rights to assistance. Thus, the right to the control over one's body that is secured by the right to noninterference cannot ground or be taken as equivalent to freedom to dispose of one's body parts or one's genetic material as one chooses. Nor does it automatically secure a right to assistance to enable one to express one's reproductive preferences, for example, for a child of a particular sex or with specific intellectual or physical capacities.[9]

Many maximal choice arguments work by appealing to some notion of bodily ownership to effect a slippage from the negative right to bodily noninterference to extensive positive rights to bodily self-determination. For example, in defending a regulated market in human eggs, David Resnik states:

> All people, it may be argued, have the right to control their bodies. People have the right to freedom of speech and movement, the right to acquire and transfer property, and the right to be free from harm or invasion of personal space. Because most of our free choices presuppose some control over own bodies, these liberty interests imply that people may even sell parts of their body, if they so desire. If we think of ownership of an object as a collection of rights to control the use of that object, then autonomous individuals own their bodies, body parts, and body products.   (Resnik 2001, 14)

Similarly, in an article defending a current market in organs, James Stacey Taylor claims that "because it is accepted that persons should be allowed to exercise control over their bodies, they should be allowed to sell their organs. Allowing a current market in human organs, then, will enhance personal autonomy through removing a prohibition that currently restricts person's control over their own bodies" (Taylor 2002, 275). Not only do these claims slide without further justification from a right to noninterference, or respect for bodily integrity, to the claim that we have a right to dispose of our bodies and body parts however we choose; problematically, they also ground both rights in the notion of bodily ownership.

The notion of bodily self-ownership has its origins in the Lockean tradition.[10] This approach to understanding the normative significance of the person-body relationship has been criticized by Kant and, more recently, by Paul Ricoeur. Ricoeur makes a distinction between two senses in which something can be said to belong to me or be "mine" (Ricoeur, 1992, study 5). In one sense of belonging, something belongs to me or is mine if I own it or possess it. In this sense, my books, my car, or my house belong to me. In this sense, the moral relationship between me and what belongs to me is appropriately expressed through the notion of ownership, and what I own is appropriately thought of as my property. In another sense of belonging, however, the moral relationship between me and what is "mine" or what belongs to me is more appropriately understood through the notion of constitution, that is, as constitutive of who I am. It is in this constitutive sense, Ricoeur argues, that we should understand the way in which our bodies belong to us. They are "ours" because they are expressive of our agency, or our person. Our bodies belong to us in the sense that we are embodied in them, we express our agency and intentions through them, and we experience the world from the perspective of our particular embodied points of view.

The constitutive view is broadly consistent with a phenomenological approach to embodiment. On the phenomenological view, our bodies and bodily capacities structure perception and consciousness at a prereflective level. One's body is the background or point of view from which one perceives and engages with the world. Consciousness is thus not separable from the body; rather consciousness and the body are a unity (Merleau-Ponty 1945/1958). The bodily ownership view, in contrast, represents the person as separate from her body and as only contingently unified with it. The constitutive view is also more in tune with understandings of the significance of embodiment that have been articulated by feminists and disability theorists. In emphasising the way in which different kinds of bodies give rise to qualitatively distinct lived experiences of the world, of bodily intentionality, and of agency, these approaches to embodiment highlight the unity of body, consciousness, and agency (Young 1990, 2005; Toombs 2001; Scully 2004).

I agree with Ricoeur that the notion of bodily ownership misconstrues the sense in which a person's body belongs to her. It cannot therefore provide an adequate normative grounding for the rights to bodily noninterference and bodily self-determination, which must rather be grounded in the constitutive view of bodily belonging.

Ricoeur's distinction between belonging as ownership and belonging as constitutive of identity echoes Kant's critique of property rights in the body. Kant argues that the body and body parts cannot be construed as property and cannot be bought and sold in the marketplace because "the body is part of the self; in its togetherness with the self it constitutes the person" (Kant 1963, 166). Respect for the body, whether our own body or the body of another, is thus integral to respect for the self and for moral personhood. Now one might agree that this is true with respect to the whole body, because the whole body is inseparable from the person. In fact, it may even be conceptually incoherent to regard one's whole body as one's property or as a commodity. But does it follow that it is also incoherent to regard one's body parts as commodities or tradeable resources? And does it follow that regarding one's body parts, or the body parts of other persons, in this way is inconsistent with respect for moral personhood? After all, we feel no compunction about disposing of some parts of our bodies, such as hair and nail clippings, as we see fit. In doing so, we do not feel as though we are violating ourselves. Why should we not adopt the same attitude to our blood products or to a single kidney that may fetch a high price in the marketplace?

What Kant himself says about why it is impermissible to sell body parts is not particularly helpful in answering such questions, because he does not distinguish selling from donating, or renewable from nonrenewable body parts.[11] Nor does he distinguish organs that are indispensable for functioning and survival (for example, the heart, the lungs, the brain) from those parts that may not be renewable but whose loss does not destroy the organism (for example, a limb, teeth, a single kidney). However, a plausible Kantian view would accept that while some body parts are not essential to our moral personhood, the body is an integrated, organic whole whose various parts all contribute to its functioning. Further, because a person is inseparable from her body, indeed because she expresses her moral personhood through her body, we cannot treat body parts that are integral to the functioning of the organism as items that are morally separable from the person (Cohen 1999). How we treat the bodies of others or our own bodies has implications for our moral attitudes toward others and ourselves. The basic Kantian objection to regarding body parts as commodities is that to do so degrades persons and their bodies, undermining human dignity by treating persons as objects or things and so reducing the value of humanity, which has unconditioned worth, to something with a market price. It also undermines self-respect, or a consciousness of one's inner moral worth that derives from the capacity for moral agency (Munzer 1993).

Now the usual response to this kind of argument is to insist that selling one's body parts need not undermine one's dignity as a person or compromise one's sense of self-respect as a moral agent. This same kind of response is also given to feminist objections to commercial surrogacy.[12] However, this response misses the point. The issue is not just whether an individual feels personally degraded by selling her body parts or what are euphemistically called reproductive services. The issue is what effect an institutionalized *system* or market for body parts would have, or does have, on our collective attitudes toward human dignity and on our sense of the respect we owe to others and ourselves as moral beings.[13] The attitudes of the buyers in such a marketplace to the sellers is also at issue. The worry expressed in the Kantian view is that in such a system, the sellers are likely to be invisible as human beings and regarded only as sources of body parts. In Stephen Frears's film *Dirty Pretty Things,* the asylum seekers and illegal migrants in London who trade body parts for false passports, often at serious risk of death, are invisible in just this way to the buyers of their organs. The upshot of this argument is not just that the right to bodily self-determination is justifiably constrained by other moral considerations; it is also that the notion of bodily self-ownership is normatively flawed.

In addition to these problems, maximal choice views are based on two questionable assumptions about autonomy. First, they mistakenly assume that increasing a person's options for disposing of her body as she chooses automatically enhances her autonomy. This is to treat all options as on a par, both morally and in terms of their effects on autonomy. What this view ignores is that some options are unjust and function to entrench or extend existing inequalities, such as those based on socioeconomic status, gender, ability, or citizenship. Adding these options to a person's choice set may simply increase the opportunities for others to exploit her, rather than increasing her autonomy, as the existence of the black market in organs functions to exploit the desperation of the asylum seekers and illegal migrants in Frears's film. Such additional options may also function as constraining options, pressuring a person to pursue an option she would not otherwise have chosen, and that may further her disadvantage. For example, had there been reasonable alternative options for the sellers in Frears's film, none of them would willingly have traded their organs at serious risk to their health and even their lives.

In response, defenders of an unrestricted right to so-called freedom of choice might argue that it is up to individuals to determine whether or not they are willing to take these risks. Whether individuals do have rights to take on any risks they choose is debatable. But this response also points to the second problem with maximal choice views, namely that they are excessively individualistic and reduce autonomy to the expression of individual subjective preferences. The problem with this view is that it overlooks the fact that individuals do not make choices in a relational and social vacuum. Our preferences, values and choices are shaped by social relationships and by powerful social forces, such as educational institutions, the law, media, governmental agencies, and corporate entities. The options that are available to us are determined by, and reflective of, the institutional structure of the society in which we live as well as by our place within that structure, for example, by gender, class position, ethnicity, ability, or disability. Further, our individual choices have social impacts. The need to take into account both the social dimensions and impacts of individual choices, as well as concerns about distributive justice—about who benefits from and who suffers the burdens of certain options—reveals the ethical limitations of equating autonomy with the expression and satisfaction of individual preferences.

The problematic individualism of maximal choice approaches is particularly evident in the way the notion of reproductive liberty is understood simply as a right of adults to dispose of their bodies, or the bodies of their offspring, as they choose. For reproductive choices do not just concern individual self-determination. Reproductive choices affect the lives of many others, including those who are brought into existence by these choices. To focus only on the rights entailed by reproductive autonomy is to overlook or trivialize the responsibilities and obligations that arise from the exercise of that autonomy, in particular weighty parental responsibilities for the flourishing and moral education of children.[14] For example, markets in human gametes institutionalize a system in which the biological, ethical, and social relationship between parents and their children is treated as a fungible commodity. In doing so, they encourage the attitude that reproductive liberty is all about the right to control one's body and to express one's personal preferences, rather than also involving serious corresponding responsibilities for the welfare of future persons.[15]

Similarly, somatic genetic interventions cannot be justified simply by reference to parental preferences but must also take into account the needs, perspective, and vulnerability of the future child. Genetic therapies that aim to cure painful or progressive genetic diseases or impairments are, at least arguably, driven by such concerns. In contrast, the type of genetic enhancement permitted by liberal eugenics, assuming it ever becomes technologically possible, would permit the irrevocable intervention of parental determination into the very conditions of the child's identity formation. In response to the argument that parents already intervene to direct the course of their children's lives through environmental influence and enhancements, I would agree with Habermas that eugenic genetic intervention is significantly different. Parental intervention that takes place through the socialization process is interactive. Ideally, it is responsive to the child and his or her personality and needs, but even in nonideal interactions the child may at some point contest the direction the parents are intending for his or her life. In contrast, as Habermas puts it, eugenic genetic intervention would involve "a one-sided act for which there can be no well-founded presumption of consent, disposing over the genetic factors of another in the paternalistic intention of setting the course, in relevant respects, of the life history of the dependent person. The latter may interpret, but not undo or revise this intention" (Habermas 2003, 64).

Further, somatic genetic interventions do not just affect the future person who is shaped by those interventions; they have broader social effects and implications. The decisions of individuals can have large-scale cumulative social impacts, as is evident from sex-selection practices in India. Genetic interventions may also affect what are taken to be disabilities in a particular society and how people with disabilities are treated. Further, they raise complex issues about distributive justice, such as who has access to genetic interventions, for example, whether distribution is based on need or on capacity to pay, and whether they not only entrench but also may increase social and natural inequalities.[16] And they raise normative issues about whether we should be intervening to alter the shape of human nature. To leave decisions about all these issues to the vagaries of individual preferences and market forces is to ensure that genetic technologies will exacerbate existing social injustices.

Relational Autonomy

Feminist relational theories offer an alternative interpretation of autonomy that has important implications for many debates in bioethics.[17] Relational theories acknowledge the importance of individual autonomy and bodily self-determination. However, they argue that individual autonomy is socially constituted. Individualistic conceptions of autonomy regard persons as only incidentally or contingently social beings, think of social relationships as voluntary associations, and treat responsibilities to others as side constraints on the exercise of autonomy. In contrast, relational theories start from the premise that our identities and self-conceptions, including our attitudes toward and experiences of our bodies, are constituted in relationships of interdependence and embedded in complex social structures. Relational theories acknowledge that while some of our significant relationships may be chosen, many may be nonvoluntary biological relationships with family members. These situate us within networks of nonvoluntary responsibilities and obligations that shape our lives, our choices, and the competences and capacities necessary for autonomy. At a broader macro level, relational theories attend to the fact that our preferences, values, and self-conceptions, and the choices and opportunities available to us, are structured by the socially available alternatives and by powerful social and political forces. In turn our individual choices can have cumulative social effects and consequences.

Relational theories are particularly attentive to the effects of power relations on individuals' choices, opportunities and capacities—both within intimate and familial relationships and at the level of social structures. Some social relationships enhance autonomy, fostering its development and exercise within the context of respectful and reciprocal relationships involving mutual responsibilities. However, social and familial relationships can also be coercive, repressive, and authoritarian, exposing individuals to harmful, disrespectful, or degrading treatment and constraining the development and exercise of autonomy. Similarly, the opportunities available to an individual may be enhanced or constrained by her social position. For example, an individual's class, race, gender, ethnicity, sexual preference, religion, ability, or disability will strongly influence her sense of the options available to her and her capacity to conceive of, or even imagine alternatives. Relational theories therefore argue that to ignore these power structures and operate with a conception of individual self-determination that assumes that all persons are similarly situated and have similar options and capacities, or to think that autonomy is constrained only by overt coercion, is to operate with a theoretical abstraction that fails to account for the complex interpersonal and social realities that shape people's lives. Similarly, equating respect for autonomy simply with the satisfaction of individual preferences risks entrenching inequalities and protecting only the autonomy of those who are most socially powerful.

By building into the conception of autonomy recognition that selfhood is relational, relational theories do not posit autonomy and interdependence, individual liberty and responsibilities to others as inevitably opposed. Similarly, by attending to the effects of oppressive or unequal social structures on individuals' preferences, choices, and capacities, they do not set up an opposition between autonomy and considerations of social justice. This is not to say that within the framework of a relational approach tensions between individual autonomy and obligations toward others or between individual liberty and social regulation are simply dissolved. But a relational approach configures these tensions differently, not as intrinsic to the exercise of autonomy but usually as effects of repressive or dysfunctional social relationships and oppressive and unjust social structures.

Conclusion

The widespread equation of autonomy with maximal choice in Anglophone bioethics, and the associated conception of bodily autonomy as bodily self-ownership, oversimplify and distort bioethical debate. Reconfiguring autonomy as relational is unlikely to result in moral consensus concerning current and emerging contested technologies and practices, including those discussed in this chapter. However, it may result in less polarized, more thoughtful bioethical debate about the scope and limits of individual autonomy, moving beyond the simplistic oppositions between autonomy and paternalism, consent and coercion, individual liberty and state interference that structure the way maximal choice theories frame moral issues. Sex selection; prenatal diagnosis; the commodification of body parts and gametes; and genetic intervention, whether therapeutic or enhancing; as well as most other issues in bioethics, involve complex moral, social, legal, and metaphysical issues. Framing these issues in terms of an opposition between, on one hand, state regulation and paternalistic interference with liberty, and on the other hand, the freedom of individuals to dispose of their bodies as they choose, limited only by the sophistication of the available technology, the opportunities made available by the market, and the individual's purchasing power, radically oversimplifies these complexities.[18]

NOTES

1. Although I accept that the concept of race has no biological foundation and racial categories are socially constructed, these categories are nevertheless highly socially significant in contexts where alleged racial differences have been used to justify the differential treatment of certain social groups. The term *ethnicity* refers to social group identities based on cultural, historical, linguistic, or geographical affiliations.

2. On the importance of "significant options," see Raz (1986) and Sen (1992).

3. In her work, Donna Dickenson (1997, 2001, 2002) discusses the implications of conceptions of the body as property and trends toward increasing commodification for women's control over their reproductive labor and over the products of that labor (eggs, embryonic and fetal tissue, stem cells, babies). She argues that commodification is unlikely to increase women's control over reproduction; in fact, the reverse is more likely to be the case. Margaret Radin (1987, 1996) has also criticized the commodification of the body in relation to commercial surrogacy, prostitution, and markets in body parts.

4. These concerns about a current market in organs have been raised by a number of authors. See, for example, Manga (1987), Chadwick (1989), and Zutlevics (2001).

5. For an argument along these lines, see, for example, Taylor (2002).

6. Results from the 2001 Indian census showed that sex ratios had dropped over the decade since 1991 from 945 females per 1,000 males to 927 females per 1,000 males. In some regions, such as Haryana and Punjab, the ratio of males to females is even higher. The Regulation and Prevention of Misuse of Diagnostic Techniques Act, banning the use of prenatal testing and selective abortion for sex-selection purposes, was introduced in India in 1994. However, the widespread use of prenatal diagnostic technologies, such as ultrasound and amniocentesis, and the willingness of many health care professionals to defy the law and use these technologies at their patients' request to determine fetal sex and perform sex-selective abortions effectively enables the law to be bypassed. More recent preconception technologies (such as sperm sorting) have also provided another avenue for sex selection. Amartya Sen (2003), who coined the term "missing women" to refer to the deficit of women arising from sex biases in cultural practices and health care, argues that since the mid-1990s the substantial reduction in female infant mortality rates in parts of India has been counterbalanced by

sex-specific abortions. For a broader discussion of the social and political context of sex selection and reproductive rights in India, see, for example, Shanthi (2004).

7. For a feminist argument along these lines, see Warren (1999). See also Zilberberg (2004, 2007). For incisive responses to this kind of argument, see, for example, Moazam (2004) and Rogers, Ballantyne, and Draper (2007). For an overview of the feminist debate, see Bubeck (2002).

8. See also Savalescu (2001), who argues that parents actually have a moral obligation to genetically select for intelligence in their children. For a detailed critical response to Savalescu, see, for example, Birch (2005). For a detailed overview of the current debate concerning genetic enhancement, see Baylis and Robert (2004).

9. For a more detailed argument to this effect, see O'Neill (2002, chap. 3).

10. Donna Dickenson (1997) argues that the Lockean tradition is actually based on a rather loose interpretation of Locke. On her reading, Locke's view is that we own our labor, not our bodies. In their discussion of limb transplants, Dickenson and Guy Widdershoven (2001, 114) raise some similar concerns to those raised here about arguments that appeal to the notion of bodily ownership to justify rights to dispose of one's body as one chooses.

11. Nicole Gerrand (1999) argues that commentators who have appealed to Kantian arguments against a market in body parts have failed to recognize that Kant's arguments would rule out not only selling one's body parts, but also all forms of organ donation. Jean-Christophe Merle (2000) rejects this claim, arguing that on a plausible reading of Kant's text donation of renewable organs and tissues would be not only morally permissible, but also morally required. My interpretation of Kant is influenced by Merle, as well as by Munzer (1993) and Cohen (1999).

12. The classic feminist objections to surrogacy include Anderson (1990), Pateman (1988), Radin (1987, 1996), and Satz (1992).

13. See Munzer (1993) and Cohen (1999) for more detailed arguments to this effect.

14. For an argument to this effect in relation to gamete donation, see Benatar (1999).

15. For a related critique of standard notions of procreative liberty, see Murray (2002), who advocates an alternative framework for approaching the ethics of assisted reproductive technologies based on the notion of human flourishing.

16. These issues are extensively discussed in Buchanan et al. (2000). However, they tend to take the standard conception of individual autonomy for granted and then argue that considerations of justice place justifiable constraints on autonomy, rather than arguing that concerns about justice and equality require a rethinking of standard conceptions of autonomy.

17. For an overview of relational approaches to autonomy, see Mackenzie and Stoljar (2000b). For more detailed explorations of different aspects of relational theories, see the essays in Mackenzie and Stoljar (2000a). For applications of relational theories to bioethics, see, for example, Dodds (2000), Donchin (2000, 2001), McLeod (2002), and Sherwin (1998).

18. There are some commonalities between relational approaches to autonomy and Raz's liberal perfectionist approach to autonomy (Raz 1986). It is beyond the

scope of this chapter to explore this issue. However, for a discussion of autonomy in genetic and reproductive ethics that is influenced by Raz, see Clayton (2002).

REFERENCES

Agar, N. 1995. Designing babies: Morally permissible ways to modify the human genome. *Bioethics* 9 (1): 1–15.

———. 1998. Liberal eugenics. *Public Affairs Quarterly* 12 (2): 137–55.

Anderson, E. 1990. Is women's labour a commodity? *Philosophy and Public Affairs* 19:71–92.

Baylis, F., and J. S. Robert. 2004. The inevitability of genetic enhancement technologies. *Bioethics* 18 (1): 1–26.

Benatar, D. 1999. The unbearable lightness of bringing into being. *Journal of Applied Philosophy* 16 (2): 173–80.

Birch, K. 2005. Beneficence, determinism and justice: An engagement with the argument for the genetic selection of intelligence. *Bioethics* 19 (1): 12–28.

Bubeck, D. 2002. Sex selection: The feminist response. In *A companion to genethics*, ed. J. Burley and J. Harris, 216–28. Malden, Mass.: Blackwell.

Buchanan, A., D. W. Brock, N. Daniels, and D. Wikler. 2000. *From chance to choice: Genetics and justice.* Cambridge: Cambridge University Press.

Chadwick, R. 1989. The market for bodily parts: Kant and duties to oneself. *Journal of Applied Philosophy* 6 (2): 129–39.

Clayton, M. 2002. Individual autonomy and genetic choice. In *A companion to genethics*, ed. J. Burley and J. Harris, 191–205. Malden, Mass.: Blackwell.

Cohen, C. 1999. Selling bits and pieces of humans to make babies: *The Gift of the Magi* revisited. *Journal of Medicine and Philosophy* 24 (3): 288–306.

Dickenson, D. 1997. *Property, women and politics.* Cambridge: Polity Press.

———. 2001. Property and women's alienation from their own reproductive labour. *Bioethics* 15 (3): 205–17.

———. 2002. Who owns embryonic and fetal tissue? In *Ethical issues in maternal-fetal medicine*, ed. D. Dickenson, 233–45. Cambridge: Cambridge University Press.

Dickenson, D., and G. Widdershoven. 2001. Ethical issues in limb transplants. *Bioethics* 15 (2): 110–24.

Dodds, S. 2000. Choice and control in feminist bioethics. In *Relational autonomy: Feminist perspectives on autonomy, agency and the social self*, ed. C. Mackenzie and N. Stoljar, 213–35. New York: Oxford University Press.

Donchin, A. 2000. Autonomy and interdependence: Quandaries in genetic decision making. In *Relational autonomy: Feminist perspectives on autonomy, agency and the social self*, ed. C. Mackenzie and N. Stoljar, 236–58. New York: Oxford University Press.

———. 2001. Understanding autonomy relationally: Toward a reconfiguration of bioethical principles. *Journal of Medicine and Philosophy* 26 (4): 365–86.

Gerrand, N. 1999. The misuse of Kant in the debate about a market for human body parts. *Journal of Applied Philosophy* 16 (1): 59–67.

Habermas, J. 2003. *The future of human nature*. Cambridge: Polity Press.

Harris, J. 1998. *Clones, genes and immortality*. Oxford: Oxford University Press.

Kant, I. 1963. *Lectures on ethics*, trans. L. Infield. Indianapolis, Ind.: Hackett.

Mackenzie, C., and N. Stoljar, eds. 2000a. *Relational autonomy: Feminist perspectives on autonomy, agency, and the social self*. New York: Oxford University Press.

———. 2000b. Introduction: Autonomy refigured. In *Relational autonomy: Feminist perspectives on autonomy, agency and the social self*, ed. C. Mackenzie and N. Stoljar, 3–31. New York: Oxford University Press.

Manga, P. 1987. A commercial market for organs? Why not. *Bioethics* 1 (4): 321–38.

McLeod, C. 2002. *Self-trust and reproductive autonomy*. Cambridge, Mass.: MIT Press.

Merle, J-C. 2000. A Kantian argument for a duty to donate one's own organs: A reply to Nicole Gerrand. *Journal of Applied Philosophy* 17 (1): 93–101.

Merleau-Ponty, M. 1945/1958. *The phenomenology of perception*, translated by C. Smith. London: Routledge & Kegan Paul.

Moazam, F. 2004. Feminist discourse on sex screening and selective abortion of female foetuses. *Bioethics* 18 (3): 205–20.

Munzer, S. 1993. Kant and property rights in body parts. *Canadian Journal of Law and Jurisprudence* 6 (2): 319–41.

Murray, T. 2002. What are families for? Getting to an ethics of reproductive technology. *Hastings Center Report* 32 (May–June): 41–45.

O'Neill, O. 2002. *Autonomy and trust in bioethics*. Cambridge: Cambridge University Press.

Pateman, C. 1988. *The sexual contract*. Cambridge: Polity Press.

Radin, M. J. 1987. Market inalienability. *Harvard Law Review* 100:1849–1937.

———. 1996. *Contested commodities: The trouble with the trade in sex, children, body parts and other things*. Cambridge, Mass.: Harvard University Press.

Raz, J. 1986. *The morality of freedom*. Oxford: Clarendon Press.

Resnik, D. 2001. Regulating the market for human eggs. *Bioethics* 15 (1): 1–25.

Ricoeur, P. 1992. *Oneself as another*, trans. Kathleen Blamey. Chicago: University of Chicago Press.

Rogers, A., A. Ballantyne, and H. Draper. 2007. Is sex-selective abortion morally justified and should it be prohibited? *Bioethics* 21 (9): 520–24.

Satz, D. 1992. Markets in women's reproductive labor. *Philosophy and Public Affairs* 21 (2): 107–31.

Savalescu, J. 2001. Procreative beneficence: Why we should select the best children. *Bioethics* 15 (5/6): 413–26.

Scully, J. L. 2004. Normative ethics and non-normative embodiment. Paper presented to International Association of Bioethics / Feminist Approaches to Bioethics Conference, Sydney.

Sen, A. 1992. *Inequality reexamined*. Cambridge, Mass.: Harvard University Press.

———. 2003. Missing women—revisited. *British Medical Journal* 327: 1297–98.

Shanthi, K. 2004. Feminist bioethics and reproductive rights of women in India: Myth and reality. In *Linking visions: Feminist bioethics, human rights, and the developing world,* ed. R. Tong, A. Donchin, and S. Dodds, 119–32. Lanham, Md.: Rowman & Littlefield.

Sherwin, S. 1998. A relational approach to autonomy in health care. In *The politics of women's health: Exploring agency and autonomy,* ed. Feminist Health Care Ethics Research Network, 19–47. Philadelphia: Temple University Press.

Taylor, J. S. 2002. Autonomy, constraining options, and organ sales. *Journal of Applied Philosophy* 19 (3): 273–85.

Toombs, S. K. 2001. Reflections on bodily change: The lived experience of disability. In *Handbook of Phenomenology and Medicine,* ed. S. K. Toombs, 247–61. Dordrecht: Kluwer.

Warren, M. A. 1999. Sex selection: Individual choice or cultural coercion? In *Bioethics: An anthology,* ed. H. Kuhse and P. Singer, 137–42. Oxford: Blackwell.

Young, I. 1990. *Throwing like a girl and other essays in feminist philosophy and social theory.* Bloomington: Indiana University Press.

———. 2005. *On female body experience.* New York: Oxford University Press.

Zilberberg, J. 2004. A boy or a girl: Is any choice moral? The ethics of sex selection and sex preselection. In *Linking visions: Feminist bioethics, human rights, and the developing world,* ed. R. Tong, A. Donchin, and S. Dodds, 147–56. Lanham, Md: Rowman & Littlefield.

———. 2007. Sex-selective abortion for social reasons: Is it ever morally justified? *Bioethics* 21 (9): 517–19.

Zutlevics, T. L. 2001. Markets and the needy: Organ sales or aid? *Journal of Applied Philosophy* 18 (3): 297–302.

CHAPTER FIVE

Trust, Method, and Moral Progress in Feminist Bioethics

JESSICA PRATA MILLER, PH.D.

Bioethics and feminist ethics share several themes. Their interest in the practical effects of method has led them to be skeptical of the claims of abstract, universalistic moral theories to adequately capture the richness of moral life. They have had to develop new strategies for analyzing morally problematic social institutions and public policies. Both have sought to construct forms of ethical theory that are grounded in the complex experiences of moral agents so that they may effect beneficial change in actual lives. This urgent practical impetus, wedded to keen attention to empirical (including personal, institutional, social, and political) details and to the complex moral psychology of ethical decision making and ethical action, has led both bioethics and feminist ethics to reject the search for an overarching theory of the good and the right, favoring instead a more piecemeal, contextual approach.

Given these affinities in method and aims, one might think that feminist bioethicists, many of whom draw on feminist ethical theory, would not find it difficult to make significant inroads in bioethics. This might seem especially likely, given that the concept of trust is central to both discourses. However, this is not the case. The concept of trust, which feminist ethicists have used as a wedge to radically critique the ontological and epistemological assumptions of dominant ethical systems from the ground up, is rendered, in mainstream bioethics, an apoliticized, uncritically celebrated moral good or, worse, just the other side of the coin of patient autonomy.

This chapter traces the relationship of feminist ethical theory to feminist bioethics and then explores the difference between feminist accounts of trust and those in mainstream bioethics. Feminist bioethicists are especially well placed to reorient the terms of the discussion of trust in medicine. To make moral progress, feminist bioethicists must push harder on the front of method, in particular by paying more attention to trust and distrust as moral categories.

Feminist Ethical Theory, Bioethics, and Feminist Bioethics: Convergences and Divergences

As internally diverse but identifiably distinct social movements, bioethics and feminism have intersected at various points: the women's health movement is the most obvious example. Many of the defining moments in the birth of bioethics were about reproductive issues, and a major focus of feminist theorists has been the effect of patriarchy on women's bodies. Feminism and bioethics are also both skeptical about traditional ethical theories, but for different reasons.[1]

Bioethics has always been closely tied to a relatively discrete, if complex, social institution, the health care delivery system, and so has had the reformist goal of eliminating injustice in the practice of medicine. Initially, many bioethicists hoped that they could apply standard ethical theories to moral issues in health care: the correct ethical theory would specify principles that generated duties that would, in turn, dictate the proper moral response in individual situations.[2] However, seemingly intractable disagreement at the theoretical level and problems with application led bioethicists to abandon the so-called engineering model. A glance at major titles in bioethics and tables of contents in bioethics textbooks suggests that bioethicists actually proceed from thick concepts, such as informed consent, generated from morally problematic medical practices, which are tested against midlevel ethical principles, such as autonomy, beneficence, and justice. Bioethical reasoning, especially in the clinical setting, is responsive to context and is well suited to narrative structuring, including particulars about individuals, their histories, and their relationships.

In contrast, feminist criticism of traditional moral theory centers on its deleterious effects, especially on women, in an unjustly gendered society. Carol Gilligan's articulation of care theory galvanized contemporary feminist ethics (Gilligan 1987a, 1987b, 1995). As is by now well known, Gilligan rejected the idea that there is only one correct form of moral reasoning, discerning a valuable alternative form, which uses not abstractions and universal principles but skills commonly associated with femininity, including a wide emotional repertoire, attunement and attention, and an ability to home in on significant moral particulars. Gilligan, and feminist moral philosophers she influenced, criticized dominant moral philosophy for constructing real women's lives as beyond the moral pale. From the feminist perspective, the practical effects of dominant moral theories, and the social and historical contexts in which they are devised, are as important as their internal coherence.

Their defining commitments to health and to the status of women, respectively, have led bioethicists and feminist ethicists alike to appreciate the moral significance of trust. Bioethicists are concerned with relationships among parties unequal in power and vulnerability, especially health care providers and patients, but also medical researchers and human subjects, and well as health care distribution systems and their beneficiaries. Feminists also, of course, are interested in relationships between social groups unequal in power. Whether and when trust (or distrust) is reasonable becomes a major concern in such relationships. Trust implies dependence, is often unconscious and slow to build, has emotional and affective components, and is best grasped by attention to particular details of concrete relations among the parties. In contrast, dominant moral theories take relations among abstract rational actors equal in power as their paradigm. It follows that the dominant emphasis in ethical theory on the rationality of impartial, independent moral actors tends to place most forms of trust on the margins of morality.

One might think that such convergences in subject matter and method of bioethics and feminism would prime feminist bioethics to have a major impact on mainstream bioethics. Initially, feminist bioethics might best have been defined as feminist attention to women's issues in contraception, abortion, and reproduction. However, feminist bioethics quickly moved *Beyond Reproduction*, as the subtitle of Susan M. Wolf's edited 1996 volume attests. In that collection, contributors address issues ranging from euthanasia to biomedical research to equity in health care, many using the tools of Gilligan's ethics to do so.[3] Susan Sherwin's *No Longer Patient*, published in 1992, provided the first book-length account of the relevance of feminist ethics to bioethics. There Sherwin pointed to the narrowness of the field of health care ethics and its lack of reflexivity on the questions of what counts as a moral dilemma in health care and which persons count as moral actors. According to Sherwin, feminist method in bioethics is grounded in a relativized social epistemology that recognizes that one's perspective makes a difference to one's experience of reality, and thus emphasizes the importance of democratic process and the uncoerced participation of moral agents from various socioeconomic locations (Sherwin 1992, 64). Appearing in 1997, Rosemarie Tong's *Feminist Approaches to Bioethics* acknowledges the diversity of feminist bioethical thought but contends that a focus on gender—in particular, on "the woman question"—constitutes the core of feminist method in bioethics (Tong 1997, 90). Sherwin and Tong insist that to be truly feminist, an ethic of care must attend to power differentials and to the question of who gives care and to whom. Anne Donchin, in her 2004 entry on "Feminist Bioethics" for the *Stanford Encyclopedia of Philosophy,* sums up the current state of the field: "A growing contingent of feminists think a framework that incorporates universal principles should constitute one dimension of an adequate bioethical theory providing its principles are formulated in nonexclusionary terms that reflect the relational context of individual lives. They draw on two themes in feminist theory. The first stems from attention to an ethics of care and the second from reflections on the sources of women's subordination in patterns of domination and oppression."

One might expect that the interventions of feminists—who have been involved since its start—would have a significant impact on the concerns and methods of bioethics as a new and still developing field. Yet Hilde Lindemann (writing as H. L. Nelson 2000) claimed that, with a few exceptions, "feminist bioethicists' contributions to ethical theory have been practically nonexistent" (494). One way to determine whether this is the case is to look at how bioethics is being taught. Most bioethics textbooks authored by philosophers begin with a discussion of ethical theory in which feminist theory is presented last, typically as a new twist on an old theory (such as virtue ethics), as a women's concern of limited interest, or as too diffuse to be useful.[4] Following this overview of ethical theory, most bioethics textbooks launch into thematically arranged sections divided into chapters that focus on discrete bioethical topics. Chapters on physician-assisted suicide, cloning, and research ethics offer an array of rival viewpoints. Because all ethical theory is abandoned at this point, in favor of the coherentist or bottom-up approach employed by bioethicists, feminist ethics fares no worse than its rivals. But, as Lindemann notes, feminist bioethicists "haven't the luxury of that sort of pragmatism, because it is the business of feminism to be deeply suspicious of the standing political and moral theories" and to create new theories that deconstruct and analyze medicine as the powerful hegemonic discourse it is (Nelson 2000, 496). Even on topics typically framed as "women's concerns," feminist perspectives represent an astonishingly small fraction of contributions in the leading textbooks.[5] If what counts as worthy of transmission to the next generation of bioethicists is the primary indication, feminist method and feminist concerns remain marginalized.

Of course, there are many factors to consider in addition to textbooks, and the question of the overall impact of feminism on bioethics is too large to attempt to answer here. As with ethical theory, to the extent that the basic players in bioethics (physician, patient, researcher, subject, policy maker, citizen) are decontextualized "neutral" actors, feminist concerns will be considered "special," "extra," and, thus, "optional." Moral agents that are gendered female tend to be overlooked. Nurses are overlooked not just in mainstream but also in feminist bioethics (Andre 2006). And the most potent symbol of femininity in the Western world, the pregnant woman, is completely invisible in debates over reproductive cloning or other genetic and/or reproductive interventions. The similarities to the lack of consideration for the unwillingly pregnant woman and her fate should abortion be criminalized (an all-too-real worry in the United States, and a reality in many other countries) are almost too obvious to mention.

Feminist bioethicists, like Sherwin and Tong, who have made incursions on the front of theory have tended to focus on problems with principlist approaches. And as with feminist ethicists, one of the most significant principles to receive attention from feminists has been respect for autonomy. As important as this is, feminist bioethicists must also take on some of the thick ethical concepts at the very heart of medical practice. Trust is especially significant because feminist ethicists have contended that acknowledging its place determines in part not only how ethical theory is done but also what things we take to matter morally. It is closely associated with care theory, the most developed component of feminist bioethical theory. Trust is also crucial in mainstream bioethics, for very different reasons: it has been viewed as a key good in medicine, whether on the micro level (the physician-patient relationship) or the macro level (public trust in medicine), and loss of trust is a major concern in bioethics. In the second half of this essay, I investigate the uses of trust and distrust at the intersection of feminist theory and mainstream bioethics.

Trust at the Intersection of Theory and Method in Feminist Bioethics

Trust came to be a major topic in feminist ethics with the work of Annette Baier, who, in her earlier writings on trust (Baier 1995), self-consciously views her project as taking up the implications for ethical theory of Gilligan's work on the ethic of care. Taking her cue from Hume, Baier seeks to naturalize morality, to find its wellspring in actual social practices. For Baier (as for Hume), the most compelling argument against the "moral rationalists" (including Locke, Hobbes, and, later, Kant), who attempt to ground a universal morality in reason-produced general principles, is that close observation and careful description of concrete human activities, in all of their complexity and richness, belies the distorting neatness of modern moral theory. In particular, looking at human practices requires recognizing that we begin as infants and only gradually become adults capable of abstract moral theorizing. Any adequate moral theory will have to make sense of both the disjunctions and the continuities between infants and adults. And this is likely to include passions, feelings, dispositions, and other elements not featured in rationalistic accounts of morality.

Against mainstream philosophers who have either ignored trust or privileged its most attenuated hyperrational forms, Baier claims that moral life is rife with those forms of trust that are less than fully conscious, voluntary, or explicit—paradigmatically, trust between parents and children. Baier also argues that contracts can be conceived as foundational to moral life only when their background conditions, and especially the work of women care providers, are ignored. For Baier and feminists who have taken up her call to make the questions of whom we trust, with what, and why central to ethical inquiry, trust is not a voluntary ability: trust is confident reliance on another's capacity and willingness to care for an entrusted item. It is a kind of attitude, specifically, a feeling of confidence and security, in the face of one's vulnerability to another in the attempt to pursue one's good. Trust is vitally important to moral life not only because "all moral virtues—those possessions of the morally lucky—contribute to a climate of trust" but also because "a climate of trust must first exist before we can expect the virtues that sustain it" (Baier 2004, 180).

It is important to place Baier's work, and the work of other feminists who have since addressed the topic of trust in ethical theory, in its proper context.[6] Several feminists have taken up Baier's call to develop an ethic of trust and have pushed trust theory in interesting and sometimes critical directions. Feminists working on trust have not yet settled the finer points of the philosophy of trust, including the question of what counts as trust; whether we should look for necessary and sufficient conditions, paradigmatic cases, or family resemblance to determine this; whether trust implies good will, integrity, or some other moral attitude on the part of the trustee; the logical relation of trust to distrust (contraries or contradictories?); the question of whether nonpersons such as organizations can trust; and to what extent, if any, trust may be willed. But for feminists, recognition of the importance of trust as a substantive moral concept—a recognition that has until recently eluded moral philosophers except in certain highly specified forms—such as trust in God and the limit case of highly rationalized trust in fellow contractors—is only possible when some central features of traditional models of moral theory are rejected. In particular, feminists' interest in nonconscious forms and affective aspects of trust stems from the acknowledgement of the problematic disconnect between abstract, argument-based moral theory and concrete, not fully rational moral life (Baier 1997). Putting trust at center stage in ethical theory forces a recognition that the implicit epistemology and metaphysics of most mainstream ethical theories—roughly, "individualism" in reason, intention, autonomy, and judgment—is inaccurate and misleading, failing as it does to take account of the complex social conditions for the very existence of these mental states.

Methodologically, the feminist foregrounding of trust is a major theme in the articulation of what Margaret Urban Walker, in an attempt to conceptualize themes in feminist ethical theory, has called the "expressive-collaborative" model of moral theory, which "pictures morality as a socially embodied medium of understanding and adjustment in which people account to each other for the identities, relationships, and values that define their responsibilities" (Walker 1998a, 61). Being a moral agent is being familiar with the media of moral understanding. It involves ongoing social negotiation of moral equilibria between people. Moral knowledge is a kind of know-how, inclusive of any skills required for the maintenance of interpersonal acknowledgment, and takes as its object not a highly general core of moral knowledge but anything relevant to getting around in the moral environment (Walker 1998a, 66). Moral resolutions are acceptable in this model not because they satisfy deductive or logical demands of first principles but because they sustain or enhance the moral integrity (defined not as being impervious to external temptations but as a kind of reliable accountability) and interrelationships of actual persons. The problem of justification is not the worry that there may be no object of moral knowledge (the skeptical threat) but rather, because moral knowledge is generated and embodied in communities, the question of the credibility of people's claims to moral knowledge, a question that cannot be answered except by understanding who it is that is claiming to know (Walker 1998a, 74).

In this model, trust is not a second-best policy in a world where individuals are sometimes unreliable and/or controls on them are insufficiently effective, nor a simple rational response to trustworthy behavior. If moral life is a cultural product, an ability of people to share a stable sense of themselves as they live in community, then trust is vitally important for morality to go on. And because feminist method broadens the scope of ethical theory, it creates room for the recognition of trust as a moral good, in a manner similar to that by which Gilligan's work spurred the recognition of mothering and other forms of caring as moral goods, rather than as merely instinctive labor or monotonous drudgery.

But, just as with the concerns about an apolitical celebration of care leveled by Sherwin and Tong, these claims should not be confused with the notion that trust is a moral good *simpliciter*. In fact, a major advantage for feminists of looking at morality through the lens of trust is that it persists in unequal relations, both just and unjust, thus shifting the focus of ethical theory away from relationships among mutually disinterested agents of equal moral status and inviting investigation of morally problematic social contexts of trust (Miller 2002).

For feminist theorists, staking a claim to the importance of trust represents a challenge to the *status quo* in moral philosophy. In bioethics, in contrast, trust has long been viewed as a key component of a well-functioning physician-patient relationship. Bioethical interest in trust has surged in recent years as a result of changes in the physician-patient relationship that seem to threaten patient trust.[7] The rise of the contract model of physician-patient relations in the latter half of the twentieth century, with its emphasis on patient autonomy and informed consent, was driven in part by increasing distrust of physicians, insurers, and related health care institutions as patients realized that many factors might serve to place physician and patient interests in tension. Bioethicists have sought to reconceive the ideal physician-patient relationship as a partnership, while at the same time recognizing the irreducibility of trust in encounters between persons unequal in vulnerability, knowledge, and power. If trust was once based on close acquaintance with a physician as fellow community member, perhaps now it could be based on confidence in a system of credentialing and licensure, together with state and local laws, review boards, and professional codes. Bioethicists view as an important task the project of defining and facilitating a nonpaternalistic form of trust in medicine in an era of simultaneous patient empowerment and institutional control.

The "crisis of trust" in medicine has been seen mainly as the problem of getting patients to trust their health care providers, especially physicians. This requires not only trustworthy physicians but also trustful patients, for distrust can be misplaced as easily as trust. Contractual devices, such as advance directives and informed consent documents, and consequences for breach, such as lawsuits, professional sanctions, bad publicity, and loss of reputation, may help to prevent or at least penalize some of the worst abuses, and more positively, may even help to initiate important but difficult discussions and clarify roles and responsibilities. Nevertheless, few would contend that they can replace trust as a key element of a functional physician-patient relationship.

The trusting physician-patient relationship has seemed important because well-placed patient trust enables good outcomes: patients who trust physicians are more likely to seek care at the first sign of trouble, to communicate important information about their symptoms and feelings, to reveal any fears or concerns that could sabotage treatment, to comply with medical recommendations, and in general, to experience less anxiety around issues of health. The kinds of discussions about medical and nonmedical values and life plans that many bioethicists now recommend as necessary for effective diagnosis and treatment could hardly occur in an atmosphere of fear and mistrust.

For these reasons, most bioethicists deplore the erosion of trust in physicians and health care more generally and advocate more trust. The majority focus on the physician virtues that would promote patient trust. Edmund Pellegrino contends that, because a kind of wary ethics of self-defense is an unacceptable alternative, violating, as it does, the phenomenology of the fiduciary relationship, in which trust in professionals is presupposed ("to seek professional help is to trust"), a new form of trust must replace paternalism-based trust. Pellegrino takes a virtue ethics approach, asserting that, given the intimacy and personal nature of the medical relationship, trust must be grounded in the personal qualities and character of the physician (Pellegrino 1991). Chalmers Clark develops Pellegrino's analysis, casting trust as a key item of exchange in the social contract between medicine and the public (Clark 2002). Patricia Illingworth argued that trust is a form of social capital, a genuine public good that greases the wheels of sociality, promoting social engagement and connectedness, and that the doctor-patient relationship is a "vessel of trust," protected by higher fiduciary duties (Illingworth 2002). According to Illingworth, trust is good for individuals and the community, as it enhances cooperative activity, which in turn has economic benefits, increases empathy toward others, and aids in protecting liberty. Finally, along the same lines, Rosamond Rhodes concurs that medicine is a profession that implies special obligations beyond the minimal noninterference requirements of ordinary morality. These obligations, summarized in the broad injunction to promote the patient's good, require core characteristics that include intelligence, ability, responsibility, honesty, caring, and respect. According to Rhodes, "All reasonably farsighted physicians must recognize that in order to practice medicine, they must *seek trust and deserve it*" (Rhodes 2001, 495).

In contrast, Onora O'Neill (2002) offered a Kantian perspective on trust in bioethics. Her *Autonomy and Trust in Bioethics* is the first book that attempts a philosophical grounding of the importance of trust in bioethics. To her credit, O'Neill grapples with the problem of misplaced trust and misplaced mistrust, prevalent phenomena that are rarely faced in simple "more trustworthiness = more trust" equations. O'Neill wonders why, in an era of increased patient autonomy, trust has faltered. She concludes that the going conception of autonomy, "individual autonomy," amounts to little more than a philosophically untenable desire-based model of agency, which is in practice operationalized as informed consent requirements, namely, the right of competent adults to choose or refuse offered treatments. O'Neill suggests substituting Kantian principled autonomy, "the attempt to act on principles on which all others could act," a constraint on practical reason that would ground moral principles that in turn generate rights and obligations (O'Neill 2002, 94).

Not surprisingly, given the feminist analysis of trust sketched above, O'Neill does not offer a satisfactory account of trust. Trust ends up being a byproduct of principled autonomy: because principled autonomy forbids deceit and coercion, doctors and medical researchers should be trustworthy; this in turn, will generate trust. In keeping with the tendency of modern Kantians to downplay Kant's rigorism, O'Neill asserts that these are not exceptionalness obligations but rather "strong commitments," and she allows that applying Kantian principles requires not algorithms but a kind of practical judgment akin to solving a design problem with several constraints (O'Neill 2002, 98, 127). Utterly missing is an account of the moral role or value of trust, other than as a rational response to perceived trustworthiness. O'Neill frequently confuses cooperative behavior with trust, typically understood as an affective attitude, so that it is not clear at all, in fact, what distinguishes trust from mere cooperation under duress. At other points, trust amounts to predictions that it would be rational to cooperate with a medical provider, thus making it indistinguishable from other rational predictions (that the sun will rise tomorrow) or kinds of nonmoral or immoral reliance (that if I do not cooperate, things will go badly for me).

The virtue ethics approach fares little better from a feminist point of view. Rhodes, Pellegrino, Clark, and Illingworth offer apolitical accounts of what feminists see as unjustly gendered, raced, and classed features of moral life. For example, they appreciate economic context—in particular the impact of managed care on the practice of medicine—but ignore political contexts. They focus on relationships, particularly the physician-patient relationship, but do not infuse this with consideration of other social features of actual physicians and patients, and as a result focus exclusively on dyadic trust rather than the complex webs of trust that better capture moral agency. They articulate the importance of character, but not of the gendered and raced notions inherent in social conceptions of virtue and vices. Perhaps most tellingly, while current proponents of trust in medicine disavow the paternalistic model, they do not question the power of medical authority or the patient vulnerability that makes trust in providers so central, and so fraught.

A major lesson about trust from feminist ethics is that it is not always to be trusted. Trust implies expectations about the trusted, but these are different from mere predictions. Rather, they are invested with moral meaning tied to social status, roles, and personal histories. The legitimacy of expectations is embedded in moral norms, which partly determine the extent to which it makes sense to trust in others. That these norms may be consciously or subconsciously accepted by the parties to a trust relationship is neither necessary nor sufficient for judging them to be fair or just.

Viewed as a branch of ethics, bioethics has an unusually high sensitivity to power differentials and to the vulnerability they entail, due to its emphasis on the physician-patient relationship. But absent is the crucial claim that trust, when viewed politically rather than merely psychologically (as a benevolent attitude), can have deleterious effects. And so a determination of whether trust meets morally salutary ends depends on more than the assessment of the motives and intentions of the individuals in a dyadic trust relationship. It also depends on the structure of the roles and the socioeconomic locations and institutional setting in which the trust relationship takes place. To put it starkly: from a feminist point of view, there is no reason to think that a decline in patient trust in physicians or in health care institutions represents a "crisis," especially not one to which the solution is "more trust." What the bioethicists who advocate trust in physicians are really talking about is "well-placed" or "reasonable" trust, yet no work has been done on the question of what that means for different moral agents in varied medical contexts. That patients, especially in acute or emergency settings, have no choice but to accept their vulnerability to medicine does not entail that they trust (i.e., take the moral attitude of hopeful expectation of good will or integrity on the part of the trustee).

For feminists, a conscientious, competent, and caring physician may remain untrustworthy in important respects, as the following examples suggest: A plastic surgeon fails to question whether small breasts evidence a lack of health that needs medical remediation, and his patient's comment that her self-esteem will flourish and her life improve with larger breasts is accepted without further discussion. A hospitalist does not wonder whether a female patient who appears to be "scamming" him for opioids may not be one of the many women undertreated for mental illness who attempts to obtain drugs via unverifiable reports of chronic pain, nor does he consider her relationship to the unidentified male who always accompanies her visits, or whether she is one of the many women who obtains drugs under pressure from addicted male lovers, brothers, or fathers. A pediatrician worries that a child's head injury may indicate abuse because his parents have tattoos, smoke, and live in a cramped trailer home. An oncologist does not question whether rapid acquiescence to a husband's demands that his wife's do-not-resuscitate order be rescinded reflects patriarchal attitudes about authority in families.

In one sense, mutual trust between caregiver and patient, or webs of trust that include the patient's family, will grease social wheels, making all of these scenarios move along—for better or worse—with some speed and finality. And this ability of trust to get cooperative ventures going and keep them moving is one of the features that has caused social theorists from diverse backgrounds and eras (consider the political divide between Robert Putnam and Frances Fukuyama, or, more philosophically, between John Locke and Thomas Hobbes) to praise it. A certain basic level of trust, or at least lack of distrust, is probably required to enter into any social interaction whatsoever. But beyond that truism, if feminist bioethicists are right that not just health care and health care delivery but conceptions of medicine, health, and illness are thoroughly implicated in patriarchy, the rational default position for feminists toward physicians in particular, and medicine in general, may well be distrust.

Conclusion

Feminist bioethical theory has developed to the point where it converges on a commitment to foregrounding gender and related social constructs, to ending oppression of all types, and to reasoned rejection of some major commitments of standard ethical theories in order to gain critical purchase on mainstream bioethics and suggest new topics and avenues of exploration. Thus, feminists are uniquely well placed to interrogate the received view in bioethics that less trust is bad and more trust is good, and to explore the ways in which trust and distrust trace and can sometimes disrupt social fault lines. However, to do this adequately, we must pair Baier's Humean recommendation to begin moral inquiry into the economic, historical, and psychological facts with Michele Moody-Adams's contention that "moral inquiry can change our moral understandings, and constructively enlarge our grasp of moral concepts, only if it can alter some of the constituent beliefs and associations that structure important patterns of situational meanings" (Moody-Adams 2004, 261). Shaking up these patterns of salience and interpretation requires novel strategies. Among the strategies Moody-Adams recommends to this end are attention to ignored empirical facts, the articulation and investigation of seemingly problematic and irrational emotions, and the use of metaphor or other imaginative techniques to reshape our conception of a particular phenomenon. Along these lines, Diana Meyers (2002) contends that entrenched cultural figurations, especially of the maternal, hamper feminist theory.

And Hilde Nelson (2001) analyzes the emancipatory potential of "counterstories" for resisting demoralizing master narratives. In bioethics, the entrenchment of the controlling image of a trust-infused physician-patient relationship—illustrated by photos of a caring (usually white male) physician and worried patient featured on the cover of many bioethics texts and much commercial medical literature—is a central feature of degrading master narratives that serve to shore up existing power structures. Part of the solution is cultural transformation to "free up our moral and political imagination," thus creating a space for new models of the patient and the health care professional.

We might disrupt the dominant view of trust by focusing on cases where trust is not warranted or by focusing on nonparadigmatic cases of reasonable trust, such as that of an unhealthy or sick doctor and his or her relation to healthy patients. Or we might focus on other types of trust that are routinely overlooked, such as physician trust in patients, or patient trust in physicians as triangulated via intermediaries such as family members or nurses.

In thinking about trust in medicine, feminists might give more attention to nurses, the majority of whom are female, to resist the trap of making trust parasitic on rational assessments of trustworthiness and defining trustworthiness as keeping one's explicit promises. Nurses recognize their unique positions "in the middle," especially in hospitals, where they take on fiduciary responsibilities to multiple parties (Hamric 2001). For nurses, trustworthiness requires negotiating complex interrelationships with managers, physicians, families, patients, third-party reimbursers, and administration. This requires "shuttle diplomacy," which implies the sort of integrity and responsiveness that undergird feminist accounts of trust. Being trusted by so many diverse parties, while having limited agency to respond to that trust, precipitates "moral distress" in many nurses, and this situation provides another set of trust cases that are immune to blanket injunctions to trust more or less.

To resist the co-opting and deradicalizing of terms like *trust*, feminist bioethics must be willing not just to theorize about but also to take up the kinds of novel, nonintegrated, diverse methods in bioethics that they and feminist ethicists have so ably defended in the last twenty years. In the case of trust, we need more than a questioning of whether some cases count as reasonable trust from a feminist point of view (although that would be a start), we need to interrogate what trust is and why it matters and to resist the urge to foreclose debate about how these questions are best approached. Trust might mean different things to people differently placed with regard to medicine and health, for example. The scrutiny of medicine practiced by feminist bioethics requires new tools: narrative, autoethnography, fiction, memoir, metaphor, might all be helpful in this endeavor. Trust, because it is linked to vulnerability and hope, can be a poignant moral emotion, and creative expression often captures trust in its fullness in a way that prose does not.

Feminist bioethicists must interrogate central concepts like trust, which can serve to shore up traditional patriarchal, classist, and racist understandings of health, disease, and medicine. And because so many of us work in the settings that we are theorizing about, we are well placed to use nontraditional historicized, contextualized, imaginative, interdisciplinary methods in our research. Because of this, there is—or should be—even less of a divide in feminist bioethics between theory and practice than in feminist theory more generally. Greater attention to method, by its very definition, implies greater application of feminist method, as trust itself evidences: trust is both a substantive more concept and a central term in a radical feminist reorientation of ethical theory. In short, greater critical attention to this still-undertheorized phenomenon is an overlooked, but important, element in moral progress in feminist bioethics.

NOTES

1. For extended comparison, see Sherwin 1992b.

2. This remark is representative: "Bioethics is not a new set of principles or maneuvers, but the same old ethics being applied to a particular realm of concerns" (Clouser 1978, 532).

3. See also Holmes and Purdy (1992), which devotes one of its five sections to care ethics.

4. For example, Tom L. Beauchamp and LeRoy Walters (2002), in a short overview of care theory, present it as nonfeminist, failing to mention gender even once in the description. Ronald Munson criticizes feminist ethics as relativistic and non-action guiding, noting that "even asking a feminist doesn't seem to be of much use, because they differ among themselves on how such questions should be answered" (Munson 2000, 54). Given that virtually every other ethical perspective summarized by Munson has its share of competing interpretations, it is interesting that only feminist ethics is subject to this particular test.

5. For example, in the section on "The Global AIDS Epidemic" in Beauchamp and Walters, no essay takes a feminist perspective or even focuses on gender, despite the fact that women account for 50 percent of the 40 million adults living with AIDS worldwide, are particularly vulnerable to heterosexual transmission of HIV, have gender-specific manifestations of HIV, and disproportionately bear the burden of HIV and AIDS as caregivers (Beauchamp and Walters 2002).

6. See, for example, Govier 1992, McLeod 2000, Friedman 2004, and Walker 1998b.

7. See, for example, Davies 1999, Anders 1996, Angell 1993, and Mechanic 1996.

REFERENCES

Anders, G. 1996. *Health against wealth: HMOs and the breakdown of medical trust.* Boston: Houghton Mifflin.

Andre, J. 2006. Remember the nurses. *American Philosophical Association Newsletter on Feminism and Philosophy* 5 (2): www.apaonline.org/documents/publications/vo5n2_Feminism.pdf.

Angell, M. 1993. The doctor as double agent. *Kennedy Institute of Ethics Journal* 3: 279–86.

Baier, A. 1995. *Moral prejudices.* Cambridge, Mass.: Harvard University Press.

———. 1997. *The commons of the mind.* Chicago: Open Court.

———. 2004. Demoralization, trust, and the virtues. In *Setting the moral compass: Essays by women philosophers,* ed. C. Calhoun. Oxford: Oxford University Press.

Beauchamp, T. L., and L. Walters. 2002. *Contemporary issues in bioethics.* Belmont, Calif.: Wadsworth.

Clark, C. 2002. Trust in medicine. *Journal of Medicine and Philosophy* 27 (1): 11–29.

Clouser, K. D. 1978. Bioethics. In *Encyclopedia of bioethics,* ed. W. Reich. New York: Free Press.

Davies, H. T. 1999. Falling public trust in health services: Implications for accountability. *Journal of Health Services Research and Policy* 4 (4): 193–94.

Donchin, A. 2004. Feminist bioethics. In *The Stanford encyclopedia of philosophy,* ed. E. N. Zalta (Fall 2004 edition), http://plato.stanford.edu/archives/fall2004/entries/feminist-bioethics/.

Friedman, F. 2004. Diversity, trust, and moral understanding. In *Setting the moral compass: Essays by women philosophers,* ed. C. Calhoun. New York: Oxford University Press.

Hamric, A. B. 2001. Reflections on being in the middle. *Nursing Outlook* 49:254–57.

Holmes, H. B., and L. M. Purdy, eds. 1992. *Feminist perspectives in medical ethics.* Bloomington: Indiana University Press.

Gilligan, C. 1987a. *In a different voice: Psychological theory and women's development.* Cambridge, Mass.: Harvard University Press.

———. 1987b. Moral orientation and moral development. In *Women and moral theory,* ed. E. F. Kittay and D. T. Meyers. Totowa, N.J.: Rowman & Littlefield.

———. 1995. Hearing the difference: Theorizing connection. *Hypatia* 10 (2): 120–27.

Govier, T. 1992. Trust, distrust, and feminist theory. *Hypatia* 7 (1): 16–32.

Illingworth, P. 2002. Trust: The scarcest of medical resources. *Journal of Medicine and Philosophy* 27 (1): 31–46.

McLeod, C. 2000. Our attitude towards the motivation of those we trust. *Southern Journal of Philosophy* 38 (3): 465–79.

Mechanic, D. 1996. The impact of managed care on patients' trust in medical care and their physicians. *Journal of the American Medical Association* 275:1693–97.

Meyers, D. 2002. *Gender in the mirror: Cultural imagery and women's agency.* Oxford: Oxford University Press.

Miller, J. P. 2002. A critical moral ethnography of social distrust. In *Social philosophy today,* vol. 16, ed. C. Hughes. Charlottesville, Va.: Philosophy Documentation Center.

Moody-Adams, M. 2004. The idea of moral progress. In *Setting the moral compass: Essays by women philosophers,* ed. C. Calhoun. New York: Oxford University Press.

Munson, R. 2000. *Intervention and reflection: Basic issues in medical ethics.* Belmont, Calif.: Wadsworth.

Nelson, H. L. 2000. Feminist bioethics: Where we've been, where we're going. *Metaphilosophy* (October): 492–508.

———. 2001. *Damaged identities: Narrative repair.* Ithaca, N.Y.: Cornell University Press.

O'Neill, O. 2002. *Autonomy and trust in bioethics.* Cambridge: Cambridge University Press.

Pellegrino, E. 1991. Trust and distrust in professional ethics. In *Ethics, trust, and the professions: Philosophical and cultural aspects,* ed. E. Pellegrino, R. Veatch, and J. Langan. Washington, D.C.: Georgetown University Press.

Rhodes, R. 2001. Understanding the trusted doctor and constructing a theory of bioethics. *Theoretical Medicine* 22:493–504.

Sherwin, S. 1992a. *No longer patient: Feminist ethics and health care.* Philadelphia: Temple University Press.

———. 1992b. Feminist and medical ethics: Two different approaches to contextual ethics. In *Feminist perspectives in medical ethics,* ed. H. B. Holmes and L. M. Purdy. Bloomington: Indiana University Press.

Tong, R. 1997. *Feminist approaches to bioethics: Theoretical reflections and practical applications.* Boulder, Colo.: Westview Press.

Walker, M. U. 1998a. *Moral understandings: A feminist study in ethics.* New York: Routledge.

———. 1998b. Ineluctable feelings and moral recognition. In *The philosophy of emotions,* ed. P. A. French and H. K. Wettstein. Vol. 22 of *Midwest studies in philosophy.* Notre Dame, Ind.: University of Notre Dame Press.

Wolf, Susan M., ed. 1996. Feminism and bioethics: Beyond reproduction. Oxford: Oxford University Press.

CHAPTER SIX

The Right to Life

Rethinking Universalism in Bioethics

MARY C. RAWLINSON, PH.D.

> Social justice, and especially sexual justice, cannot be achieved
> without changing the laws of language and the conceptions of
> truths and values structuring the social order. Changing the in-
> struments of culture is just as important in the medium to long
> term as a redistribution of goods in the strict sense. You can't
> have one without the other.
>
> *Luce Irigaray, "How to Manage the Transition from Natural to*
> *Civil Coexistence?" in Democracy Begins between Two, 2000*

In October 2003, the General Conference of the United Nations Educational, Scientific, and Cultural Organization (UNESCO) decided that it was "opportune and desirable to set universal standards in the field of bioethics with due regard for human dignity and human rights and freedoms, in the spirit of cultural pluralism inherent in bioethics" (32 C/Res. 24, 46–47). A committee of seven, composed mainly of scientists, physicians, and lawyers and including two women and two philosophers, drafted the "declaration of universal norms in bioethics." Between January 2003 and October 2005, consultations with U.N. member states were conducted, and the draft declarations were debated at meetings in Paris to which observers from nongovernmental organizations and other interested parties were invited.[1]

On October 19, 2005, the General Conference of UNESCO adopted the *Universal Declaration on Bioethics and Human Rights.*[2] The document identifies bioethics narrowly, as "ethical issues raised by the rapid advances in science and their technological implications" (preamble). The problems of bioethics, the document insists, result from *progress* in science and technology and are the unfortunate side effects of an immense good. Given its focus on research and the value of new knowledge, the document defines the protection of individual autonomy and the conditions of consent as the central issue of bioethics, invoking, as a guiding principle, maximizing benefit and minimizing harm. The website of the Bioethics Section of UNESCO, under whose auspices the document was formulated and promulgated, aggressively reinforces this definition of bioethics as limited to issues raised by scientific experimentation, scientific practice, and the use of new technologies in the life sciences. The paradigm problems of bioethics for UNESCO's Bioethics Section are "stem cell research, genetic testing, cloning."

The section's introduction to the *Universal Declaration on Bioethics and Human Rights* is more ambiguous, citing obliquely the development of bioethics beyond its core issues in the life sciences to include "reflection on societal changes and even on global balances brought about by scientific and technological developments." This recognition of the complicity of scientific progress in social injustice is, however, left behind in favor of an abstract summary of these "new" questions under the heading of the "relationship of ethics, science, and freedom."

The document explicitly addresses member states of the United Nations and is meant both to promote and to guide the operation of national bodies regulating scientific research and medical practice. The website gives an excellent history of the meetings and activities of the various committees involved in promoting the declaration, especially through the formation of national bodies charged with applying its provisions. Clearly, the purpose of the document, and of the whole project, is to shape the discourse of bioethics around narrowly focused issues in the life sciences, while consigning to the margin issues of health and social justice, particularly those raised by scientific and technological progress. By refusing to make issues of health and social justice central to bioethics, the project shies away from any effective critique of infrastructures of subjection that are inimical to health, substituting for such a critique abstract proclamations on "freedom" and "dignity."

The declaration insists on the "fundamental equality of all human beings in dignity and rights," as well as the necessity to "ensure that they are treated justly and equitably" (article 10). Invoking the "interests and welfare of the human person," the document argues that the rights of this abstract entity "should prevail over the sole interest of science or society" (article 3). The document specifically insists that the right to "the enjoyment of the highest attainable standard of health" is a *human* right, "without distinction of race, religion, political belief, economic or social condition" (article 14). These differences are to make no difference in a consideration of "norms for bioethics." The article does not mention gender, as if human bodies were "beyond" gender and unmarked by its differences.

At the same time that it embraces the rights of "the person" and an abstract equality, the declaration refers to cultural diversity only as a possible threat to human rights. Twice the draft document articulates respect for cultural diversity, only to qualify it by the injunction that such diversity may not be "invoked to infringe upon human dignity, human rights and fundamental freedoms, nor upon the principles set out in this Declaration" (preamble, article 12). The problem of health and justice in a global context becomes a conflict between human rights and scientific progress on the one hand and "cultural diversity" on the other.[3] This clarifies the summary on the bioethics website of problems related to "social change" or "development" as conflicts of ethics, science, and freedom. It anticipates the deployment of cultural diversity only as an argument *against* the universal, not as a source of it. The declaration implies that valid norms for medical practice and research can be articulated only by abstracting to a generic "human person."

Yet, the generic "person" of human rights and bioethics is not innocent. The concepts of universality, rights, persons, and equality on which UNESCO's declaration relies did not fall from the sky, as from some *topos noetos*. They belong to a particular conceptual tradition and history and are generated in the context of specific conceptual commitments. The "human person" and his rights depend on the fiction of the "state of nature" and derive from mythological accounts of the origin of human society. These concepts ineluctably invoke the logic of fraternity and philosophies of "man's" common sense.

Within this conceptual history, women have been defined not as agents, but as property, the medium of exchange through which the bonds of brotherhood are elaborated, as both Freud and Levi-Strauss demonstrate. From Aristotle's account of her as a "nutritive medium" to Hegel's sequestering of her in the family, apart from public life, where she tends the body, this tradition renders "woman," at best, a supplement to "man's" agency, lacking the self-consciousness and rational capacities necessary for autonomous, self-directed activity. Moreover, "woman's" fate provides a paradigm of subjection that is deployed on other identities. These concepts of universality, equality, and dignity install the hegemony of particular racial and cultural, as well as sexual, identities.[4]

By failing to pay attention to this conceptual history, the UNESCO project puts forward abstract concepts of equality that hide the real inequities that characterize contemporary ethical urgencies. Ethical challenges tend to arise in relations that are *unequal*: doctor/patient, teacher/student, parent/child, boss/worker, or between the politically and economically powerful and those who are poorer, weaker, and disenfranchised. By asserting the "fundamental equality of all human beings in dignity and rights," UNESCO, no doubt, *means* well, but the *Universal Declaration on Bioethics and Human Rights* marginalizes the essential logical and historical links between the abstract discourse of rights and inequities of wealth and power. Under the abstract discourse of rights, many subjects do *not* enjoy an equality of dignity and rights. A person who cannot vote or drive in her own country, a person who is condemned by her village council to be raped to settle a dispute among men, a person whose children die of dysentery in the twenty-first century, for example, is not "fundamentally equal," or such equality is so abstract as to be unreal. By marginalizing structural (as opposed to merely accidental) inequity, UNESCO's discourse of abstract rights seems counterproductive. It aims "to promote equitable access to medical, scientific, and technological developments… [particularly in developing countries]" but fails to center its analysis on the intertwining of health and wealth in developed, as well as developing countries (article 2). Article 14 on "social responsibility and health" quickly identifies "the promotion of health" as the responsibility of individual governments, thus forestalling any global circulation of that responsibility. The connections among health, poverty, political status, and education are invoked only to insist that "progress in science and technology should advance… access to quality health care [and the other conditions of life]; elimination of the marginalization and exclusion of persons on the basis of any grounds; and the reduction of poverty and illiteracy" (article 14). Thus, while the document defines itself as addressing ethical problems arising from progress in science and technology, even these are limited to issues of individual autonomy and consent. The complicity of scientific progress with inequities of power and wealth is relegated to the margin by the *Universal Declaration on Bioethics and Human Rights,* along with the link between those inequities and the discourse of rights. The document stipulates that these inequities "should" be ameliorated by scientific progress.

In this way, the document is not so much a call to action as a "reassuring drug" (Irigaray 1994, xi). Indeed, the document exhibits the very features criticized by Luce Irigaray in her analysis of the 1948 *Universal Declaration of Human Rights.*

- By stating emphatically and repeatedly that human "persons" *are* equal, the document forecloses the recognition of structural inequalities that would be necessary to any treatment of social justice.
- By insisting on abstract human rights, it marginalizes gender inequity in

the discourse of ethics and fails to recognize gender difference as irreducible in human experience.

- Its articulation of abstract goals of access and shared benefits from scientific research belies the way in which scientific and technological development frequently contribute to social and economic inequity. It ignores the fact that the results and benefits of much of this research are private property.
- In insisting on the figure of the generic human, it not only denies to women any consideration of the specificity of their experience as it relates to the articulation of a civil identity, but also denies to men and women the resources of women's experience and bodies as points of departure for the moral imagination.

In the *Universal Declaration on Bioethics and Human Rights*, as in the *Universal Declaration of Human Rights,* sexual difference has been aggressively neutralized. As Irigaray remarks, "I cannot feel that this 'universal' charter includes me unless I renounce my sex and its properties, and also agree to forget all the women who do not enjoy the minimal civil liberties that I do." The "egalitarian slogans" of these declarations, Irigaray argues, "promote a totalitarian ideology" (Irigaray 1994, xi). Their proclamations of equality and equal access to social goods support the posture of virtue, while rendering invisible relations of subjection and the differences of power and wealth they produce. Rhetoric matters; and what matters more in the declaration than the abstract language of equality and human rights is what remains unsaid.

Indeed, the history of these abstract rights of the "human person" reveals their complicity with the history of property and their production as safeguards of the privilege of property. The mythological accounts of society's origin in a voluntary contract obscure the way in which these rights were instituted precisely to establish the validity of ownership and to secure inequities of wealth. The rhetorical strategies of rights—the fiction of the "state of nature," the myth of the voluntary social contract, the abstraction of the "person," the recreation of man as a generic, the ideology of equality, and the institution of fraternity as a figure of the social bond—install a social logic that legitimates inequities of wealth as well as the subjection of certain classes of human as the servants of that wealth.

In failing to articulate the reality of our ethical urgencies, UNESCO's *Universal Declaration on Bioethics and Human Rights,* in effect, makes them more opaque and more subjected to an absolute voice. What is implicit in the abstract language? Its proclamations of equality and equal access distract from the vast and increasing inequities of wealth and power that obtain within and across societies, just as its focus on progress in science and technology covers over the role of global development in the dislocation and dispossession of peoples as well as the degradation of the Earth.

A critique of the rhetoric of rights, persons, and equality and of fraternity as a social figure opens up the possibility of reconfiguring the concept of justice, so as to take account of structural inequity and to deploy the subjected as new figures of moral agency. Such a critique reveals the impossibility of approaching the issue of health apart from that of social justice. Human health turns out to be a lever of intervention that disrupts the function of discourse on rights, at the same time that it implies a way of figuring moral agency as socially constituted rather than a property of an autonomous "person."

Moreover, a consideration of the necessity of gendered rights, and of *women's* right to health, reveals not only the complicity of the discourse of the rights of man in histories of subjection but also the positive possibility of refiguring our position in the world as moral agents in ways that may improve our health. This critique re-evaluates "cultural diversity" and the specific difference of gender, not as a threat to "freedom" or "ethics," but as a resource that might respond to the inadequacies and complicities in the rights of man. From Aristotle to Hegel, the subjection of woman has been identified with the subjection of nature, and the rhetoric of rights marks the transition from nature to civil society. In our time, however, as Irigaray often reminds us, we live on a polluted Earth of diminishing resources under the threat of nuclear annihilation (Irigaray 1993). We live with disease-inducing noise at an unsustainable pace, subject not to the rhythms of our own hearts, but to the circulation of global capital, which concentrates the privileges of ownership even as it engulfs populations in the logic of commodification. In the developed world, inequities of wealth are widening dramatically, while social securities are undermined. In the developing world, environmental integrity and local institutions are sacrificed in the name of an economic prosperity that touches only the already privileged, the educated who have the skills required by globalization. Perhaps, using woman as a lever of intervention, and particularly, her right to health, it is possible to tell a different story of how we stand on the Earth together.

Following Irigaray, my chapter develops a critique of the discourse of human rights, demonstrating its complicity with concepts of property and propriety that sustain inequalities of wealth and power. Second, I explicate Irigaray's claim for the necessity of gendered rights and show how beginning from women's experience reorients the discourse of rights around the right to life rather than the right to property. Finally, this reorientation of moral thinking around the right to life suggests a new figure of justice, focused on imagining "livable futures" rather than on settling accounts.

The Mythology of Rights: Installing the Inequalities of Property and Propriety

> The true founder of civil society was the first man who, having enclosed a piece of land, thought of saying, "this is mine."
> *Jean-Jacques Rousseau, Discourse on Inequality, part II, 1755*

> On whom has oppression fallen in any quarter of our Union? Who has been deprived of any right of person or property?
> *James Monroe, First Inaugural Address, 1817*

> The emergence of "human rights" is coterminous with the emergence of what are commonly referred to as structural inequalities—that is, with the emergence of forms of inequality that are independent of personal attributes and instead derive from modes of economic, political, and cultural organization.
> *Anthony Woodiwiss, Human Rights, 2005*

The discourse of rights depends on mythmaking. The concept of right derives directly from the myth of origin developed in social contract theory. Philosophers, Hobbes and Rousseau for example, fabricate stories about the origin of civil society to demonstrate that rights are both *necessary* and *natural*, on the one hand, and the result of a *voluntary* contract or convention, on the other. The institution of right joins instinct to liberty.

Hobbes, understandably shaken by the chaos of civil war, hypothesized a "state of nature" before the advent of civil authority in which each one's right is absolute and guaranteed only by his own power. In this "war of every man against every man," each one is justified in doing whatever is necessary to his own "self-preservation," and he is both constantly subject to the fear of aggression and entirely reliant on his own strength. Thus, it is in man's own interest and, hence, *natural* that he should contract with other men to form civil society, laying down his absolute right for the limited but socially guaranteed rights of a political community.

While in Hobbes's myth of origin it would be unnatural, contrary to his own interest and instinct for self-preservation, for man to persist in the state of nature, the legitimacy of civil authority depends on man having freely accepted constraints on his liberty. A man may be forced into servitude, but he cannot be constrained into citizenship. Only if, following the dictates of his own reason, he voluntarily accepts the authority of the state's sovereign power, can he be legitimately subject to its judgments and justice. Yet, the voluntary promise is forthcoming only because it is consistent with the laws of nature, necessitated by self-interest and the intolerable insecurity of the state of nature. Thus, the institution of right installs a chiasmatic relation between natural necessity and self-legislating reason, a complicity that belongs to its origin in the idea of nature as a state of absolute war.

The contract takes place in a mythical time, and with respect to actual human history, always *will have been*. Because it is the natural counterforce to nature as war, the contract will always already have taken place. One will always already have assented. In Hobbes's account the installation of a governing sovereign power cannot be undone, for any revolution would constitute a return to nature as war. In principle, sovereign power cannot be illegitimate because it is the condition of legitimacy. The contract and the rights it establishes cannot be rescinded. The contract prescribes legitimate relations among actual human and nonhuman bodies.

Hobbes argues that only the "voluntary transferring of right" institutes property as a legitimate ownership guaranteed by civil authority rather than mere force. As with right in general, the validity of the paradigm right to property depends on the myth of origin in the idea of nature as war. Only after each one has laid down his absolute right to the goods of nature and agreed to accept limitations on his liberty in return for a guarantee of peace and safety, are specific civil rights, first and foremost the right to property, installed as conditions of judgment and punishment. The right to property is just as natural and necessary as the contract that establishes it and the primary counterforce to nature as war.

Though Rousseau directly challenges Hobbes's account of the state of nature and the emergence of civil society, his method is no less mythological and just as clearly identifies the emergence of civil right with the advent of property. Indeed, the chief distinction between his account and Hobbes's is that he imagines man in the state of nature as solitary and subject only to the immediacy of his own physical needs. Rousseau's analysis centers on the idea that, as men come into association, a natural division of labor produces conflict and inequality. Some accrue wealth, while others are not so skilled, applied, or lucky. Some possess, while others are possessed. To secure property in the legitimacy of right, rather than by the mere force of possession, requires civil law.

Language introduces the capacity for reflection and the ability to make comparisons, giving rise to the logic of esteem, "on the one side, to vanity and scorn, and on the other to shame and envy" (Rousseau 1992, 60, 80). Thus, the equality of man in the state of nature gives way to the inequality of civil society in three phases: first, the difference of property between rich and poor; second, the difference of power between those able to enforce their claims and those dependent on them; and, finally, the difference of liberty between masters and slaves, between property owners and those men who become property themselves.

The solution to the inequities that arise with civil society is hardly its dissolution; rather, Rousseau concentrates on distinguishing good from bad government and on identifying the appropriate structures of authority to ensure liberty and happiness. While in Hobbes's *Leviathan*, the topic of women, gender, or sexual difference appears only in a passing discussion of the marriage of priests, Rousseau makes sexual difference essential to man's identity and the conceptual key to good government.

Rousseau not only valorizes the heterosexual family as the basic social unit but also embraces it as the paradigm of good government. Paternal authority, unlike the despotic power of bad government, "looks more to the advantage of him who obeys than to the self-interest of him who commands." And it is fitting that the child obey the man, but "only as long as [his] help is needed and that beyond this point [father and son] are equals" (Rousseau 1992, 73). While the wife and daughter remain, according to their nature, subservient to paternal power, paternal authority is exercised over the son only in order to bring him to manhood. Thus, fraternity or a society of equals, from which women are excluded, necessarily evolves from paternal authority. While critiques of women's subjection often focus on patriarchy, it is, in fact, fraternity that secures the authority of man's civil rights and his hegemony over other bodies, including woman's. The familial hierarchy of paternity is set within and guaranteed by the lateral filial network. Freud and Hegel tell still more violent stories of the father's overthrow and the subjection of the patriarchal family to the lateral exchanges of goods and power among brothers, in which the paradigm unit of exchange is the daughter's/sister's body.

Within this context, woman not only serves as the paradigm of property, providing the body whose exchange establishes the brothers' bonds. She also preserves for the brother the domain of the heart and blood, so that he is free to be the man of reason and to participate in the discursive domains of science, politics, and philosophy. Thus, in the discourse of fraternity and the rights of man, woman has no civil status of her own. She does not participate in the mutual recognition that comprises the relations of fraternity, and her identity as a supplement to her husband has no integrity of its own.

On this account, woman's nature requires her subjection to man, and her subservience to him is essential to the happiness and well-being of both. Rousseau interprets sexual difference as the original division of labor in nature. Thus, the figures of man and woman in Rousseau's analysis are sanctioned by nature, even as they will require a vast and complex social apparatus for their maintenance and regulation. In the state of nature man was "solitary," but women will always have been dependent on men. Men, naturally independent, may become dependent, but it is woman's nature to be subject to man.

> For this reason, the education of the women should be always relative to the men. To please, to be useful to us, to make us love and esteem them, to educate us when young, and take care of us when grown up, to advise, to console us, to render our lives easy and agreeable: these are the duties of women at all times, and what they should be taught in their infancy. So long as we fail to recur to this principle, we run wide of the mark, and all the precepts which are given them contribute neither to their happiness nor our own.   (Rousseau 1979, 106)

From infancy, woman must be taught to tend the body, to subject her will to another, to dedicate herself to the happiness of others, to trade respect for love. If she does not play her role, man will have trouble sustaining his.

Citing certain animal behaviors, such as the reluctance of a horse to trample any living body underfoot, Rousseau argues that nature has endowed man with pity to "bolster his reason" (Rousseau 1992, 46). Yet, this natural pity is extinguished by the education and reflection that characterize civil society. Thus, the philosopher cares only for the abstraction of "society as a whole," and "someone may with impunity slit the throat of a fellow man under the philosopher's window, and the philosopher need only put his hands over his ears and argue a bit with himself to prevent nature, which is rebelling inside him, from making him identify himself with the man being murdered… It is the ill-bred rabble, the market-women, who separate the scufflers and prevent decent people from tearing each other to pieces" (Rousseau 1992, 47).

It is not accidental that Rousseau here refers to the rabble as "market-*women*," for it is the natural destiny of woman to supplement man's rational nature with the "sweetness of her temper." Together they constitute a "moral person," a figure in which woman's autonomy is submerged and reduced to the feeling of sympathy and an ability to "read the hearts of men." (Rousseau 1979, 160).[5]

Thus, not only are rights modeled on the right to have, that is, the right to property, but they also invoke standards of what is proper to each sex. These proprieties are established in the context of the family and serve the installation of fraternity as a system of power. While legal theories establish the "suspension" of the woman's existence in marriage, social contact theory prescribes duties and traits specific to her, just as it prescribes a specific form of sexuality as both natural and normative. The enormous armamentarium of laws, institutions, and practices required to produce and enforce this heterosexism might suggest otherwise. The privileging of the dimorphism of sex can no longer be sustained given this critique of its production as well as the practical disconnection of sex and reproduction through new reproductive technology. No doubt there is more than one way to satisfy the human need for companionship and physical intimacy, as well as more than one solution to the problem of human reproduction and childrearing. Yet, the discourse of rights depends on this commitment to a fraternity of patriarchal families.

Thus, the discourse of the *equality* of rights does not address the problem that these rights derive from concepts of ownership and identity that do not reflect women's identity and experience. Within what Irigaray calls the "framework of familio-religious relations in which the woman is the body to the man's head," the assertion that "men and women are now equal or well on the way to becoming so has served almost as an opiate of the people for some time now" (Irigaray 1993, 77). To embrace equality as a guide for political development is "very problematic," insofar as such a strategy accepts as fixed the concepts of rights produced by fraternity's concern with property and propriety. It ignores the possibility that a narrative of women's experience or the logic of women's bodies might be a source of rights unheard of in fraternity. While the idea of equality may secure women wider rights in the domain of acquisition and the ownership of property, it does not address her lack of agency in the context of fraternity, nor the rights that might be necessary to discover and secure a distinctively female agency (Irigaray 1993, 72).[6]

The discourse of equality is to be rejected on two counts. First, proclamations of the equality of men and women are empirically false in virtually every register. Women are structurally disadvantaged with respect to men economically, politically, and civilly. Poverty is "feminized" and women's labor underpaid. In many parts of the world women enjoy limited, if any, real property rights. Women are drastically underrepresented politically in almost every part of the globe. Most important, as it is a condition of women's agency, the figure of woman is not recognized as a figure of the universal. Thus, women are denied the experience of themselves as a site of the universal, the subject of science, politics, and philosophy.

Second, we must ask with Irigaray: equal to what? These declarations of rights do not take into account the differences in the bodies and experience of the two sexes. Inevitably, they reinscribe fraternal power, as if the lack of attention to the conditions of female identity and agency did not matter, as if man could indeed speak for all. "The *Universal Declaration of Human Rights* [*La Declaration universelle des droits de l'homme*]" requires that "I renounce my sex and its properties." It assumes that I will "forget all the women who do not enjoy the minimal civil liberties that I do" (Irigaray 1994, viii–ix; brackets in the original). The Declaration depends on a forgetting of the fact that sexual difference has been forgotten, rendered null and void in the context of ethical value.

If, as Article 21 of the declaration insists, "Everyone has the right of equal access to public service in his [*sic*] country," then, why are there so few women in leadership positions around the globe? If everyone has the "right to the security of his [*sic*] person" and "no one should be arbitrarily deprived of his [*sic*] property," then how are we to understand the difference between the way this culture of rights treats the bodies of men and those of women? Is the traffic in women's bodies and the exploitation of the female body in media, advertising, and pornography an "act of disrespect of my physical or moral person" that would require a "national tribunal" to provide me an "effective remedy?" Does this not constitute the "degrading treatment" of which the declaration speaks? How does this declaration of rights assure the "security of my person," if the state can intervene in my intimate decisions about reproduction? Does its emphasis on civil rights in the public sphere not leave untouched the violence that takes place within the family?[7] Does the declaration not fail to recognize the specificities of woman's body, history, and identity, so that the articulation of abstract human rights, in fact, reinscribes both her subjection and the invisibility of her identity within the fraternal order?

Women's Rights, Human Rights: The Right to Life

Man seems to have wanted, directly or indirectly, to give the universe his own gender, as he has wanted to give his own name to his children, his wife, his possessions.

Luce Irigaray, "Women's Discourse and Men's Discourse,"
je, tu, nous: Toward a Culture of Difference, 1993

Redefining rights appropriate to the two sexes to replace abstract rights appropriate to non-existent neutral individuals, and enshrining these rights in the law, and in any charter constituting some sort of national or universal declaration of human rights, is the best way for women to hold on to rights already gained, have them enforced, and gain others more specifically suited to female identity.

Luce Irigaray, "Introduction," *Thinking the Difference* (1994)

There is no mention in the philosophical history of rights or in these contemporary declarations of rights, not even in the declaration concerned with health, of the right to decide one's own destiny in relation to human reproduction. This reflects both the differences in embodied possibilities that comprise men and women and the appropriation of women and children as property within the discourse of rights. By refusing woman this right, the state denies her agency and indicates that *women cannot be trusted with this decision.*

This job [mothering] requires more subtlety and intelligence than any other. It would certainly be done better if women had the full benefit of their identity. But, to date, those who engender and protect life don't have a right to it. In an incredibly distrustful maneuver, it's suspected that they would no longer want to protect life the moment they themselves have a right to it. Women are often nothing more than hostages of the reproduction of the species. Their right to life requires them to have legal authority over their body and their subjectivity.   (Irigaray 1993, 78)

Within the discourse of rights, where man claims to be the absolute figure of the universal, even this distinctively female possibility must be administered for her. Not only does she lack a political and civil identity that reflects her own experience and her own body, but also her body itself is laid open to state regulation. The "right to life" in contemporary political discourse refers, not to the bodily integrity and agency of the one on whom life depends for its reproduction and care, but to the subjection of that integrity and agency to the fraternal power of the state. Irigaray argues that women are "enslaved" by not being in charge of their own reproductive destinies. Under the "tutelage" of the state and the church and subjected to their decisions, "woman... does not yet have the right to manage her own nature for herself" (Irigaray 2000, 42–43). Women's civil identity depends on her being sovereign in her own body and entrusted by the state with the decisive power over reproduction.

The necessity of this sovereignty to her civil identity derives from the fact that the body is the site of the universal, as well as the necessity of social forms, codes, and institutions that recognize and sustain her agency. Only through his embodied performances in the context of collective practices and institutions can the scientist or the politician experience himself as freely participating in a universal project. Similarly, proclamations of women's rights are empty without the elaboration of social forms that recognize a woman's sovereignty in her own body and sustain her authority with men in defining the future. "The universal cannot be reached outside the self; it is not a sum of individuals, a multiplicity of cultures, an accumulation of possessions" (Irigaray 2000, 28). To realize its universality, its solidarity with other human beings, each human body, male and female, requires codes and institutions that support the practices and performances through which each one collaborates with the others in a future. "Justice in the right to life cannot be exercised without a culture of humankind comprising men and women, and written law defining civil rights and obligations that correspond to their respective identities" (Irigaray 1993, 80). Social justice, then, depends not only on "changing the laws of language" and redistributing wealth but also on the collaborative authorization of social forms appropriate to sustain women's agencies. Her citizenship remains abstract and unreal unless the state recognizes her sovereignty in her body and her authority over her reproductive destiny free from its tutelage.

As Irigaray notes, even in those states where a woman is accorded "reproductive rights," these are generally reduced to the right to have an abortion. While insisting on the necessity of resisting any compromise of abortion rights, Irigaray links the right to life and the bodily sovereignty of women to virginity, to the decommodification of the female body, and to motherhood. Against the historical position of women as property and the commercial use of their bodies and images, Irigaray proposes virginity, not as a literal state, but as a figure of physical and moral integrity not convertible to money. Irigaray argues that women's health suffers "above all" from the lack of formal, institutionalized structures recognizing and securing this bodily integrity: "Without this dimension, [a body] is bound to be ill, ill in many ways, unable to keep itself together, with no suitable medical cure. Resorting to an exclusively somatic treatment might well give it even less chance of true healing" (Irigaray 1993, 105). The failure to entrust women with authority over reproduction and to respect their right to choose whether to be pregnant and the number of pregnancies undermines women's sense of themselves as agents and deprives them of that affirmation of their subjectivity and agency by which "they can unify their corporeal vitality" (ibid.). This sense of agency, Irigaray argues, is essential to health, for a body "is bound to be ill" unless it is animated and organized by a personal or spiritual project, unless it experiences its universality through the value of its agency in defining a future among and with other men and women.

The agency and health of women also depends on the codification of specific rights that recognize the authority and obligations of women as mothers. While children have historically been viewed as the property of the father, subject to his authority and recognized only in his name, the actual work of caring for and rearing children has always been the responsibility of women. The realization of women's agency requires the elaboration of new civil rights that recognize this responsibility. Irigaray suggests that, just as women ought to be free to manage their own reproductive destinies without civil and religious tutelage, so too it should be the mother who registers the child's birth with civil authorities and is identified by law as the guardian and authority in her children's lives. Changing legal codes in this way would require new forms of negotiation and news ways of relating among men and women. While proclamations of abstract rights and equality abet the continued hegemony of the male gender, these changes in law and social forms would precipitate a redistribution of power between the genders and invest women with the possibility of real agency in their reproductive destinies.

The installation of man as the figure of the human denies to women any relation to the universal, as if her body and her experience were not a site for its production. Public discourse and social forms reflect this lack and fail to provide the opportunities and images through which women might understand their solidarity within their own gender. Thus, in specifying the new civil rights that need to be articulated to support women's agency and identity, Irigaray regularly insists on "women's right to their own specific culture" (Irigaray 1994, xv). Identity and agency are formed in social institutions and mediated by the images that circulate in our culture. As long as women's bodies are exploited commercially, in advertising, pornography, and prostitution, women's agency and identity will be undermined. Thus, new civil rights protecting the integrity of women's bodies in these domains are needed. Similarly, the identification of the family with patriarchy and the social and political space with fraternity eviscerates women's agency and identity. The patriarchal family provides no recognition of women as responsible citizens. The subjection of women renders the family a scene of violence, and this domestic violence supplies the paradigm for the public violence that occurs between man's states, armies, religions, and tribes. Providing civil rights for women is not only a matter of justice for women but also promises to open up new ways of relating that may improve human health.

Livable Futures

> We should not delude ourselves that History can redeem all our mistakes. This sort of dreaming is no longer valid: humanity, particularly industrial capitalism, has put the planet itself in danger and there will not be a future unless we make the salvation of the Earth itself our immediate concern.
>
> What brings greater happiness than the return of spring?...
> All this happiness which we receive for nothing should be given priority protection by a politics which is concerned with the well-being of each and everyone of us. It is a simple happiness, a universal happiness, a happiness which does not involve competitiveness or aggression, but, on the contrary, favors a rational and sensible sharing at both the national and supranational levels.
>
> *Luce Irigaray, "Politics and Happiness," in*
> *Democracy Begins between Two, 2000*

The critique of man's false transcendence, his fallacious claim that his gender supplies the absolute figure of the human, displays the link between philosophy and health. Man's hegemony has produced not only the subjection of women but also a world that is inimical to our health. The universalism of fraternal rights hides its own origin in a system of concepts linking the right of property to war, the mastery of nature, and social inequity. In the *Critique of Judgment*, for example, Kant defines man's moral vocation as "the mastery of nature and the mastery of nature in man." It is man's destiny to subject nature to his rational purposes. In explicating this vocation, Kant valorizes the warrior character as the most noble and insists on the necessity of war as a formative activity. War solidifies the identity of a people and demonstrates the necessity of a sovereign power to security and to a liberty at once limited and guaranteed by the law. "Prolonged peace debases the way of thinking of that people" (Kant 1790/1987, 263). Moreover, under the sublime project of mastery, the development of culture requires, in addition to war, real social inequalities. Some serve so that others will have the leisure for science and art; the latter keep the former in a "state of oppression, hard labor, and little enjoyment" (432). And, this difference of class is gender marked. In fact, the edifice of culture, its institutions, practices, and artifacts as well as its history, science, and philosophy, depends on the subordination of one gender to the other.

The discourse of the rights of man absolutizes forms of life that belong to one gender, and even to a group within this gender that also bears other markings of race and wealth. Its operation in complicity with regimes of power invested in war and the mastery of nature has produced an almost uninhabitable world that undermines our health in at least three ways:

(i)   Its emphasis on progress fails to recognize the fragility of nature and installs a negative relation to nature that in our time threatens the Earth itself, which is the necessary condition of our health. The threat of nuclear disaster demonstrates, against the assumptions of philosophers,[8] the mortality of the Earth, even as global warming demonstrates our capacity to make our own Earth uninhabitable for us. The very scientific and technological progress invoked by UNESCO's *Universal Declaration of Norms for Bioethics* produces a world that is too noisy, fast, and polluted to be conducive to human health.

(ii)   In the era of global capital man's built environment often proves inimical to human flourishing. (Thus, in the competition to build the world's tallest building, architects regularly encounter the problem of how to transport people up and down within the space without causing inner ear damage.) Man's technologies of transportation and communication insist upon a speed that is out of proportion to human life. Built spaces isolate, alienate, and frustrate, when they are not, as they have so often been in human history, strategies of subjection.

(iii)   The discourse of rights legitimates war as a political strategy and renders historically necessary its catastrophic human and environmental results. Nowhere is the duplicity and immorality of the abstract discourse of rights more evident than in the sophistries used to justify war.

> Huge amounts of capital are allocated to the development of death machines in order to ensure peace, we are told. This warlike method of organizing society is not self-evident . . . it has a sex. . . Patriarchal culture is based on sacrifice, crime and war. It is a culture that makes it men's duty or right to fight in order to feed themselves, to inhabit a place, and to defend their property, and their families. (Irigaray 1994, 4)

This ideology of the political necessity of war takes life, inflicts suffering, and forestalls the elaboration of more effective forms of social negotiation.

(iv)   Finally, in installing man as the univocal figure of the human and denying the difference of gender, the fraternal discourse of abstract rights
provides the paradigm for the reduction of all difference. Actual human
beings are rendered mere units in a social process or mere instances of
some general form: worker, consumer, citizen. This reduction of difference sets the stage for the "unconditional power of money," which serves
as the measure of all things. It provides the single scale with respect to
which all entities can be measured and to which all differences of value
can be reduced. Thus, the universalism of fraternal rights produces a
social focus on consumption. As Wordsworth remarked, "Getting and
spending, we lay waste our powers." Social relations tend to be mediated
by wealth, and social activities tend to focus on spending, consumption,
and acquisition. Women's bodies play a significant role in this social
economy. A woman's body, more or less naked, sometimes angelic, sometimes lewd, not only serves as a marketing tool but is also commodified
and itself marketed. These representations do not install her as a subject in
the social space but reinforce her definition as property. (The ubiquity of
capital as a conceptual standard is reflected in UNESCO's declaration of
universal norms for bioethics: after defining autonomy and informed consent as if ethics were a matter for abstract individuals, it cites only cost-
benefit analysis as a principle of decision making, as if all the goods and
values that are in play in health and sickness, from my bodily motility to
my relations with others, could be arrayed like units on the same scale.)

Thus, the abstract discourse of human rights is complicit with practices and
strategies that undermine our health rather than contributing to our personal
and collective happiness, just as it depends on the enforcement of the gender
division of labor and identity.

The universalism of fraternal rights authorizes forms of social life that do violence to our identities and our ways of being together, as well as to the rhythms
of our natural being. The forms authorized by fraternal rights do not accommodate women in their specific identity or sociality, nor do they acknowledge the
specific rhythms of the female body. The *New York Times* reported on a trend
among women at Ivy League institutions. Contrary to what might be expected,
an increasing number plan not to work outside the home after marriage. Many
have decided, citing the experience of their mothers, that it is impossible to successfully combine work and the care of children. They report a desire to avoid the

pain and heartache that comes from compromising performance in both areas (Story 2005).

Some of the most talented women in the United States, who would be entering the world of work at a privileged rank, have decided that these hard-won opportunities are not worth the cost to themselves as mothers, demonstrating clearly the painful structural incompatibilities in current social forms. As Irigaray remarks, "The incentives that exist for women to go back into the home have a good chance of success, not necessarily among the most reactionary women, as is too readily believed, but also among women who wish to try to become women" (Irigaray 1993, 85). Outside these ranks of privilege women continue to labor in the care of the body, whether in the family, where the labor is often hard, or in the "service industries," which involves them in the same conflicts that their more privileged sisters have encountered, but without the same means of escape. As Irigaray observes, allowing women the choice to get married, to have children, *and* to work is not a recognition of them as women (Irigaray 2000, 146).

The public discourse within which our being together must be negotiated, when it is not drowned out by the surfeit of media and "communications," concerns almost exclusively questions of war or money. In the United States, as in many nations, issues of security and consumption are coupled with an effort to enforce and reinforce the fraternal figure of the family in its subordination of women and the subjection of women's reproductive destiny to state regulation. In many parts of the world, the institutions of women's subjection are more explicit and more complex in their penetration of women's experience. In some countries, women are killed for learning to read or are raped in settlement of a tribal dispute or are murdered for being raped or are disfigured by acid for refusing an arranged marriage. Given environmental crises, the ubiquity of social and state-sanctioned violence, extremes of social inequity, the sophistry of public discourse, and the explosion of "lifestyle" illnesses, such as addiction, heart disease, or diabetes, related to habits and stress, it is not surprising that in reflecting on our time, Irigaray often strikes an apocalyptic tone.

Her analysis focuses us, however, on the project of collaboratively producing a livable future. The critique of the universalism of fraternal rights calls for a public conversation about these matters, instead of a continued reliance on proclamations of abstract equality and dignity. (Irigaray remarks that we might start by "letting women do half the speaking.") The discourse of human rights needs a new nonmythological origin. It needs to begin from a critique of current structural inequities and the hegemony of certain identities and forms of life and to make possible a new relation to nature and new forms of social negotiation. It might begin by considering the continuity of women's bodies with the natural world in order to rethink a relation to the Earth as our home. It would find a nonbellicose originary nature in the relation of mother and child. Pregnancy provides a paradigm of human respect and solidarity that ought to inform our social and political life. While, as Irigaray notes, our culture has "blindly venerated" the mother-son relation, it has not appreciated the political significance of pregnancy as the "toleration of the other's growth within." Our culture has failed to reflect on "the meaning of this economy of respect for the other" (Irigaray 1993, 45). A discourse that begins from this "model of tolerance" would directly counter the ideology of war and social inequity at the heart of the rights of man.

Conclusion

Irigaray's critique of human rights suggests a new methodology for moral and political philosophy. Perhaps, rather than focusing on the rational calculation of rights and duties, philosophy would better serve human health and happiness by developing a moral imagination focused on the production of "livable futures." Let us imagine a world in which each man and woman enjoys the "right to life": "to air, to water, to light, to the heat of the sun, to the nourishment of the Earth. Rescuing the planet Earth means, too, being concerned about happiness, as much for ourselves as for others. Happiness of this kind does not cost much, has nothing to do with economic calculations—or, at least, it should not have—but is, perhaps, the highest form of happiness if we learn how to perceive it, to contemplate it, and to praise it" (Irigaray 2000, 168).

Orienting ourselves around an immediate concern for the "salvation of the Earth," addresses the need for a new relation to nature to nourish human health and happiness. Moreover, actively imagining and pursuing a world in which each one enjoys this right to life will necessarily produce new forms of association, negotiation, and solidarity.

While the tradition of rights, persons, and equality is not absolute and is marked by its origins in fraternity, other traditions and experiences offer resources for generating new concepts of justice and society. Women long ago learned to hear themselves in "man." The experience of women, of other races, of cultures other than that of "man," who is, after all, a white Anglo-European, can be universalized too. The differences in our experiences matter: they produce different images of the good, justice, and society, and we enrich our concept of the universal by thinking it from multiple perspectives. Figures of universality ought to operate as images and concepts that call for and sustain solidarity without reducing the specificities of experience to a general form such as "man" or "woman." *For his own sake,* if for no other, "man" ought to come to hear himself in the experiences of women, for he will find new figures through which to address the persistent problems of his particular version of moral and political life. Until we begin to generate concepts of the universal, of justice, and of social life from perspectives other than that of "man," our thought will continue to be too impoverished to answer to the ethical urgencies that beset us.[9]

NOTES

1. I was able to attend the meetings as an observer sponsored by the International Association of Bioethics. Many thanks to Alex Capron and Leonard deCastro for arranging the invitation. My views should not be attributed either to them or to the association.

2. http://portal.unesco.org/shs/en/ev.php-URL_ID=1883&URL_DO=DO_TOPIC &URL_SECTION=201.html. Earlier drafts of the document, as well as an excellent account of the process, are also available on the UNESCO Bioethics Section website.

3. To its credit, the Bioethics Section gives ample access to the debate between the Andean countries, who argued that the connection between social justice and health was central to bioethics, and an array of others led by Germany and the United States, whose narrow definition of bioethics held sway. See http://portal.unesco.org/shs/en/ files/8037/11169295721Summary-informal_meeting_en.pdf/Summary-informal%2B meeting_en.pdf.

> The fundamental underlying conceptual divergence seems to be the extent of the notion of bioethics as applied to this declaration. There are two schools of thought: a broader one that locates bioethics in its social and environmental context and another one that restricts the concept to the ethical issues arising from medicine and life sciences. This basic divergence permeates the entire text of the draft declaration but it shouldn't be irresolvable. The Chair hopes that it could be dealt with in the Use of terms and Scope articles, therefore facilitating the negotiation of the remaining articles.

4. Hereafter, man and woman, without quotation marks. These terms refer to the concepts articulated in philosophy and science that install and maintain gender norms, as distinct from the actual men and women subjected to those norms. They function as logical figures, authorizing and regulating social infrastructures, as well as individual identities.

5. Cf. Blackstone (1765, I.XV.430): "By marriage, the husband and wife are one person in law: that is, the very being or legal existence of the woman is suspended

during the marriage, or at least is incorporated and consolidated into that of the husband, under whose wing, protection, and *cover*, she performs everything."

6. Irigaray specifically distinguishes two "women's liberation movements": the first, organized around the idea of equal rights, emphasizes equality in the possession of goods; the second, advanced by her own work, promotes an individual and collective "*subjectivity*" that is valid for women and insists on the necessity of different rights for male and female subjects.

> 7. Gender discrimination was so taken for granted by the authors of the UDHR and the Covenants that no one realized there was a problem about confining the applicability of human rights to the public sphere of courts, politics, work and welfare, until this was pointed out by feminist scholars . . . Moreover, once the private sphere of relationships and families was opened up to interrogation in terms of human rights, it was discovered that women's problems were not reducible to instances of discrimination in the public sphere . . . but included not just sui generic private abuses such as domestic violence and those associated with reproductive issues . . . but also sui generic public sphere issues that follow from women's 'special' status in many cultures as mothers, wives and daughters.   (Woodiwiss 2005, 123)

The Convention on the Elimination of All Forms of Discrimination against Women represents a countermovement within human rights discourse in its recognition of the necessity of conceptualizing rights in relation to gender. www.un.org/women watch/daw/cedaw/.

8. Hegel describes the Earth as the "eternal individual"; while Kant insists on the immortality of nature. This failure to recognize the mortality of the Earth is essential to their logic of fraternity. It authorizes their arguments for the necessity of war, as well as the violence associated with social inequity.

9. UNESCO's own strategy of "gender mainstreaming" runs counter to the rhetoric of the rights of man and insists on the necessity of approaching all problems from the perspective of sexual difference. See Walby (2003).

REFERENCES

Blackstone, W. 1765. *Commentaries on the laws of England.*
Irigaray, L. 1993. *je, tu, nous: Toward a culture of differences*, trans. Alison Martin. New York: Routledge.
———. 1994. *Thinking the difference*, trans. K. Montin. New York: Routledge
———. 2000. *Democracy begins between two*, trans. K. Anderson. London: Athlone Press.

Kant, Immanuel. 1790/1987. *Critique of Judgment*, trans. Werner Pluhar. New York: Hackett.

Rousseau, J.-J. 1755/1992. *Discourse on the origin of inequality*, trans. D. A. Cress. Indianapolis: Hackett.

———. 1762/1979. *Emile, or: On education*, trans. A. Bloom. New York: Basic Books.

Story, L. 2005. "Many women in elite colleges set career path to motherhood," *New York Times*, September 20.

Walby, S. 2003. *Gender mainstreaming: Productive tensions in theory and practice.* Social politics: International studies in gender, state and society, doi:10.1093/sp/jxio18. Available at: http://portal.unesco.org/shs/fr/ev.php-URL_ID=7057&URL_DO=DO_TOPIC&URL_SECTION=201.html.

Woodiwiss, A. 2005. *Human rights.* London: Routledge.

PART THREE

From Theory to Method

JACKIE LEACH SCULLY, PH.D.

The previous section explored how feminist theory engages with some of the major philosophical building blocks of mainstream bioethics. We saw there examples of how this intersection has resulted in dynamic theoretical approaches that enrich the identification and analysis of bioethical problems. In addition to a distinctive take on *theory*, feminist bioethics is characterized by commitment to certain *methodologies*—that is, the ideas about how to conduct research, how to frame the arguments, or how to decide between competing claims that lie behind the choice of method.

Admittedly, it can sometimes be harder to recognize methods or methodologies as specifically feminist than theoretical contributions. Those who teach feminist methodology in courses on ethics, social science, epistemology, or politics are familiar with this problem in the form of the *so what?* response. This happens as we introduce concepts or approaches that feminism first brought to a discipline but that have now been seamlessly incorporated into its repertoire. When we describe a familiar methodology as feminist, the reaction is often bewilderment. Students have a hard time seeing what is specifically feminist about these approaches because they know them as just the ones the discipline uses. Those of us who have had this experience will recognize the mixture of satisfaction, irritation, and unease that goes with it. Satisfaction because broad acceptance of feminist thinking and praxis within the academy was, after all, the original goal; irritation because of the ahistorical approach to the discipline's antecedents, whereby feminism's contribution is rarely acknowledged; and unease because such incorporation provokes the question of whether a once-subversive movement, in becoming legitimate and having its methods taken up by the establishment, inevitably loses its radical force.

So let's take a look at feminist methodology in bioethics. Shared feminist methodologies arise from a commonality of theoretical and political commitments: Rosemarie Tong summarizes this as asking "the so-called woman question to raise women's (and men's) consciousness about how gender oppression distorts and hinders women's personal and professional lives, and, in one way or another, [engaging] in forms of practical reasoning aimed at moving gender-aware persons from thinking about gender oppression to doing something about eliminating it" (Tong 1997, 91). Note that the distinctive thing about this description of an academic discipline is the transformative imperative undergirding feminist bioethics' practical choice of methods and frameworks.

It is crucial to realize that a methodology is not feminist by virtue of its focus on "women's issues." Some mainstream bioethicists have dismissed feminist bioethics as marginal, not because it responds to the claims of a socially marginalized group but because these bioethicists believe it must necessarily be methodologically as well as theoretically concerned with only limited areas of bioethics—those that are uniquely or at least particularly relevant to women and not to men. These issues are generally assumed to be reproductive health, children and family relationships, or the "caring" aspects of medical practice. In reality, feminist methodology extends into any and all existing areas of bioethical interest; it also, as we shall see, exposes new topics of concern. Therefore, what distinguishes feminist bioethics is not the topics addressed but the inclusion of a combination of the following methodological biases: (1) focusing on experience; (2) consciously linking the personal/private with the public/political; (3) attending to relationships of social, political, or epistemic power; and (4) a commitment to social and political change.

Focusing on Experience

However elaborate its theorization becomes, feminism is rooted in the simple observation that the experiences of women differ in significant ways from the experiences of men. For most feminists today, this is a social and contextual claim rather than an ontological one: they would say that women's experience differs from men's at least as much because of contingent social arrangements as because of biologically determined differences between the sexes. Feminist methodologies therefore are primed to exploit a number of methods that introduce experience, suitably problematized, into philosophical, sociological, or political reflection. And because feminism starts by noting and validating differences in experience, in its choice of methods it strives to retain an awareness of differences within the experiences of women and between classes, ethnic and cultural groups, sexualities, and so on.

Feminist ethics sometimes draws on empirical data or uses phenomenology or narrative accounts to "ground" theory in lived experience in ways unlike traditional moral philosophy (Nelson 2001). In recent years, however, mainstream bioethics also has experienced what some observers have called a *sociological* or *empirical turn*, a move toward incorporating empirical or experiential material into bioethical analyses (Borry, Schotsmans, and Dierickx, 2005; De Vries et al. 2007). Empirical approaches can be highly descriptive, such as ethnographic studies, or they can generate data for an ethical critique of biomedical practices or to enrich normative ethical reflection. Clearly, the impetus for this turn in mainstream bioethics did not come solely from feminist methodology—among the other influences was a social science critique of the practices of bioethics itself (Haimes 2002; Hedgecoe 2004). Nevertheless, feminist bioethics is the most influential strand so far within the field to give "naturalized bioethics" (Lindemann, Verkerk, and Walker 2008) a central place in bioethical engagement. In this context, naturalized bioethics means one that is grounded in the natural, social, political, and institutional worlds.

Lori d'Agincourt-Canning's chapter exemplifies one approach to a naturalized epistemology in bioethics. She uses empirical data as the basis from which to explore how knowledge is influenced by social location and individual subjectivity, in the case of individuals from families with hereditary cancer. As she notes, genetic testing has received a lot of scrutiny from feminist theorists, but little attention has been given to the ways in which a family/personal history of cancer affects both the experience of testing and the epistemic claims made about the body and the self. In classic feminist style, this work is rooted in the methodological commitment to take seriously the lived experience of women, but retain a critical stance, not giving in, as Lorraine Code puts it, to the "tyranny" of experience (Code 2002, 164). D'Agincourt-Canning differentiates two forms of subjective knowledge of cancer in her participants' accounts: "empathetic knowledge," derived from close associations or emotional ties with others with cancer, and "embodied knowledge," derived from one's own bodily experience. With this dual perspective on forms of experience, she can examine the effect of a long family history of genetic disease on individual understandings of it. As a result, it becomes clear that bioethics' normal focus on a narrow range of theoretical issues (the right to know or not know about genetic status, privacy, confidentiality of genetic information, and the threat of genetic discrimination) excludes areas that are in fact of intense ethical concern to patients in this situation.

Linking the Personal/Private with the Public/Political

Feminist bioethics' acceptance of narrative and other personal accounts as legitimate epistemic resources also reflects its methodological commitment to destabilizing, or at the very least questioning, the conventional separation of personal and private issues from public and political ones. Indeed, second-wave feminism has long argued that this segregation allows the voices of women and minorities to be excluded from serious consideration, as important features of their lives are labeled as private or personal troubles and thereby consigned to areas with which bioethics (or politics, economics, or philosophy) should not concern itself.

In this section, Fiona Utley's chapter exemplifies two things: the way that feminist methodology pushes the limits of what falls within bioethics' catchment area, and how feminist methods place highly personal, individual concerns within broader frameworks of theory and the moral responsibilities of communities. Using narrative as source material, Utley considers how women's narratives of rape reveal failures in health care practices specifically, and more generally in the practices of support provided by society to traumatized individuals. She draws on phenomenology to describe the effect of rape as a destruction of the bodily narrative. By asking whether bioethical analysis can in some way contribute to improved practice, she puts the social world and bioethics in a relationship of mutual responsibility in a way that is uncommon in mainstream bioethical discourse.

Attending to Power Relationships

Both medical ethics and bioethics take the interaction between the medical profession and patients to be of central concern, and in doing so have always placed *certain kinds* of power relations under scrutiny. Medical ethics delineates the responsibilities of the doctor to patients, fellow doctors, and the community, while bioethics largely focuses on operationalizing the principle of autonomy of the individual patient through procedures of informed consent in clinical practice and research. Feminist bioethics, however, approaches power relations along a different methodological trajectory. First, feminist investigation starts from the experience of social structures that are oppressive or disadvantageous to women; and second, feminist methodologies are devised so that these organizations and practices, often taken for granted or obscured, can be disclosed and scrutinized. This methodological approach is less a set of defined procedures than it is a cognitive stance or a habit of asking certain kinds of critical questions in a rigorous, systematic way.

Feminist bioethics therefore extends the range of power relations that are up for critical examination beyond the doctor-patient dyad. The context moves out of the clinic, and beyond the health care system, to take into account the wider social and global economic arrangements that maintain patterns of domination. As one example: feminist bioethics examines stem cell research not only in terms of the moral status of the embryo, nor even of the asymmetry in the power relationship between stem cell researchers and individual women donating embryos for research, but also through the social and political forces that bear unequally on poorer women and make them especially vulnerable to ethically problematic trades in oocytes or embryos (Dickenson 2002, 2004).

Unlike d'Agincourt-Canning, Janice McLaughlin's chapter does not use empirical data. Instead, she gives a feminist critique of a paper by Greenberg and Bailey (2001) justifying the use of reproductive technologies to avoid the birth of a homosexual child. The justification is based on a familiar liberal argument of the right to procreative liberty. As she notes, the "obvious" centrality of this right prevents fundamental questions about freedom and constraints on choice being raised. At the core of Greenberg and Bailey's argument is what McLaughlin identifies as an assumption that "parental liberty is a fundamental right, so significant, so sacrosanct, that it can only be challenged by overwhelming proof that its exercise will lead to significant harm." McLaughlin mobilizes a feminist critique of liberalism and of the liberal notion of the family. It could be argued that the well-recognized liberal arm of feminism might itself present a different critique. Nevertheless, McLaughlin's methodology is characteristic of feminist approaches more generally in terms of its attention to the (mis)use of power and authority, in this case not only the relationship between parental and legislative authority in the reproductive domain but also the epistemic blind spots created by the intellectual authority of liberal bioethical arguments.

Commitment to Social and Political Change

Feminism is fundamentally an activity combining both theory and practice. Having developed into an academic discipline out of / alongside a social movement, feminist scholarship now lives with the tension between its allegiance to the demands of academic legitimacy (detachment, objectivity, clarity, rigor) and to its ethical traditions and strategic goals of global justice and equality, especially but not solely in the lives of women. Again, this is not a feature that inheres to any specific kind of method, but it does entail a methodological desire to carry analysis beyond simple diagnosis of a problem and on into social and political change, even if only incrementally.

In consequence, feminist bioethics is often distinguished by its pragmatism. One criticism leveled at mainstream bioethics, and not only by feminist critics, is that its analysis of ethically questionable practices and recommendations for improvement will turn out to be simply ineffective. By ignoring the details of real moral lives—the social, economic, psychological, or spiritual parameters that support moral understandings (Walker 1998) and within which ethical recommendations have to be implemented—bioethics often falls short of the mark. Although it presents other kinds of problems, the fact of feminist bioethics' foundational allegiance to a broad agenda of social progress means that it is better at avoiding the trap of irrelevance. Feminist bioethicists can never avoid asking the question, *how does this work in the lives of real women and men, and in the current political frameworks in which we exist?*

This pragmatism is reflected in a tradition of interdisciplinary collaboration between theorists and health care practitioners that characterizes some work in feminist bioethics. And although mainstream bioethics itself has an interdisciplinary and collaborative tradition, and while not all feminist work is interdisciplinary, feminist methodologies favor projects of the kind exemplified in Ilhaam and Gaskin's chapter. This collaboration between a philosopher and a midwife starts by "troubling" what they see as the comfortable relationship between the medical profession and bioethics, exemplified in the absence of bioethics perspectives from public health issues. From their collaboration they identify ethical difficulties in clinical practices around birth that were hitherto taken for granted. While they note in passing feminist critiques of autonomy and gendered theories of selfhood that might account for the empirical data about elective cesareans, they are avowedly more concerned with using their analysis to improve women's understanding of childbirth and provide realistic improvements to future practice, "developing transdisciplinary, nonhierarchical collaborative models in the production of knowledge about ethics and childbearing." This collaboration between an academic and a practitioner raises further methodological challenges, those of professional situatedness. The anecdotes and general claims about birth outcomes derive from personal narration and stories, which can flesh out and give substance to theoretical discourse. It has been suggested that the language and knowledge claims of midwives, which stem from the intuitive and/or anecdotal realm, are taken by them to be as substantive as any other epistemological position. When a midwife says that medical mistakes are chronically underreported and that nurses inform her about practices that cannot be documented, she is describing the conditions through which knowledge claims are made legitimate and is in fact interrogating the notion that what is "documented" is "true." In the recent trend toward more empirical and "evidence-based" scholarship, this appeal to the intuitive and/or narrative may seem less legitimate as a method of inquiry.

We can't hope to illustrate every feminist method within the constraints of this section. Nevertheless, the diversity of these four contributors exemplifies the methodological richness and vitality of contemporary feminist bioethics, and its contribution to mainstream bioethical work. There is a thread of critique (of the mainstream) and self-critique running through all four chapters, and this critical strength provides one response to the question of the co-opting of feminist bioethics' radical edge.

REFERENCES

Alcoff, L., and E. Potter. 1993. *Feminist epistemologies*. New York: Routledge.

Borry, P., P. Schotsmans, and K. Dierickx. 2005. The birth of the empirical turn in bioethics. *Bioethics* 19:49–71.

Code, L. 2002. Narratives of responsibility and agency: Reading Margaret Walker's *Moral Understandings*. *Hypatia* 17:156–73.

De Vries, R., L. Turner, K. Orfali, and C. Bosk. 2007. *The view from here: Bioethics and the social sciences*. Oxford: Blackwell.

Dickenson, D. 2002. Commodification of human tissue: Implications for feminist and development ethics. *Developing World Bioethics* 2:55–63.

———. 2004. The threatened trade in human ova. *Nature Reviews Genetics* 5:167.

Greenberg, A. S., and J. M. Bailey. 2001. Parental selection of children's sexual orientation. *Archives of Sexual Behavior* 30 (4): 423–37.

Haimes, E. 2002. What can the social sciences contribute to the study of ethics? Theoretical, empirical and substantive considerations. *Bioethics* 16:89–113.

Hedgecoe, A. 2004. Critical bioethics: Beyond the social science critique of applied ethics. *Bioethics* 18:120–43.

Jagger, A. M. 2007. *Just methods: An interdisciplinary feminist reader*. Boulder, Colo.: Paradigm.

Lindemann, H., M. Verkerk, and M. U. Walker. 2008. *Naturalized bioethics*. New York: Cambridge University Press.

Nelson, H. L. 2001. *Damaged identities, narrative repair.* Ithaca, N.Y.: Cornell University Press.

Tong, R. 1997. *Feminist approaches to bioethics: Theoretical reflection and practical applications.* Boulder, Colo.: Westview Press.

Walker, M. U. 1998. *Moral understandings: A feminist study in ethics.* London: Routledge.

CHAPTER SEVEN

Bodies, Connectedness, and Knowledge

A Contextual Approach to Hereditary Cancer Genetics

LORI D'AGINCOURT-CANNING, PH.D.

The connection between embodied experience and legitimate knowledge has increasingly become a focus of feminist inquiry. Contrary to traditional epistemology, where authoritative knowledge is deemed to be universal, objective, and free from outside influence, feminist scholars have argued that the structure and experience of human activity has a direct influence on what may be known and how it is known (Hartsock 1987; Smith 1987; Code 1991; Harding 1993). The conviction that knowledge is influenced by social location and individual subjectivity gives rise to a more reflective approach to epistemology. It also motivates empirical inquiry to examine how subjective and situated experiences contribute to knowledge claims.

Based on empirical data, this chapter sets out to describe the ways in which individuals from families with hereditary cancer experience and construct knowledge about breast/ovarian cancer. I further aim to assess the intersection between experience, construction of knowledge about cancer, and construction of risk and risk-identity. Understanding women's use of experiential knowledge in relation to their bodies and hereditary breast/ovarian cancer is particularly important with the advent of individualized genetic testing for this disease. This technological development (and the promise of many more genetic predisposition tests) has raised serious ethical questions regarding privacy, confidentiality of information, and the potential for genetic discrimination. Feminist scholars as well have cautioned that through genetic testing and the ideology of geneticization,[1] women's bodies will be subject to increasing forms of intervention, social governance, and control. Yet, while genetic testing has received detailed treatment by feminist theorists, the associated viewpoints of those seeking testing have received little feminist attention. Even less attention has been paid to *how* a family/personal history of cancer affects the ways in which the body—and self—

are experienced and known. Because people from families with hereditary cancer have experiences of health, illness, and embodiment that likely differ from those who do not have histories of this disease, my question is how these differences shape knowledge about cancer and ultimately choices about genetic testing.

Certain points need to be made before I proceed, however. Lorraine Code posed hard questions about the privileged standing given evidential experience and what the subject claims to know. The problem, as she puts it, is: "A moral epistemology that is committed to counting experiences as 'evidence' has to guard against replacing an entrenched tyranny of expertise deaf to experience with a new tyranny of experience" (Code 2002, 164). She cautions that "neither tellers nor listeners" can take experience as incontestable. Rather, experience, and hence knowledge derived from it, is mediated by the location of experiencing persons within a specific time, place, culture, and material environment. Along similar lines, poststructural critics argue that experience is not a purely subjective act but is shaped by culturally and historically specific networks of practices (Oksala 2004).

I agree with Code that narrative accounts are not themselves transparent windows on how the "self" experiences the world. I too do not view representations of "experience" as unadulterated truth. Yet as Margaret Walker reminds us, experiential accounts are of central importance in that they provide insight into how situations seem and feel in everyday life (2002, 181). In other words, attention to lived experience is part of the effort to understand how individuals construct knowledge about that experience in making sense of the world. Lived experience alludes to the process in which individuals describe and give meaning to what happens to them. It is found in the stories that people tell about themselves and about the things that matter to them. Yet, as others have so clearly stated, it reflects, reproduces, and recreates our social world.

Thus, this work is based on the premise that experience with hereditary cancer leads to certain kinds of knowledge about the disease. It does not ask whether this experiential knowledge is medically accurate; nor does it claim that knowledge gained from study of personal experience should supplant the usual modes of feminist analysis. Rather, this project's main objective is to explore how hereditary breast/ovarian cancer is experienced and known, and in doing so, to broaden ethical analysis of genetic testing to include the voices of those the technology most directly affects.

This chapter is organized into four sections. The first section begins with a background review of hereditary cancer genetics. Next, I present my research methodology, followed by narrative accounts given by women/men from families with hereditary cancer regarding their experiences. In the third section, I use these findings to explore the connection between experiential knowledge and constructions of risk and risk identity. I conclude by discussing the particular nature of knowledge construction and the implications of study findings on feminist theorizing about genetic testing.

Background

The detection of mutations in two genes, BRCA1 and BRCA2, offers the opportunity to identify women who have inherited a strong disposition to develop breast and ovarian cancer (Muto 1997; Burke and Press 2006). Current data indicate that women who inherit a mutated copy of either gene have a 45 to 65 percent risk of getting breast cancer by 70 years of age (Antoniou et al. 2003). The same mutations increase a woman's lifetime risk of getting ovarian cancer to 11 percent (BRCA2) and to 39 percent (BRCA1). These inherited mutations are also associated with a 59 percent risk for premenopausal breast cancer and an increased risk for second primaries (new breast and/or ovarian cancers in a person with cancer, as opposed to recurrent disease) (Easton et al. 1995). In contrast, the corresponding population risks for North American women to develop breast cancer and ovarian cancer are 10 percent and 1.4 percent, respectively (Greene 1997; Foulkes and Narod 1998).The incidence of breast cancer in male mutation carriers is extremely low, with mainly BRCA2 mutations posing an elevated risk of 6 percent (Easton et al. 1997; Sverdlov et al. 2000).

Genetic testing for breast/ovarian cancer susceptibility offers the potential to reduce cancer morbidity and mortality from these diseases. Knowledge of a positive mutation status may encourage identified carriers to engage in cancer surveillance, avoid exposure to triggering mechanisms, or make decisions about other options such as prophylactic surgery and/or chemoprevention (Burke et al. 1997; Eeles 2000; USPSTF 2005). There is fair evidence now that prophylactic surgery (mastectomy and/or oophorectomy) can significantly reduce the incidence of breast/ovarian cancer in women with known BRCA1/2 mutations (Rebbeck et al. 2004; Warner et al. 2004). Tamoxifen appears to decrease breast cancer risk for women with BRCA2 mutations but not for those with BRCA1 mutations (Narod 2002). Accordingly, the potential benefits of genetic testing for those with strong family histories of these diseases is substantial (USPSTF 2005; Burke and Press 2006).

Methodology

The work reported here was part of a larger ethnographic study designed to explore women's moral and social experiences with genetic testing for hereditary breast and/or ovarian cancer (d'Agincourt-Canning 2003). The research comprised in-depth interviews with 53 participants, 45 women and eight men. Participants were recruited through the Hereditary Cancer Program (HCP) at the British Columbia Cancer Agency, Vancouver, where they had been referred to genetic counseling for breast/ovarian cancer because of their personal and/or family histories of the disease. Of the 45 women who participated, 17 women had been affected by cancer already, and the remainder were cancer-free but were considered at high risk based on family history. The interviews were tape recorded with prior consent of all participants and transcribed verbatim. Analysis entailed an iterative process of moving back and forth between data collection, dialogue with participants, coding, and conceptualization of common themes.

Themes

Thematic analysis revealed two broad categories of experiential knowledge—empathetic knowing and embodied knowing—as ways of coming to know cancer as a familial disease. I follow Abel and Browner's (1998) lead in characterizing "empathetic knowledge" as knowledge derived from close associations or emotional ties with others experiencing a particular event. Empathetic knowledge enables individuals to give authority to their own understanding of disease, which has been generated by connectedness to and knowledge of other family members' experiences. "Embodied knowledge," on the other hand, refers to subjective knowledge derived from bodily experience (Abel and Browner 1998), in this case, of having cancer oneself. In what follows, I present and explain each of these two forms of experiential knowledge using quotations from the interviews as data.

Empathetic Knowledge

Empathetic knowing appeared to exist along a continuum from weakly held to strongly held convictions based on close ties with others. Of the 53 participants, more than two-thirds (n = 39) came to genetic testing aware of their strong family history of the disease. For the majority of participants, these histories included living with someone with breast cancer or witnessing the deaths of relatives. Lorraine's story is typical in this regard.

> My Auntie P., who married my dad's brother, was the first one in that family to get diagnosed with cancer, and she died of breast cancer at the age of 37. Then, the next sister was Auntie F. She had breast and ovarian cancer, I believe, and she was 47. Then mom's younger brother, Uncle J. got diagnosed with a brain tumor, and he was about age 50 when he died. So it always seemed like we were going to funerals and people were sick when I was a kid growing up… And then about five years ago now, my mother, well she died about five years ago, but she was diagnosed six years before she died with ovarian cancer. So she had surgery, and then she had chemo, and then she had chemo again… I took time off work and looked after her for about three months with my father. She died at home.

Indeed, many participants had difficulty in distinguishing clearly the age at which they first learned about the existence of cancer in the family. It was just something that was always there. One of Barbara's earliest childhood memories was waiting in a car outside a hospital while her father visited his sister. Her aunt was being treated for breast cancer and died soon after at age 31. A few years later another aunt died of breast cancer, and when Barbara was in her twenties, several cousins were diagnosed with the disease. Then one of Barbara's sisters (one of a set of twins) developed breast cancer when she was 39 years old. She died three years later, and her twin developed cancer one year after that. This sister fortunately has just reached the five-year-survival mark.

In addition to being aware of their family cancer history at an early age, many of the women interviewed had provided care for mothers or other family members who had the disease. These women drew on experiences of caring for others to construct knowledge about breast/ovarian cancer and the course it might take in their lives. The more complex the trajectory, the more difficult the lived experiences became. Vicki talked about the pain of watching her mother suffer from ovarian cancer and get progressively worse over time. This was made harder for Vicki by the fact that she herself had breast cancer 10 years earlier.

> Mom died of cancer at 56, you know. So she kept believing that the Lord was going to heal her like he did me, but it never happened and it was really hard watching my mom go through this just a few years after I had gone [through it] … It was I think like five years or something after I had it. She had ovarian

cancer and then she fought it for a long long time and then she just gave up. I saw her.

As the preceding passages suggest, the kinds and intensity of lived experiences shaped the manner in which participants came to know and understand cancer. The experience of watching and caring for relatives with cancer had a strong impact on how they perceived the disease. Other participants' recollections were shaped by what they perceived as the relentless progression of the disease trajectory. Marlee was seven when her mother was first diagnosed with breast cancer, and the disease has been a backdrop to her life ever since.

[My mother] was thirty-seven when she was first diagnosed with breast cancer, and since then it's been ongoing... Five years later she got ovarian cancer and we thought we were going to lose her. They said she wasn't going to live. I was very close to my mom, very close, and so it was hard... Like I said, it's just been ongoing. She's had ovarian—I think three or four times it's recurred—and the breast cancer, and then she had [cancer] in her lymph nodes in her neck. And of course scares along the way, so it's been very emotional and up and down.

Recent Knowing

The extent to which individuals are aware of hereditary conditions depends not only on communication within the family but also on the temporal course of cancer within the family (Richards 1996). Indeed, for Kate, knowledge that cancer "ran in the family" was a new discovery. Up until her generation, the family apparently had been cancer-free. Both her mother and father, although elderly, were in relatively good health. Grandparents and older relatives had died of unknown or unrelated causes. There was no documented diagnosis of breast cancer in either immediate or extended family. Thus, the issue of hereditary risk did not arise until two of her four sisters developed breast cancer. Her older sister was diagnosed with breast cancer at the age of 43 and her younger sister at age 39. Kate was in her early 40s at the time.

Oh, I must say, I really didn't think that much about it when Margaret was diagnosed, but when Kim was diagnosed, like the first thing that comes to your mind is *who's next?*

One participant learned about her family history purely by chance. Sara's parents had divorced when she was very young, and her mother had lost contact with her father's side of the family. Long after Sara had left home, her mother ran into her former husband's cousin at a local store. They recognized each other, and the cousin, who had been tested for the BRCA1 mutation, told her about the program. The cousin, through Sara's mother, invited Sara to participate. This was the first Sara had ever heard about either genetic testing or the family history of breast and ovarian cancer. Several times during our interview, she spoke about how this discovery disturbed her.

> I think it was just overwhelming… for me, to sort of realize that hey, there's all these people that I am related to, all of the sudden there is this realization that something's happening in the family and it could have affected me or could affect me. And I didn't have a clue about it… And I do realize that because even with my dad and his parents and stuff there was a lack of communication, so I can see why it happened. But it is kind of frightening when you look on paper at all these people and you're going wow, I don't even *know* them.

A genetic test yields results that extend beyond the individual, affecting all members of a shared biological descent. Sara's words suggest that her concern about getting cancer was made more difficult by the lack of communication with family members and uncertainty about her past. She had lived her life divorced from these other family members and unaware of her family's history of cancer. In learning about this history, Sara was compelled to renegotiate her identity both in terms of a newfound family and knowledge about a disease for which she was at risk.

Embodied Knowledge

While the previous group of women used family history, the experiences of caring for others, and family stories to construct their understandings of cancer, others also drew on embodied knowledge. This group is distinguished from the previous participants by having had cancer already. "Embodied knowledge" referred to women's actual experiences with breast cancer, with chemotherapy and radiation, and with surgery. It reflected knowledge gained by living with the disease, including ongoing physical and emotional changes.

Participants' embodied knowledge typically began with the diagnosis of breast cancer. Some participants found the lump themselves. For others, detection occurred during a clinical exam, and for others still, by mammography. Embodied knowledge was influenced by disease extent (localized disease versus lymph node involvement) and the effect of cancer therapy on women's bodies. Women reported diverse physiologic responses to their cancer and cancer treatment. Overall, however, surgery (e.g., lumpectomy or mastectomy) did not seem to pose as much of a physical challenge to participants as did chemotherapy and radiation treatment. Similar to other studies in the breast cancer literature (Potts 2000), some women talked about hair loss (following chemotherapy) as being a direct challenge to their experience of self. Complications related to surgery posed a challenge for others. For instance, Margaret talked at length about the impact that lymphedema (resulting from axillary node dissection) had made on her life.

> I have had a fair bit of trouble with lymphedema… and my quality of life has somewhat changed. I mean I used to be the one that mowed the lawn and we used to have a huge garden where that camper sits right to the back here. And I remember coming home from physio and saying to [my husband] that the physiotherapist said like I shouldn't be doing that hard of work with my lymphedema and the heat. So we planted cement. That was a little hard to take.

The comment above illustrates how the physical reality of the body is integral to daily life, agency, and self-identity as well as how individuals construct knowledge about the effects of a particular disease. As Abel and Browner (1998) stated, embodiment affects how we see ourselves, how we live our lives and the decisions we make. Selves are not separable or identical to bodies but "are created and sustained by the establishment of particular sorts of interconnections" (Church 1997, 88). Thus cancer (and ensuing treatments) may set limits on or reveal new possibilities for the self through the body.

From Cancer Knowledge to Risk Identity

For many women in this study, cancer evoked a common story and shared identity that connected the individual self to others. Perceptions of risk for future disease were grounded in personal illness as well as the experiences of others. This knowledge of shared identity also had implications about cancer risk for daughters, granddaughters, and future family. Without exception, all parents diagnosed with breast/ovarian cancer expressed concern that their children were now at increased risk for cancer. Concern was frequently raised about risk for siblings and other family members as well. In Margaret's words:

> I am scared for them. I don't want them to have to go through what I went through. I really don't want them to have to have cancer. I don't want them to have to go through all the chemotherapy and all the horrendous experience that it causes.

Participants who were cancer-free also drew on the experiences of other family members to construct perceptions of whether or how cancer might affect them. Just as their knowledge of breast cancer was shaped by family history and caring for loved ones with the disease, so too were their beliefs about personal cancer risk. Participants used their experiential knowledge as a basis for constructing risk identities. Vulnerabilities were triggered by knowledge gained through connectedness to others and by personalizing life experiences of family members affected by the disease. Gillian's initial awareness of cancer began with her mother's diagnosis of breast cancer, although she did not think of it as a family disease until both her aunt and sister were diagnosed with breast cancer several years later. Her mother's first cancer was treated with a lumpectomy. Several years later, however, she developed breast cancer in her other breast. She elected to have a double mastectomy, at which time a third cancer was found behind the lumpectomy scar. This was quickly followed by two episodes of ovarian cancer. As a result of observing her mother, Gillian views cancer as a disease that is unyielding. Her mother's experience has also made Gillian concerned about her own risk.

> I was just really scared because I thought, geez, it is so relentless. You know, this cancer is just, won't go away . . . I was just really scared for her, but also, like, angry, you know, why, why it just won't stop. And also then I, I got nervous about myself like, you know, what my risks were. They're pretty high.

As this comment suggests, Gillian drew on her mother's experiences to construct knowledge about cancer. She incorporated her mother's experiences into her own evolving sense of risk and self-identity. As Elliott (1999) observes, "Illness and health, disability and difference, cure and enhancement: it is a mistake to think there can be rigid distinctions here. This is because illness, health, disability and difference all are connected to a person's identity, her sense of who she is" (48).

Disease that is passed from generation to generation bears an enormous familial significance. It creates distinctive vulnerabilities that arise from being part of this group. Women who resembled mothers, sisters, or other relatives afflicted with breast or ovarian cancer felt especially vulnerable about getting the disease. In addition to family resemblance, the age at which close family members were first diagnosed with cancer acquired particular salience for some participants. They worried more, and their sense of vulnerability increased as they neared the age when others in their family had developed cancer.

Interestingly, this sense of vulnerability was not held exclusively by women.

Although male participants did not fear breast or ovarian cancer per se, they did express concern about developing some form of cancer around the same age that a close relative had it. Ross was 14 years old when his mother died of breast cancer. When I asked him whether he ever worried about getting cancer himself, he put it this way:

> My mom was sick for quite a while but played quite an important role in our lives when we were younger. And there is probably hardly a day that goes by that you don't think about her... I guess you asked the question did I worry about it at times? Well I guess the period of worrying about it was when my children were young and I was the age of my mother when she died and thinking you know God, what she went through with three boys and knowing that she was dying of cancer. Like I guess that is a time where you start to worry about it you know, like a little bit. [But] that period passed.

Women used their experiential knowledge not only to construct notions of personal risk but also to override physicians' advice when it seemed wrong. The medical recommendation most commonly rejected was that they were too young for mammography. Frequently participants were told that breast cancer was a disease of older women and that they did not need this kind of surveillance. Despite the women's family histories, physicians did not always support their concerns or take action. Many of the younger participants said they had to complain and pressure their physicians to obtain these services. They looked to medical technology (in particular, mammography) as the best hope for early cancer detection and improving their chances of survival. In the following account, the participant talks about pushing her family physician to refer her for annual mammography following her sister's diagnosis at age 37. The participant was 33 when her sister got cancer.

> It's not that they were offering, I was asking for them [mammograms]. And saying, you know, I want that, and [they said] well you're too young... I just said, I want one and I want it within the week.

Leslie pressed her surgeon to remove a lump she found in her breast. She considered herself at high risk for breast cancer based on her experiential knowledge. Multiple family members, including her mother and sister, had been afflicted with cancer. Although the surgeon knew her family history and suspected that there might be a genetic mutation in the family, she was reluctant to do the lumpectomy. Leslie was told that in women of her age, most breast lumps are benign. Yet she sought medical technology and expertise to deal with her own way of knowing.

My surgeon suspected that I was a gene carrier. And she still didn't want to give me my lumpectomy… Well, I had to tell them, you know, I'm 27 years old, I'm not an idiot, you know. I have a big lump sitting in my chest and if you don't cut it out, I will take a steak knife and take it out myself. I don't care. It's coming out. And I shouldn't have to do that.

From the vantage point of power, the behavior and responses of these individuals can be read as a challenge to authoritative knowledge and medical networks of power. The conflict between experiential knowledge and professional knowledge frequently played out in access to medical resources for younger women. In these two cases, the participants were asking for services that paralleled the screening recommendations made by genetic counselors based on their family history. In fact, Leslie was later found to be a BRCA1 mutation carrier. It is important to note, however, that not all participants experienced such confrontational interactions with their medical providers. Many felt fully supported by family physicians who took their concerns about family history seriously and supported their decision to have mammography.

Discussion

Experience has long occupied a central role in feminist theorizing about knowledge. Critical of positivist interpretations of objectivity, feminist work in epistemology has drawn attention to the importance of understanding women's diverse experiences and the power structures that shape them in developing theoretical accounts of knowledge (Keller 1985; Longino 1990; Code 1991, 1993). My purpose has been to explore the kinds of knowledge that result from living with hereditary cancer in order to introduce further reflexivity into current debates about genetic testing. I maintain that attention to women's experiences with hereditary disease is critical to discussions about the potential harms and benefits of new genetic technologies.

The findings presented represent my interpretation of how knowledge about hereditary cancer is derived from different ways of knowing and experiencing the disease. I have drawn on Abel and Browner's (1998) characterization of experiential knowledge as embodied and empathetic to further explore the issue. In this study, embodied knowledge referred to the situated knowledge of having cancer and receiving cancer treatment. Participants' accounts revealed that embodied knowledge is far more than discrete biological or physical events, but is a way of knowing based on the individual's ability to integrate contextual and personal meanings with bodily responses (Raingruber and Kent 2003). Embedded in this way of knowing are issues of self, reality, and agency. In addition, embodied knowing speaks to the social character of knowledge. For example, cancer can remove individuals from their social roles and activities (family, work, social life). For many women, this has profound implications on the way they conceive their selves and their bodies, as well as their selves as embodied. Beyond this, embodied knowledge is set within the context of the family's broader story (past and ongoing) and changing medical information.

Empathetic knowing is also a social enterprise. Fox Keller (1985) describes empathy as "a form of knowledge of other persons that draws explicitly on the commonality of feelings and experiences in order to enrich one's understanding of another in his or her own right" (117). In this research, family members acquired empathetic knowledge of cancer—its particular manifestations, the side effects of treatment, and the likelihood of survival—from personal experiences in living with or caring for relatives who have had the disease. I also expanded this concept to include knowledge acquired about particular others (with whom one shares a biological connection) that is obtained through less direct means. For example, some participants came to know cancer through family stories passed down from one generation to the next. Although far less personal, this form of empathetic knowledge is also likely to be important in shaping meanings about hereditary cancer. I suspect that it will give rise to distinctive vulnerabilities (constructions of personal risk) that come from being a member of this specific family. Emotional involvement may be less, but it still entails interpretation of cancer risk based on connections to others.

As Abel and Browner (1998) point out, although one type of knowledge derives from "direct sensory experience" (315) and the other from emotional bonds between individuals, uniting these two types of knowledge is their particularity. Particularity brings to bear the strong role that subjectivity, social location, context, and experience play in knowledge claims. For more than two decades, feminist theorists in philosophy and other disciplines have stressed the significance of particularity of context and the "specificity of the knowing subject" (Code 1993) in the development of knowledge. It has been argued that interpersonal experience is necessary for individuals to have beliefs and to know (Bleier 1984; Code 1991; Nelson 1993). This view purports that knowledge is not an objective activity based on rationality and self-interest but is a process that emerges and is constructed in dialogue with others. It is relational and interactive (Alcoff and Potter 1993). Indeed, in this study we see that knowledge of cancer is obtained within the context of the individual's story as well as within the family's broader story. Based on experience, family members construct and share their knowledge about a particular disease as well as knowledge that the disease is familial.

Although the characterization of experiential knowledge as embodied and empathetic serves a useful heuristic function, the distinction is not rigid. Empathetic knowledge may shape how embodied knowledge is interpreted, and embodied knowledge may shape how empathetic knowledge is interpreted (meaning that my embodied experience of cancer may be influenced by how I saw the disease play out in my sister's or mother's life). Especially for families with hereditary disorders, the two are often intertwined, as they contribute to experiential knowledge that extends across generations and evolves over time. Further, neither category is static. Each may be revised to reflect insights gained from new experiences or new understandings about the disease. Although some might view embodied knowledge as more valid, I would argue that in the case of hereditary cancer (and I suspect other illnesses) empathetic knowledge can be just as poignant. The intensity of that knowledge derives from the fact that it is grounded in relationships. As many participants articulated, the situation of having one's sister, mother, and grandmother have breast/ovarian cancer is emotional and extremely difficult.

While this chapter has focused on the familial context of knowledge production, it is important to recognize that individuals' experiential knowledge of cancer is also shaped by external knowledge. As feminist scholars remind us, individuals and families are socially and historically located (Meyers 1997). Knowledge about the disease develops within a broader community—social, cultural, and medical—that views the illness in a certain way (Good 1994). Epistemological communities are multiple (Nelson 1993). Medical information undoubtedly contributes to individuals' knowledge claims. Yet, as was seen in this study, experiential knowledge may also conflict with medical knowledge. Because breast cancer is perceived to be a disease of older women, some participants reported being denied access to mammography because of their age. But experiential knowledge is a powerful force. People view themselves as knowers and interpreters of this lived experience. Most participants used this knowledge to accept or reject clinical recommendations and to gain access to services they felt they needed. At the same time, experiential knowledge may not always be reflective or free from misconception. It is possible that experiential knowledge shaped by feelings of intense loss, for example, may override more rational approaches to a problem. Just as with external knowledge, reflection and inquiry are needed to assess the validity of experiential knowledge.

What implications do these findings have for ethical debate about genetic testing? To date, ethical evaluation of genetic testing for hereditary cancer has focused on a fairly narrow range of theoretical issues: the right to know or not know, privacy, confidentiality of information, and the threat of genetic discrimination. Feminist theorists have broadened the discussion by raising critical questions about the economic and political basis for "geneticizing" cancer, while the social causes are shunted aside (Kenen 1994; Lippman 1998). Some have questioned whether normalization of genetic testing may lead to excessive individualism and, in the future, reduce women's choices by making them feel compelled to be tested (Lippman 1998; Sherwin and Simpson 1999). Others argue that genetic testing may reignite tendencies to characterize people as "other"—to further marginalize groups already disadvantaged on the basis of supposed racial or ethnic heritage (Nelkin and Lindee 1995; Asch and Geller 1996; Davis 2000). Yet while feminist scholars have pushed the boundaries of ethical debate, feminist critiques of genetic testing have remained within a theoretical domain. In other words, ethical theorizing about genetic testing for the most part has been removed from the life context in which this technology has its moral meaning.

This study underscores the need to explore the value of genetic testing from the vantage point of those who live with hereditary disease. As we have seen, for most participants cancer was not a one-time event or a risk probability but something ever present in their lives. Extending across generations, cancer had a timeless quality. It affected people's understandings of their present and future selves, as well as their past. It affected their relationships with others and how they viewed themselves in the world. Although meanings of cancer can be evaluated through examination of social, cultural, and political ideologies, the disease had a palpable—and mostly tragic—presence here. Thus, for individuals from hereditary cancer families, the use of genetic testing may well raise different moral issues and choices than it does for other people.

For example, several studies have indicated that responsibility to others serves as a primary motivator for women and men to undergo BRCA1/2 testing (Goelen et al. 1999; Hallowell 1999; Burgess and d'Agincourt-Canning 2001; Hallowell et al. 2003; d'Agincourt-Canning 2006). Choices around testing reflected practical decisions about personal health but also intersected with responsibility to obtain this information for other family members. The duty to disclose or share this information with others served as a key feature of moral decision making and, for some, became a moral obligation that was difficult to fulfill (Burgess and d'Agincourt-Canning 2001; d'Agincourt-Canning 2001). Genetic testing has also been found to raise ethical questions regarding reproductive decision making. Specifically, should one have children knowing that there is a 50 percent chance that a BRCA mutation can be passed on to them? Thus, to view decisions about genetic testing as the choices of a single isolated agent overlooks the moral dimensions that define everyday relationships and family life. As Scully, Banks, and Shakespeare (2006) observed in another context, being a good parent—and to this I would add, being a family member responsible with genetic information—may involve a relinquishing of choice that in another setting might suggest a constraint on autonomy.

Conclusion

Empirical work provides access to the kind of knowledge that promises to enrich feminist analysis of genetic testing. Its importance lies not only in the issues it describes but also in the questions it raises. I do not suggest that empirical work is a substitute for philosophical analysis. Rather, it may help us capture something about subjective and moral experiences that escape strictly theoretical accounts. It further offers to clarify the moral issues at stake in the development of new genetic technologies and, in doing so, to enrich ethical analysis.

Acknowledgments

Some of the data for this chapter first appeared in the *Journal of Genetic Counseling* 14 (2005): 55–69. This material is used by permission of Springer Publications.

I would like to thank foremost the women and men from families with hereditary breast/ovarian cancer who so willingly shared their experiences with me. I'd also like to thank Patricia Baird, Carolyn Ells, and Jackie Leach Scully for their helpful comments on different versions of this article and to acknowledge the contributions and invaluable support of the Hereditary Cancer Program, BC Cancer Agency, Vancouver, British Columbia. This research was supported by the Canadian Breast Cancer Foundation, the Huntington Society of Canada, and the Earl and Jennie Lohn Foundation under grants held by Dr. M. Burgess, chair of biomedical ethics, University of British Columbia, and Dr. D. Horsman, director of the Hereditary Cancer Program, BC Cancer Agency.

NOTE

1. Abby Lippman (1998) coined the term "geneticization" to describe the tendency of medicine to distinguish people, behavior, and illnesses on the basis of genetics.

REFERENCES

Abel, E. K., and C. H. Browner. 1998. Selective compliance with biomedical authority and the uses of experiential knowledge. In *Pragmatic women and body politics,* ed. M. Lock and P. A. Kaufert, 310–26. Cambridge: Cambridge University Press.

Alcoff, L., and E. Potter. 1993. Introduction: When feminisms intersect epistemology. In *Feminist epistemologies,* ed. L. Alcoff and E. Potter, 1–14. New York: Routledge.

Antoniou, A., P. D. Pharoah, S. Narod, H. Risch, J. E. Eyfjord, J. L. Hopper, M. Loman, et al. 2003. Average risks of breast and ovarian cancer associated with BRCA1 or BRCA2 mutations detected in series unselected for family history: A combined analysis of 22 studies. *American Journal of Human Genetics* 72:1117–30.

Asch, A., and G. Geller. 1996. Feminism, bioethics, and genetics. In *Feminism and bioethics: Beyond reproduction,* ed. S. Wolf, 318–50. New York: Oxford University Press.

Bleier, R. 1984. *Science and gender: A critique of biology and its theories of women.* New York: Pergamon Press.

Burgess, M. M., and L. d'Agincourt-Canning. 2001. Genetic testing for hereditary disease: Attending to relational responsibility. *Journal of Clinical Ethics* 12:361–72.

Burke, W., M. Daly, J. Garber, J. Botkin, M. J. Kahn, P. Lynch, A. McTieman, et al. 1997. Recommendations for follow-up care of individuals with an inherited predisposition to cancer. II BRCA1 and BRCA2. *Journal of the American Medical Association* 277:997–1003.

Burke, W., and N. Press. 2006. Genetics as a tool to improve cancer outcomes: Ethics and policy. *Nature Reviews Cancer* 6 (6): 476–82.

Church, J. 1997. Ownership and the body. In *Feminists rethink the self,* ed. D. T. Meyers, 85–103. Boulder, Colo.: Westview Press.

Code, L. 1991. *What can she know? Feminist theory and the construction of knowledge.* Ithaca, N.Y.: Cornell University Press.

———. 1993. Taking subjectivity into account. In *Feminist epistemologies,* ed. L. Alcoff and E. Potter, 15–48. New York: Routledge.

———. 2002. Narratives of responsibility and agency: Reading Margaret Walker's moral understandings. *Hypatia* 17:156–73.

d'Agincourt-Canning, L. 2001. Experiences of genetic risk: Disclosure and the gendering of responsibility. *Bioethics* 15:231–47.

———. 2003. Experiential knowledge, moral agency and genetic testing for hereditary breast/ovarian cancer. Ph.D. diss., University of British Columbia.

———. 2006. Genetic testing for hereditary breast and ovarian cancer: Responsibility and choice. *Qualitative Health Research* 16 (1): 1–23.

Davis, D. 2000. Groups, communities and contested identities in genetic research. *Hastings Center Report* 30 (6): 38–45.

Easton, D. F., D. Ford, D. T. Bishop, and the Breast Cancer Linkage Consortium. 1995. Breast and ovarian cancer incidence in BRCA1-mutation carriers. *American Journal of Human Genetics* 56:265–71.

Easton, D. F., L. Steele, P. Fields, W. Ormiston, D. Averill, P. A. Daly, R. McManus, et al. 1997. Cancer risks in two large breast cancer families linked to BRCA2 on chromosomes 13 q12–13. *American Journal of Human Genetics* 61:120–28.

Eeles, R. A. 2000. Future possibilities in the prevention of breast cancer: Intervention strategies in BRCA1 and BRCA2 mutation carriers. *Breast Cancer Research* 2: 283–90.

Elliott, C. 1999. *Bioethics, culture, and identity: A philosophical disease.* New York: Routledge.

Foulkes, W., and S. Narod. 1998. Cancers of the breast, ovary and uterus. In *Inherited susceptibility to cancer: Clinical, predictive, and ethical perspective,* ed. W. Foulkes and S. Hodgson, 201–33. Cambridge: Cambridge University Press.

Goelen, G., A. Rigo, M. Bonduelle, and J. De Greve. 1999. Moral concerns of different types of patients in clinical BRCA1/2 gene mutation testing. *Journal of Clinical Oncology* 17:1595–1600.

Good, B. 1994. *Medicine, rationality and experience: An anthropological perspective.* Cambridge: Cambridge University Press.

Greene, M. 1997. Genetics of breast cancer. *Mayo Clinic Proceedings* 72:54–65.

Hallowell, N. 1999. Doing the right thing: Genetic risk and responsibility. *Sociology of Health and Illness* 21 (5): 597–621.

Hallowell, N., C. Foster, R. Eeles, A. Ardern-Jones, V. Murday, and M. Watson. 2003. Balancing autonomy and responsibility: The ethics of generating and disclosing genetic information. *Journal of Medical Ethics* 29:74–83.

Harding, S. 1993. Rethinking standpoint epistemology: "What is strong objectivity?" In *Feminist epistemologies,* ed. L. Alcoff and E. Potter, 49–82. New York: Routledge.

Hartsock, N. 1987. The feminist standpoint: Developing the ground for a specifically feminist historical materialism. In *Feminism and methodology,* ed. S. Harding, 157–80. Bloomington: University of Indiana Press.

Keller, E. F. 1985. *Reflections on gender and science.* New Haven, Conn.: Yale University Press.

Kenen, R. 1994. The human genome project: Creator of the potentially sick, potentially vulnerable and potentially stigmatized? In *Life and death under high technology medicine,* ed. I. Robinson, 49–64. London: Manchester University Press.

Lippman, A. 1998. The politics of health: Geneticization versus health. In *The politics of women's health: Exploring agency and autonomy,* ed. S. Sherwin, 64–82. Philadelphia: Temple University Press.

Longino, H. 1990. *Science as knowledge: Values and objectivity in scientific inquiry.* Princeton, N.J.: Princeton University Press.

Meyers, D. T. 1997. Introduction. In *Feminists rethink the self,* ed. D. T. Meyers, 1–11. Boulder, Colo.: Westview Press.

Muto, M. 1997. Genetic predisposition testing: Taking the lead. *Gynecologic Oncology* 67:121–22.

Narod, S. 2002. Modifiers of risk of hereditary breast and ovarian cancer. *Nature Reviews Cancer* 2:113–22.

Nelkin, D., and M. S. Lindee. 1995. *The DNA mystique: The gene as a cultural icon.* New York: W. H. Freeman.

Nelson, H. L. 1993. Epistemological communities. In *Feminist epistemologies,* ed. L. Alcoff and E. Potter, 121–60. New York: Routledge.

Oksala, J. 2004. Anarchic bodies: Foucault and the feminist question of experience. *Hypatia* 19 (4): 97–119.

Potts, L., ed. 2000. *Ideologies of breast cancer: A feminist perspective.* New York: St. Martin's Press.

Raingruber, B., and M. Kent. 2003. Attending to embodied responses: A way to identify practice-based and human meanings associated with secondary trauma. *Qualitative Health Research* 13:449–68.

Rebbeck, T. R., T. Friebel, H. T. Lynch, S. L. Neuhausen, L. van't Veer, J. E. Garber, G. R. Evans, et al. 2004. Bilateral prophylactic mastectomy reduces breast cancer risk in BRCA1 and BRCA2 mutations carriers: The PROSE Study Group. *Journal of Clinical Oncology* 22:981–83.

Richards, M. 1996. Families, kinships and genetics. In *The troubled helix: Social and psychological implications of the new human genetics,* ed. M. Richards and T. Marteau, 249–73. Cambridge: Cambridge University Press.

Scully, J. L., S. Banks, and T. Shakespeare. 2006. Chance, choice and control: Lay debate on prenatal social sex selection. *Social Science and Medicine* 63:21–31.

Sherwin, S., and C. Simpson. 1999. Ethical questions in the pursuit of genetic information: Geneticization and BRCA1. In *Genetic information: Acquisition, access and control,* ed. A. Thompson and R. Chadwick, 121–28. New York: Kluwer Academic/Plenum.

Smith, D. 1987. *The everyday world as problematic: A feminist sociology.* Boston: Northeastern University Press.

Sverdlov, R. S., I. Barshack, R. B. Bar Sade, R. G. Baruch, G. Hirsh-Yehezkel, E. Dagan, M. Feinmesser, et al. 2000. Genetic analyses of male breast cancer in Israel. *Genetic testing* 4:313–17.

U.S. Preventive Services Task Force. 2005. Genetic risk assessment and BRCA mutation testing for breast and ovarian cancer susceptibility: Systematic evidence review for the U.S. Preventive Services Task Force. *Annals of Internal Medicine* 143 (5): 362–79.

Walker, M. U. 2002. Morality in practice: A response to Claudia Card and Lorraine Code. *Hypatia* 17:174–82.

Warner, E., D. B. Plewes, K. A. Hill, P. A. Causer, J. T. Zubovitis, R. A. Jong, M. A. Cutrara, et al. 2004. Surveillance of BRCA1 and BRCA2 mutation carriers with magnetic resonance imaging, ultrasound, mammography and clinical breast examination. *Journal of the American Medical Association* 292:1317–25.

CHAPTER EIGHT

Stories of Innocence and Experience

Bodily Narrative and Rape

FIONA UTLEY, PH.D.

It is not uncommon to meet a woman who reveals to you that she has been raped. Her rape may have happened years before or the night before, but either way her story, I have learned, never sinks to the level of a casual conversational gambit, no matter how much time has passed between the event and the telling. Her story has layers of meaning inherent in it that can be difficult for both the listener and the teller. In my experience of listening to these stories, what has been most striking is the way that a woman's whole self communicates her experience of both herself and the world; to make sense of her words as her words, I need to listen to them as inextricably intertwined with her physical gestures and comportment. Let me begin by telling you of one such experience of listening.

It took six years after being gang raped before Dorothy[1] felt able to go to a crowded public venue without her partner walking behind her so that no one could touch her back. For Dorothy, this touch in a public place was no longer a benign accidental interaction or a respectful gesture to gain attention. This tapping of her back had been a part of positioning her to be pushed through a door where a group of males were waiting to rape "some woman." The gang rape had been brutal. Dorothy had sustained severe physical injuries and was told by the police that she was lucky to be alive.

Six years later, Dorothy was sharing a hotel room with a work colleague. She told her story of going to the casino with other colleagues the previous night and what it meant for her. As she spoke more about her trip to the casino, the story of her rape took over. She began to shudder, at the same time responding to this with attempts to control her strong bodily contractions. This continued for some time, and when it came time to go from the hotel to the airport, Dorothy became increasingly aware that this would require her to be composed in a way that she could not achieve. Her colleague ordered a taxi, and she and another friend walked on either side of Dorothy, shielding her as they left the building. Dorothy gripped her friend's hand so tightly it hurt; she leaned into her and even in the taxi was unable to release her grip. (personal experience 2002)

While this story about a rape and its aftermath is incomplete, we see two significant features of interpersonal communication: that there are times when words fail us and we are unable to put into words some aspects of our lives, and that the listeners involved were attentive to a story that was being told partly without words. The listeners were attentive to the bodily comportment of this woman *at the same time* that they attended to the words that were said or not said. The combination of both bodily and verbal aspects of the narratives *experienced* by the listeners led to "understanding" something of what was being conveyed.

It is apparent that much is going on in this story that philosophical accounts of the self will miss, primarily because the person's linguistic narrative is dealt with separately from the things that the person is doing.[2] In this chapter I set out a conception of bodily narrative as a way of making sense of how it is that *the body* narrates both message and meaning. First, I will discuss what narrative is, using Ricoeur's conception of the mimetic arc of the narrative. While this sees the narrative as a form experienced by tellers and listeners, it retains inherent limitations by speaking of it solely as a cognitive ordering principle. Second, I turn to Merleau-Ponty's conception of the doubling of consciousness and body—the intertwining of mind and body that is the body-subject—from which we can derive an extended understanding of the narrative form to include bodily narratives. I then use this phenomenological account of bodily narrative to reconceptualize the aftermath of rape in order to facilitate a deeper discussion of appropriate public responses to problems of harm.

Life and Narratives

The minimum conditions for what counts as a narrative (Lamarque 2004, 394) include: (1) a story is made, not discovered—it is a telling of something; (2) a story has at least two events that are in some way related, with this relationship having a temporal dimension; and (3) if a text is identified as a narrative this does not, of itself, imply anything about the text's context, truth, subject matter, or purpose. So, narratives can be about any subject, referring to real or imaginary events and/or entities, can serve a multitude of ends, and can be true or false in what they tell. Narration is consciousness at work, but it is how we understand consciousness that is central here.

Paul Ricoeur's work on narrative gives important insights into the relationship between life and narrative but remains committed to understanding narrative as the artifact of subjective representation that follows from experience in the world. Life is an "incipient story," not only because of the ways that the symbolic context of our actions make them a "quasi-text" with a "first readability" (Ricoeur 1991a, 434) but also because our experience has a "pre-narrative structure." This structure makes "experience as such already something like a virtual narrativity which does not proceed from… a projection of literature on life, but which makes for an authentic demand for a story" (Ricoeur 1991a, 434).

While Ricoeur remains committed to a representational model of the narrative, he recognizes mimesis as having three stages. *Emplotment*—Aristotle's *mythos*—is understood as an integrative process of creating order, a weaving together of the incongruent and dissimilar that is the productive (*poiesis*) aspect of the *mimesis*[3] of fiction. The first mimetic stage—*mimesis1*—is the stage of prefiguration of the narrative. The "pre-narrative quality of human experience" (Ricoeur 1991a, 434) is the means by which we understand the characters of stories as having motives and goals; indeed we understand everything that the plot of a narrative entails because of our preunderstanding of action that comes from living our life.[4] For this reason, Ricoeur recognizes the narrative as being a process secondary to our entanglement in stories. He says, "This 'entanglement' thus appears as a pre-history of the story told… This… is what connects the latter to the larger whole and provides it with a background. This background is built up into a living, continuous overlap of all the lived stories" (Ricoeur 1991a, 435).

We use what Aristotle calls "phronetic intelligence" to create and, at the same time, understand both our experience and the story. The creativity of the weaving together of events into the intelligible, dynamic plot as well as the refiguration of the reading uses this mode of intelligence, which is both characteristically narrative and "always already there" (Ricoeur 1991a, 428). In referring to this Aristotelian model of thought, Ricoeur recognizes that another model, such as Kant's relation between the schema and the categories that designate "the ordering principle of the mind," could do just as well as Aristotle's designation of the plot as the "well-spring of the story" (Ricoeur 1991a, 428–29), but Ricoeur's emphasis is on this narrative intelligence as the first-level intelligence from which the second-level discourse of narratology emerges. Narrative fiction, then, is an irreducible dimension of the understanding of the self in which, in recovering "the narrative identity which constitutes us" (Ricoeur 1991a, 436) we give unity, a narrative wholeness, to a life.

The second stage—*mimesis2*—is characterized in three interrelated ways: as a synthesis of multiple events organized in an intelligible, but singular, order; as the unification of diverse elements of both intentional and unsought experience; and as the synthesis of our experience of time as both flux and duration (Ricoeur 1991a, 426–27). This understanding of the narrative form sees the story not as a passive representation of the "pre-existing thing[s]" of life, but as "bring[ing] about an augmentation of meaning in the field of action, which is its privileged field" (Ricoeur 1991b, 138). In this way the story "produces what it imitates" (ibid.). Emplotment is also characterized as creating a dynamic that "does not come to fruition other than in the living receiver of the story being told" (Ricoeur 1991a, 426). The configuration of emplotment is creative, transformative, and productive. The act of refiguration—*mimesis3*—is one in which the reader exercises the freedom to experience the story as "her own"—that is, while it is about something or someone else, and the reader is thus constrained by its text, the reading of it is *her experience* and becomes part of her life. In this way, it "returns" to experience. The reader brings the work of emplotment to completion.

By exploring the way that stories have an active and open quality whereby we complete the work (Ricoeur 1991a, 432), Ricoeur brings us back to seeing stories as belonging to experience. This belonging and embeddedness in life not only provides the dynamic element but also makes intelligible everything that is the narrative form. Narration begins and ends in experience.

Bodily Narratives and Phenomenology

Maurice Merleau-Ponty refers to perception as the "original text" but also to this "text" as "[carrying] its meaning within itself" (Merleau-Ponty 2002, 24). I claim that this original text is a narration of our world. Narration is the natural emergence from the work of perceptual consciousness, and as such, the world as we perceive it is not a collection of things but a narrated world with its meaning within itself.

Understanding the notions of the body-subject and the phenomenal body "involves a profound transformation of the notions of body and consciousness" (Merleau-Ponty 2002, 409). The primacy of perception grounds Merleau-Ponty's theory of the body-subject. Perception has a synthetic activity, which means that in perception we find our "nascent logos," and hence, for Merleau-Ponty perception *is* consciousness (Merleau-Ponty 1964, 25). Perception has an "intentional arc" that subtends its being and makes it both perception and consciousness. The phenomenal body is thus underpinned by operative intentionality—our "I can"— that is our basic bodily bond with the world. For Merleau-Ponty, the phenomenal body is our anchorage in the world and our access to understanding, primarily through perception. Perception inheres in a point of view (Merleau-Ponty 2002, 44), and facts about the world are, in part, due to facts about the body-subject. The subject is implicated in all perception.

The phenomenal body is thus "inhabited by a consciousness," and experiencing this inherence of consciousness in its body *and its world* is the body-subject. This thesis of the doubling of consciousness and body takes that crucial step beyond the picture of an embodied and relational self that is nevertheless still embedded in dualistic assumptions. Consciousness, understood as characteristically engaged—dynamic rather than passive and always directed toward the world—is the other side of the lived body, also engaged, active, and directed toward the world. The body-subject "take[s] up this unfinished world in an effort to complete and conceive it" (Merleau-Ponty 2002, xxiii), and so the phenomenal body is "the potentiality of a certain world" (Merleau-Ponty 2002, 122) and is always lived "in the world."

From the opening preface to Merleau-Ponty's *Phenomenology of Perception* (2002), and throughout his work, we can find references that signal support for the notion of bodily narrativity.[5] Merleau-Ponty recognizes the activity of speech as continuous with a broader embodied expression. He sees the body as "a power of natural expression" (Merleau-Ponty 2002, 211), the spoken word as a gesture (Merleau-Ponty 2002, 214), and this linguistic gesture as "like all the rest" (Merleau-Ponty 2002, 216). He draws a parallel between a "representation of movement" and a verbal image: "I do not need to visualize external space and my own body in order to move one within the other. It is enough that they exist for me, and that they form a certain field of action spread around me. In the same way I do not need to visualize the word in order to know and pronounce it... I have only one means of representing it, which is uttering it" (Merleau-Ponty 2002, 210). Finally, he says, "The spoken word is a genuine gesture, and it contains its meaning in the same way as the gesture contains it. This is what makes communication possible" (Merleau-Ponty 2002, 213). This gives our bodies the capacity for narration, just as in speech we have this capacity.

I see Ricoeur's three stages of mimetic configuration as attempting to capture the way that consciousness is always intertwined with lived experience. Ricoeur's movement of the text as open to completion by the reader reflects the openness of the body-subject to both complete the world and to be completed by the world.

Yet consciousness in the Cartesian model has no direct access to the extension that is the world, and so Ricoeur's integrative process retains a Cartesian mind-body dualism.

Merleau-Ponty says perception has an intentional arc: "The unity of the object is based on the foreshadowing of an imminent order which is about to spring upon us a reply to questions merely latent in the landscape. It solves a problem set only in the form of a vague feeling of uneasiness, it organizes elements which up to that moment did not belong to the same universe" (Merleau-Ponty 2002, 20). While Ricoeur's mimetic arc does not overcome the mind-body dualism, Merleau-Ponty's intentional arc, when placed alongside Ricoeur's mimetic arc of narrative, can be identified as a narrative arc. While perception has no "stages," it has a rhythm, an arc of movement that is the achievement of its own being. As a first "stage," a "vague feeling of uneasiness" heralds a "problem" needing to be solved. The second "stage" is one of figuration in which consciousness draws together associations, memories, and any other elements, such as possible projects, that "belong to the same universe." The third "stage" is one of knowing and achieving the unity characteristic of perceptual experience and at that point withdrawing and resuming its own operations. Out of the tension of possibilities and expectations an "imminent order" is revealed. This intentional arc enfolds us within a movement that brings us back, always, to our body as "the pivot of the world" (Merleau-Ponty 2002, 94). Merleau-Ponty says, "We shall have only an abstract essence of consciousness as long as we refrain from following the actual movement by which it resumes its own operations at every instant, focusing and concentrating them on an identifiable object, gradually passing from 'seeing' to 'knowing' and achieving the unity of its own life" (Merleau-Ponty 2002, 44). Merleau-Ponty uses the gestalt model to have us see the indivisible complexity of perception. I claim that understanding the lived experience of perceptual consciousness and its intentional arc as narration helps us understand the indivisible complexity that is being in the world. We are the story we talk about, the "ceaseless accomplishment... which continually gathers[s] within itself its past, its body and its world" (Merleau-Ponty 2002, 110).

Rape and Its Effect on Bodily Narrative

The victim of rape *experiences* the world as shattered, exposed as illusory. After rape or trauma, the world is no longer safe. But what is it that has been shattered? Brison sees that her own postrape incapacitation was "the incarnation of a cognitive and emotional paralysis resulting from shattered assumptions about [her] safety in the world" (Brison 2002, 44). While she acknowledges that trauma memories show an "intermingling of mind and body," her conclusion is that "'traumatic memory is not narrative. Rather, it is experience that reoccurs'"(Shay 1994, quoted in Brison 2002, 44). The difference is that "they are more tied to the body than memories are typically considered to be" (Brison 2002, 45). Brison also states that traumatic memory is "articulated, selective, even malleable," thus indicating some level of control over the traumatic experience and indicating the possibility of a narrative expression. In this way, traumatic memory is "like narrative memory" (Brison 2002, 31).

Brison tells of her exaggerated startle response, jumping at the sound of what turned out to be a leaf blowing along the sidewalk behind her (Brison 2002, 80–81). This response is linked to hypervigilance, which characteristically involves our physical relationship with, and sensory awareness of, our surroundings. Sounds that might once have blended in with background noise are heard distinctly, and may mean something. Others' "facial and gestural expressivity" is observed more closely for intention. In exploring how these actions might be understood. Brison concludes that because she once hadn't jumped at these noises, it might be a sort of rewiring of her brain "caused" by the assault, even though this rewiring will still have some reference to her previous dispositions. This neurological interpretation must be seen in the context of Brison's resistance to the idea that, in a certain sense, she chooses to behave this way.

While Brison resists the "snapshot" characterization of some theorists who view traumatic memory as "bodily, fragmented, sensory, intrusive, recurrent, uncontrollable" (Brison 2002, 31), she also sees these experiences as different from "ordinary" experience that is supported by cognitive and emotional activity she now lacks. This implies that the physical comportment she often experiences post-trauma lacks the structure, continuity, and embeddedness that cognitive memory provides. Cognitive paralysis results from her memories of a safe world being challenged. The challenge comes from her experience of the world. Yet, her cognitive awareness of a safe world would also have come from her *experience* of the world as safe. That, I suggest, characterizes all memory as "experience that re-occurs" and as tied to the body, with trauma memories being "more" tied than others.

Brison's account implies a deeper narrativity that belongs to an "intermingling" of mind and body, yet she still associates personal narratives with the mind, while the body, which might "articulate," "select," and shape expression, remains primarily *the vehicle for sporadic remembering* that is the result of a lack of control at a level of cognitive narrative formation. Aftermath experiences can seem like this—fragmented and intrusive. How might we see these expressions as belonging to conscious narratives?

I want to look at one point in Brison's account of her experience and explore the patterns of association that are activated. Post-trauma, she hears, while walking, a sound that is later identified to be a leaf twirling in the breeze. Her experience of this sound stands forth with "an immanent significance." In her current experience, this ordinary sound could herald a possible attack. This is because there is now an association set up with an earlier ordinary sound—the sound of footsteps behind her. Before her rape and attempted murder, Brison "looked up from [her] berry picking... and saw a man standing in the driveway just ahead" (Brison 2002, 105). This man was her attacker, but there was nothing about his reply of "bonjour" to her greeting, which was made with eye contact, in which she saw any sign of attack. In fact, it allayed an "apprehension" that she felt, reassuring her that the situation was safe. Such exchanges are filled with meaning—they both constitute and articulate our cooperation with each other. As Brison said, if he hadn't replied as he had, that is, if she had not got the reassurance of enacted cooperation that these gestures are, she might have changed her course of action (Brison 2002, 105). But she had no "reason" to. Reassured, she walked past the man and on down the road. She *did not hear* his footsteps as he ran toward her. This sound was not picked out by Brison as meaning anything out of the ordinary. Indeed, given the cooperative gesture from the man, the sound carries the meaning of "to be trusted" and sinks into insignificance for her. The success of the attack trades on her reading of his cooperation, on her trust. Given this, it is not surprising that she now apprehends a different meaning to such sounds—what she was previously able to trust can no longer be trusted.

We encounter her post-trauma, hearing an insignificant sound—a leaf twirling—but this now recalls that earlier "insignificant" sound as a theme of knowledge, and this knowledge tells her to beware. I do not see this as disordered in any sense. There is no pathology here, only normal, ordinary—"healthy"—functioning in the world. What is peculiar is the "uncalled" nature of the experience; the way that it overwhelms the present makes it disturbing to the reader, as it is disturbing to the survivor. We need to notice the way that trust is damaged. Because we are no longer able to trust an ordinary level of being in the world, the present is no longer protected by its own meaning—its meaning cannot be established. Other possible meanings crowd the horizon, including that of our vulnerability to the world and that of a woman's particular vulnerability to rape in a society that seems to allow it. We see how this present is indeed "pregnant with meaning" and how little of it can be trusted. When this trust has been damaged, we no longer have the trust that brings forth other associations.

Significantly, even when attacked, Brison continues to find in her experience aspects resembling the ordinary cooperation of others. All of these "normalities" blend in with the horror of this normality being breached. There is the sense of a conversation going on in this attack. In response to his saying, "I have to kill you," Brison makes promises—she won't say a word about him or the attack, she will say she has been hit by a car (Brison 2002, 106). Such are the strengths of these meanings to us: her attacker calls her a liar when she "breaks her promise" by screaming when she hears a rustling on the road above her. Both Brison's response to his "bonjour" and his response to her promises speak of the meaning that, for both of them, cannot help but float around their exchanges. Crucially, though, it is the breaching of Brison's trust that is damaging to her ongoing constitution of her world. We do not hear whether her lie created problems for the rapist. What leaps out is his continued trading on a horizon of meaning whereby he could call on her expectations of herself in the world (to be trustworthy), taking the opportunity to tell her of *her* "failure" *toward him*.

Narratives of Repair

Brison describes three major obstacles (Brison 2002, 49–50) to reconstituting the self after trauma. These include the loss of one's former memories of safety in the world, which can never be recovered as they were. Additionally, one's basic cognitive and emotional capacities are radically altered, often leaving the survivor numbed. The emotional possibilities of pleasure, happiness, and hope no longer seem possible. And finally, the ability to formulate a "'rational plan of life,'" understood by Rawls to be essential to personhood (Rawls 1971, quoted in Brison 2002, 52) is at least compromised, if not entirely lost. One is unable to envisage a future.

The narrative self that Brison refers to here is the *cognitive* narrative self. For the trauma survivor to regain the capacity to construct self-narratives, Brison says we need "audience[s] able and willing to hear us and to understand our words as we intend them" and emphasizes that "this aspect of remaking a self in the aftermath of trauma highlights the dependency of the self on others and helps to explain why it is so difficult for survivors to recover when others are unwilling to listen to what they endured" (Brison 2002, 51). I agree with Brison here but want to extend this notion of narrative repair to include our bodily narratives.

Given that bodily narratives are ongoing, they are present and operative even when words fail us. So while cognitive narrativity is interrupted when we can't find words that express our experience, our bodily narrativity continues. Brison quotes one trauma survivor who could only express her deep anguish by intimating how the powerful compulsion for this expression is physical: "Only if we were capable of tearing out by the force of our pent-up anguish the greatest of all mountains, a Mount Everest, and with all our hatred and strength hurling it down on the heads of [the offenders]... this would be the only fitting reaction on our part" (Lewin 1942, quoted in Brison 2002, 51).

The body-subject imagines a powerful physical gesture to express feelings *as well as* the need for power and control in the situation. Words cannot express, but gestures could. However, this imagined gesture is controlled, thus also expressing the overriding desire to reconnect with our world. Our more mundane bodily narratives express both trust and respect toward others—these shared meanings guide us to manage such expressions for the sake of our shared moral existence. Acts of self-control express to others our cooperation. Where the rape victim has experienced another who *has not exercised* this control, the control of such imagined gestures of rage asserts the need to reconnect with our world.

Here a notion of narrative repair is expanded when we understand how the retrieval of bodily narratives focuses on the lived experience of relationship and self-repair. The woman sees the world from the position of diminished trust.[6] This diminished trust affects the way in which the victim experiences the world and herself. Previously we have trusted ourselves to deal with a trusted world, but there comes a point where fear is such that we are no longer able to trust ourselves in the same way. We do not feel confident or capable in *this* world. It is because of this that the survivor has difficulty envisaging a future.

Brison focuses on narrative repair through the shaping and reshaping of our narrative accounts of our experience. Each time this is experienced with empathic listening, we are able to exert control over our traumatic memories. This happens because empathic listening involves us in embodied listening to bodily narratives—at the same time of course, our own bodily narratives of empathy *and self-trust* are "heard" or experienced by the trauma survivor. For the woman who has been raped, both trust in the world and self-trust need to be consciously and actively established, demanding active participation from the listener. Without this, power in the world cannot be reestablished. The listener is at once of the world and also intermingled with self. The need for active participation of the other asks that the other care and express this care. This cannot happen unless the listener can demonstrate their own genuine self-trust as they listen to the woman. This means that they themselves may be affected by the exchange but are still able to extend their own self-trust toward the woman. This cannot be done if they fear the woman's bodily narrative or if they seek to judge or reinterpret this narrative for the woman. Not only for the raped woman, but also for the listener, power in the world must now acknowledge and encompass vulnerability and trust. In this way, the raped woman can reconnect with embodied trust of the world and others. If trust is not established, experiences of betrayal, fear, disconnection, and violation will continue to erupt as a demand to set this right.

Postrape, many women's processes of narrative repair are hindered or marred and remain incomplete. Often the victim carries the burden for too long, and the identity that forms has incorporated much of the violent subordination and subjection that she experienced in the rape. The telling of the story is important not only for the process of sorting and testing that the woman undergoes in this, but also because she is reaching out to the world in this gesture, and her reception needs to be such that she can begin to repair the trusting relationship at the core of this interaction. Understanding healing to be a layered process embracing both verbal and bodily narratives, we need to understand what repair of bodily narratives requires.

Unlike Brison, I remain concerned that episodes of aftermath are too easily absorbed into cultural narratives of illness—particularly that of post-traumatic stress disorder (PTSD)—that overascribe responsibility to the woman and do not pay attention to the needs we have of others in this process of narrative repair. Brison sees that a PTSD diagnosis and treatment can be empowering when it gives recognition to the woman's experience that is otherwise denied (Brison 2002, 80). This certainly emphasizes the need to listen and engage more compassionately with the process of narrative repair, but I want to explore this listening further. In thinking about how we listen to these narratives, we need to think about the ways our narratives intertwine with theirs. I believe that in wanting to retrieve the listening and affirmative aspects of the PTSD diagnosis, Brison is too hasty in her disagreement with Lamb's argument that PTSD is "[one] of the worst thieves of victim agency / victim resiliency" (Lamb 1999, quoted in Brison 2002, 80).

Too often an incomplete process of narrative repair, or indeed the further damage that occurs at this time, is attributed solely to the character or abilities of the person undergoing this process. Given the interactional nature of identities, we also need to look at how her first-person account is heard. Listening to others at this time can be difficult—the details of a violent rape are appalling and frightening. When we listen and take in what happened, even in a small way, we glimpse something of the horror of the event. We want to withdraw from its reality, even in our imagination.[7] Exacerbating this difficulty is the fact that the victim often expresses her trauma physically. As listeners we withdraw more quickly from this level of interaction. The jagged physical presence of another disturbs not only our thoughts about what the world is like but also our world itself.

While we have responsibility in our narratives through our control over them, we have no control over the other's listening. We often say at this point, "You don't understand," pointing to the other's inability to be cognizant of our story. We might try saying things again, perhaps using different words that may better convey our selves. It is here, perhaps, that we slip into illness narrative, because we find that to be better than not being heard. Jean Amery's account of being tortured by the Nazis elucidates why women might choose an illness narrative in order to be re-embraced by their communities. Bergoffen refers to his account: "What is dehumanizing about being tortured is not the physical pain and abuse, but the sudden understanding that the other is impervious to his cry for help—that there is no one he can trust. The essence of torture, he concludes, is the destruction of the trust in the other that makes the concept of humanity possible" (Amery 1986, cited in Bergoffen 2003, 130).

To pathologize this suffering merely works to incorporate suffering and its meaning into a broader cultural narrative about selves. Without questioning the cultural narrative that facilitates this move, we cannot create space for reconceptualizations that might facilitate a more complete narrative repair. Phillips sees illness narratives as vehicles to express suffering (Phillips 2003, 320, 323). When women experience postrape traumas, this suffering has the capacity to be read as illness, as acute psychopathologies that threaten to become chronic and potentially be incorporated into the woman's sense of self. Phillips refers to Kleinman's work, identifying that suffering can "become imbricated in his or her ongoing life narrative" (Kleinman, cited in Phillips 2003, 320). Phillips goes on to say that the structural devices of our cognitive metaphors (plot lines, core metaphors, and rhetorical devices) can "shape and even create experience. The personal narrative does not merely reflect illness experience, but rather it contributes to the experience of symptoms and experience" (Phillips 2003, 320). Here, the illness narrative has become part of the world that the body-subject is inhered with.

This movement toward incorporation can nevertheless be understood as part of the desire to heal. Sufferers generally want to "heal" what is "insufferable." They desire this for their own peace, which includes acceptance and inclusion in their community. However, healing often struggles against normative ideas about what a life is, what a person is, and how this person, ideally, should shape her life. These normative ideas exist as gateways to belonging to what is considered "normal" society. Illness narratives, particularly when we are talking about any form of mental illness, draw on the notion of the autonomous individual. Within the cultural narrative of illness, the individual has the responsibility to return to normal, and the individual wants this. Yet she often finds that what is normal cannot accommodate the experience of suffering; she needs to ask that what is normal find space for her.

Conclusion

Something needs to be heard from these bodily narratives, something more than poignant stories of personal suffering. They cannot simply be viewed as a failure of control on the survivor's part. To simply place the woman in a position of having to deal with these postrape traumas as if the body is an object to be controlled often results in her experiencing a sense of repeated failure. We speak of controlling our bodies, as if the body is an object over which we have an authoritative relationship. Rather, according to Merleau-Ponty, "There is a body of the mind, and a mind of the body and a chiasm between them" (Merleau-Ponty 1968, 259).

In our embodied listening, we participate in the rape victim's narrative repair, thus acting as moral agents working to complete the world. Narrative repair needs to encompass our ability to say, with some conviction and some strength, "I can"—it is thus that our intentionality is restored. This is not just a cognitive capacity to consent, but it is the lived body's experience of consent, it is expressed in the body as a situation in which we again, with some security, navigate our world. Perhaps naïve trust is impossible because of the fact that our future is unknown, but we can desire a tempered trust based on the knowledge that others respect our personhood and do not see us as an instrument of their own impossible desire.

Repairing the world in the public realm requires public acts, such as the U.N. Hague war tribunal's groundbreaking 2001 Foca verdict that ruled on rape as a crime against humanity. As Debra Bergoffen claims, "In speaking of this right [intentionality of sexual integrity] as a human right, and in tying this right to the right of consent, the court brings the phenomenologically lived body into the halls of justice" (Bergoffen 2003, 121). Bergoffen draws on Derrida, asserting that justice needs to be concerned with the heteronomy of our vulnerability. Derrida urges us to live our heteronomy virtuously through friendship, and Bergoffen similarly sees the Hague decision as belonging to a broader politics of vulnerability, where all subjects are defined by their embodied finitude and there exists "a universal human obligation to acknowledge and abide by the virtue of trust"

(Bergoffen 2003, 133). In friendship we risk our vulnerability to the other—we practice the virtue of trust in that we trust the other, we make ourselves trustworthy, and we feel a measure of self-trust.

This practice of trust differs from the tradition of the political interpretation of vulnerability as feminine and of determining a woman's situation as one of dependency and needing protection (Bergoffen 2003, 131). Within traditional liberalism, the autonomy of the social contract is not possible for women. Men, who live this autonomy, are invulnerable and authoritative in their "protection" of women, which means that protection often equates to "use." The world a woman navigates is one where she experiences the continual threat of invasion from her protectors. In this disymmetry "the question of trust is translated into the question of the sexual relationship... [and] then gets perverted" (Bergoffen 2003, 131). Thus, Bergoffen argues, "the rape of the women exposing the latent violence of a system that recognizes only one sexed body as vulnerable and allows the other sexed body to enjoy the fantasy of autonomy" (Bergoffen 2003, 131). In exploring the narrative surrounding rape and consent, Bergoffen correctly identifies the vulnerability of all bodies. She moves beyond cultural narratives about consent and violence and argues that "violation of humanity occurs... the moment when my vulnerability is used against me" (Bergoffen 2003, 121).

Brison writes that her autonomy was undermined as a result of her trust in the world being shattered. Although we may have survived this experience, our self-trust in our ability to navigate the world has also been shattered. In aftermath experiences we have not yet established a realistic self-trust. Until we do this, we are more dependent on others, not so much for their protection as for their enabling presence. Here the actions of others, which for Brison included friends walking with her, her workplace providing night lighting in car parks, the securing of a door at the gym, self-defense training, and participation in a support group were crucial to her regaining her sense of control over herself, her environment, and reconnecting with humanity (Brison 2002, 61, 63, 65). Brison emphasizes listening as part of this enabling presence. I give an account of listening as embodied and embracing bodily narrativity, necessitating that we rethink suffering as an ethical matter and reconsider the political translation of our positive and social obligations toward those who suffer. Understanding the suffering of trauma aftermath through the cultural narrative of illness—here PTSD—can ascribe undue responsibility to individuals and evade the political problem of women's need to experience the world as safe. Recognizing trauma aftermath as being bodily expressions that tell us not only about the vulnerable self but about how the world is experienced as unsafe demands that we think more deeply about ways that the public realm be made safe for women.

Understanding the nature of our embodied selves is crucial to all ethical dilemmas but most particularly to those that center on the harm of violation of the self. There are many ways that the body-subject can be violated, and humans will surely invent more. By relooking at the harm of rape and the suffering of rape aftermath through the lens of Merleau-Ponty's phenomenology, and as embodied narrative, we can add to the work imagining an alternative ethical stance in which vulnerability, trust, and dependency can be taken up again, reconstituted and recreated as part of our world. By recognizing the existence of bodily narratives that need to be heard, we better understand the importance of a politics of vulnerability.

NOTES

1. Not her real name.

2. We tend to think of understanding another's story as coming from listening to their words. Stemming from this sort of understanding, the bodily aspect might be referred to as the "body language" of the woman. Diana Meyers (2004, 292), in discussing the notion of the embodied self, says that body language—gestural expressivity—"conveys much of the meaning of people's speech, as well as their nonverbal behavior." In this characterization, however, such gestures and expressions are viewed as isolated instances of expression that can be interpreted. This characterization, however, does not do justice to the way that these gestures belong to a broader expression of self, indeed, *are* the self.

3. Mimesis in the Aristotelian sense is creative imitation—*mimesis praxeos.*

4. To properly evoke the idea of the incipient story, Ricoeur describes two examples where the story that exists in a person's "pre-history" of lived experience emerges: in each case, the story still needs to be "found." One is the case of the client who, with the aid of psychoanalysis, "draws out from these bits and pieces [lived histories, dreams, 'primitive scenes,' conflicting episodes] a story that is both more intelligible and more bearable" (Ricoeur 1991a, 435). Without such a story, the various episodes are experienced as lacking in unity and meaning. The other is the judge who works to "unravel the knot of complications in which the suspect is caught" (ibid.). In both cases the stories that emerge exist in the "prehistory" of experience.

5. In *Phenomenology of Perception,* Merleau-Ponty conceived of the *tacit cogito.* This notion retained a sense of "pure interiority" that he later abandoned, saying that "the acts of the I are of such a nature that they outstrip themselves leaving no interiority of consciousness. Consciousness is transcendence through and through" (Merleau-Ponty 2002, 438). The notion of the *tacit cogito* can be likened to the idea of pre-narrative narrativity. If we reject this, as Merleau-Ponty intended, then we have support for the immediacy of bodily narratives expressing the work of consciousness.

6. The degree of diminishment of trust could reflect the degree of shattering of self.

Those who believe they were in the wrong place at the wrong time may not experience the severe dislocation that others do. However, this is not at all straightforward.

7. To accept these accounts is to be faced with the task of how we incorporate them into our own worldview. Is this what the world is like? The likelihood of it happening to us feels too close. We have a variety of ways of protecting ourselves from what we hear, and often for the layperson (that is, anyone not possessing counseling skills), this involves some measure of judgment: that this person's world is radically different from ours, that where they live and who they associate with locate them in spheres of increased risk; and that this person is radically different from us, that their behavior at the time was pertinent to the event. These judgments on our part are often incorrect and merely reflect our need as listeners to distance ourselves from the experience. As Brison recounts, her "others," in the post-trauma phase, often found empathy difficult. Their responses perhaps expressed the ways that their need for self-reassurance overwhelmed their ability to respond to Brison's actual needs (Brison 2002, 9–11).

REFERENCES

Amery, J. 1995. Torture. In *Art from the ashes: A Holocaust anthology,* ed. L. Langer. New York: Oxford University Press.

Bergoffen, D. 2003. February 22, 2001: Toward a politics of the vulnerable body. *Hypatia* 18 (1): 116–34.

Brison, S. J. 2002. *Aftermath: Violence and the remaking of a self.* Princeton, N.J.: Princeton University Press.

Kleinman, A. 1988. *The illness narratives: Suffering, healing, and the human condition.* New York: Basic Books.

Lamarque, P. 2004. On not expecting too much from narrative. *Mind and Language* 19 (4): 393–408.

Lamb, S. 1999. Constructing the victim: Popular images and lasting labels. In *New versions of victims: Feminists struggle with the concept,* ed. S. Lamb. New York: New York University Press.

Merleau-Ponty, M. 1964. *The primacy of perception.* Evanston, Ill.: Northwestern University Press.

———. 1968. *The visible and the invisible.* Evanston, Ill.: Northwestern University Press.

———. 2002. *Phenomenology of perception,* trans. C. Smith. London: Routledge & Kegan Paul. Originally published 1945 as *Phenomenologie de la perception* (Paris: Gallimard).

Meyers, D. T. 2004. Narrative and moral life. In *Setting the moral compass: Essays by women philosophers,* ed. C. Calhoun. New York: Oxford University Press.

Phillips, J. 2003. Psychopathology and the narrative self. *Philosophy, Psychiatry and Psychology* 10 (4): 313–28.

Rawls, J. 1971. *A Theory of Justice.* Cambridge, Mass.: Harvard University Press.

Ricoeur, P. 1991a. Life: A story in search of a narrator. In *A Ricoeur reader: Reflection and imagination,* ed. M. J. Valdes. Toronto: University of Toronto Press.

———. 1991b. Mimesis and representation. In *A Ricoeur reader: Reflection and imagination,* ed. M. J. Valdes. Toronto: University of Toronto Press.

Shay, J. 1994. *Achilles in Vietnam: Combat trauma and the undoing of character.* New York: Atheneum.

CHAPTER NINE

Where's the Harm?

Challenging Bioethical Support of Prenatal Selection for Sexual Orientation

JANICE MCLAUGHLIN, PH.D.

> The proposition... that there is nothing morally wrong with
> homosexuality by no means entails the proposition that there is
> something morally wrong with trying to avoid having homo-
> sexual children.
>
> *Greenberg and Bailey 2001*

The mid-1990s saw a brief flurry of media excitement in the United States and Europe over the work of various scientists exploring the link between sexual orientation and genetics or, as it became known, the "gay gene" (LeVay 1993; Hamer and Copeland 1994). Much of this initial research has been scientifically disputed, but attempts to identify the genetic basis to sexual orientation, in particular gay male orientation, continues (Mustanski et al. 2005). If a gene appears to link to same-sex sexual orientation, various possibilities emerge, including the use of preimplantation genetic diagnosis or antenatal screening to try to avoid giving birth to a lesbian or gay child.

The possibility that (a) sexual orientation is linked to a particular gene and (b) this knowledge could be used to preselect heterosexuality (or homosexuality) raises significant ethical issues around whether society should think of sexual orientation as a genetic trait and whether prospective parents should then have the right to purposively avoid having a child who has the associated gene. The deliberate avoidance of homosexuality has been addressed by bioethicists Greenberg and Bailey (2001), who make a case for the ethical legitimacy of parents using screening to shape the family of their choice. The justification is that such choice lies at the core of parental liberty, and parental liberty is central to individual freedom in a liberal democratic society. This form of argumentation makes Greenberg and Bailey good examples of those who have become "the authorized spokespersons on reprogenetics issues" (Paul 2001, 26); that is, those who use claims to liberty and rights of privacy to justify individuals utilizing the range of genetic screening technologies to shape the offspring of their choosing. However, employing liberty and privacy arguments in bioethical debates is seen as problematic by some. Critics suggest that the "obvious" centrality of parental liberty has replaced a substantive debate about the human and social dimensions of choices and health care provision (Fox 1990; Myser 2003). It is therefore important to have such a debate and, in particular, to question whether the centrality of parental liberty is legitimate.

The aim of this chapter is to explore the arguments of Greenberg and Bailey in order to challenge the privileged and unquestioned position they give to parental liberty, drawing on feminist critiques of liberalism and broader critiques of bioethics. There are several reasons for doing this. The first is to challenge the specific notion that it can be ethically acceptable to purposively determine or attempt to determine the sexual orientation of a future child. The second is to explore the wider significance of Greenberg and Bailey's argument as an example of liberal bioethical arguments that have emerged out of U.S. political and policy culture and which have a privileged position in ethical debates on reproductive technologies. The particular style of ethical argumentation present in Greenberg and Bailey is symptomatic of an approach that minimizes the social and political context and the consequences of individual choices. I will argue that the ethical evaluation of screening technologies requires a broader landscape of interrogation than allowed for by liberal approaches.

The Right to Select

The paper by Greenberg and Bailey is in the careful and logical style of liberal ethics argumentation. Different propositions are considered in turn in the search for abstract principles that can obtain in all cases. Their paper investigates whether there is any justification for denying individuals the right to shape their family in the way they wish. Through a series of points, the grounds for denying parental liberty to determine the sexual orientation of a child are rejected. Greenberg and Bailey begin by asserting that the method of selection is irrelevant. Whether selection is before or after conception, the moral issue is the same: is it acceptable to seek to avoid a human characteristic? This claim is drawn from bioethical justifications for abortion of fetuses with congenital conditions that state there is no difference between taking extra folic acid to reduce the risk of congenital conditions and choosing abortion after a "positive" diagnosis.

Although wishing to remain "neutral" on the question of whether there is something wrong with being gay, Greenberg and Bailey argue against assuming that people seek to avoid a homosexual child out of malevolence or prejudice. They argue that the desire can be born out of love, for example, the wish to spare the child unhappiness, or to ensure grandchildren. It also can be a product of the need to bond with the future child, which they argue is more possible when parents "shar[e] the sexual orientation of their children." What could parents talk about over the dinner table if they did not share the same sexual orientation as their children?

The core of Greenberg and Bailey's argument is that the rights and wrongs of preselection involve considering the balance between parental liberty and the avoidance of harm. Those who wish to justify reducing the rights of parents to choose the child of their dreams must prove that direct or significant indirect harm is entailed. Direct harm to a person is impossible because the fetus, aborted, does not become one. Instead the focus is on indirect harm. The authors dispute any possible indirect harm, that is, that preselection for sexual orientation will harm homosexual people in general. They propose that it is *unlikely* that preselection will

1. significantly reduce the number of homosexual people born and subsequently harm the ability of homosexuals to collectively campaign against discrimination;
2. encourage homophobia;
3. express societal or individual disapproval of homosexuality; or
4. endorse the idea that removing a fetus because it is identified as homosexual is a good thing to do and is socially approved.

In each case, even if some harm is "possible," they assert that "it is by no means clear that those harms would outweigh parents' liberty interest in raising the sort of children they wished to raise" (2001, 432). This statement identifies the core of their argument; parental liberty is a fundamental right so significant, so sacrosanct, that it can be challenged only by overwhelming proof that its exercise will lead to significant harm.

Greenberg and Bailey are not the only bioethicists to make this case. Murphy (1990) makes similar arguments, in particular that one should not assume that parents' choosing to preselect for heterosexuality would be evil or immoral, particularly because "it would be odd to think of heterosexuality as an evil inflicted on a child" (130). Indeed, he suggests that the future child will be grateful that her or his parents have gone to so much trouble to ensure she or he is just like mom and dad. Like Greenberg and Bailey, Murphy focuses on indirect harm and similarly concludes that any discrimination this personal choice expresses is not significant enough to justify denying the right to express that choice. Society, he argues elsewhere (Murphy 1995), has no moral duty to guard against the number of lesbian and gay men living in society falling. For Murphy, there is a greater good to be protected, "preserving the centrality of personal moral responsibility" (1990, 139).

Greenberg and Bailey are symptomatic of a version of liberal bioethics that positions choice and the rights of the individual citizen as preeminent. This strain within bioethics continues to be strong (although not uncontested) and remains present in more recent accounts advocating the use of preimplantation genetic diagnosis (PGD) to enable gender selection and avoid disability (Savulescu 2001; Robertson 2001, 2003; McMillan 2002; Steinbock 2002). The arguments put forward by Greenberg and Bailey and Murphy raise various questions. What is parental liberty? Why does it have such status? Is it such a fundamental universal principle that any qualification must respond to burdens of proof virtually impossible to obtain? These questions can be explored by drawing on feminist critiques of liberal thinking.

Feminist Challenges

Feminists are far from alone in challenging the foundations and priorities of liberalism. The emergence of poststructuralist and queer perspectives has been particularly influential, as it has created what Okin calls "an identity crisis" (1994, 5) in theories of justice and liberal political rights (key writers here include Rorty [1989], Butler [1990], Bauman [1993, 2001], and Braidotti [2002]). Poststructuralist and queer writers propose that the sovereign individual is a social and political construct, no more than a discursive device, which allows for a particular political culture and set of values (such as universality, rationality, and reason) to operate unquestioned and to have the appearance of universal application. Feminists have also played an important role in the destabilization of liberalism. While liberal feminism was an important element of second-wave feminism, particularly in the United States, this period of feminism also marked the beginning of a sustained critique of liberal thinking. (Note that there are feminists who argue that liberal thinking and feminism are compatible; see Okin [1994], Nussbaum [1999, 2003], and Abbey [2007].)

There are three important elements to Greenberg and Bailey's argument, which we can begin to tease apart using feminist critiques of liberal rights discourse:

1. The sovereign individual is the central figure of political and social rights;
2. the private and public boundaries of societal life are clear and natural formations; and
3. the choices of the individual are private matters that carry no societal significance.

Each one will be discussed in turn.

The Sovereign Individual

Parental liberty is based on the rights of the individual. In the Greenberg and Bailey piece, the bioethical concerns center on what it is permissible to remove from the liberty of the individual. The individual as such is a construct whose rights and choices have the power to shape the scope of what is considered when examining the ethical dimensions to screening processes. What we see here is the central premise of liberal bioethical and political thought: how much can the state take from the individual, in terms of restrictions on their right to shape their own version of the good life? How much does the individual owe the state in terms of responsibility to be a good citizen?

The individual enters society to protect their and their offspring's well-being. What they seek from the state is the protection of their rights, in particular to property; in return they promise to be good, productive citizens. The human qualities of rationality and reason enable us to make the calculation that looking beyond ourselves ensures our own individual prosperity. A sovereign individual, in light of their ability to act with reason and rationality, has the right to make judgments about their property, body, and actions, including how they will raise their family. This model is premised on certain assertions about human nature, rationality, and our basic similarity in terms of needs and wants. Contracts between individuals, and between the state and the individual, protect against one individual exerting their desires over the rights of others. A shared morality maintains the contract, and where that fails the sanction of law provides penalties for those who do not live up to societal expectations. For law to be just, it must be blind to particular interests and treat all individuals the same. In Greenberg and Bailey's analysis, the presumption is that the individual can have rights restricted only if direct harm can be proven; because they argue that it cannot, they conclude the state may not interfere with the right of the individual to make choices about her family as part of her version of the good life.

Contemporary feminists have drawn on ideas from within poststructuralist and postmodern approaches to continue the challenge to liberal arguments, which began in the second wave of feminism (Tong 2007). Their critique begins with the assertion that the individual of liberal thought is a fictional and exclusionary notion. Liberalism is based on a definition of the individual as male, for the individual of liberal thought operates in the public sphere disinvested from care responsibilities and feelings of attachment and connection (Pateman 1988; Brown 1992; Cavarero 1992). Such a figure can exist only through the gendered boundaries within society, which allow for masculinity and the public sphere to take on the characteristics liberalism associates with it: "The meaning of the individual remains intact only so long as the dichotomies (internal to civil society) between natural/civil, private/public, woman/individual—and sex/gender—remain intact" (Pateman 1988, 225).

Feminists question whether the individual exists as a separate, freestanding, sovereign being. For many feminists, the answer is no, and instead what is proposed is the socially and culturally embedded nature of any individual self, who is not born preformed but instead emerges as a particular individual within particular environments that inform her development (Gilligan 1993; Sevenhuijsen 1998): "There is no presocial component because the self is always situated within a concrete set of circumstances, beliefs, and constructions. The communities that formed us not only help us shape answers to the questions we face, but they also provide form to our worlds and define the problems we recognize as important" (Rudy 1999, 48). It then becomes less clear whether we can talk about rationality and reason as human values shared by all, not least because they are values that emerged from one particular group of male actors, but also because it becomes more difficult to talk of universal understandings of rationality and reason (Haraway 1991; Harding 1993).

If there are differences among us, and these differences relate to identity as well as social position, then is it not possible that the way we define rights, justice, fairness, and morality will be influenced by who we are and where we are (Benhabib 1992)? Phillips argues that the liberal focus on the abstract individual—to ensure that particularity and difference do not contaminate conceptions of the good life—means that the individual is abstracted from the very conditions that make her unequal: "A politics that tries to transcend (read ignore) difference is one that confirms the inequalities that exist" (Phillips 1993, 43). If this is the case, then how can any political theory make a claim to objectivity or truth in its knowledge of human nature and the operation of society? This points to "the importance of grounding one's theories of justice in the value structures of the surrounding world" (Phillips 1993, 56), an argument that Haimes (2002) and Osborne (1994) make in relation to bioethics.

The more the differences among citizens are recognized, the less legitimate it is to think of rights being protected through a universal set of rules. If rights are protected only at the level of the individual, then questions of justice and citizenship are minimized. Abstract individualism is a "powerful impediment" (Phillips 1993, 115) to equality because it does not allow for a reordering of the political and societal system so that systematic inequalities can be addressed. It provides no mechanisms to address the inequalities created by lack of wealth (Lister 1997) or of recognition (Fraser 2001). Cornell (1998) argues that the abstracted conditions Rawls (1972) proposes for constructing an environment in which individuals are treated as equals are insufficient for equality to be achieved.

If lives are "inescapably part of particular communities and contexts, and the values embedded there help us to set goals for ourselves" (Rudy 1999, 48), why build a framework to abstract judgment and decisions from those communities? All such a framework does is provide a pretence of universality, leaving hidden the influence of context on the judgments made. In the process difference is trivialized or read as deviant. Brown (1993) argues that recent history indicates the liberal state has lost its "guise of universality as it becomes ever more transparently invested in particular economic interests, political ends, and social formations" (392).

If we look back to Greenberg and Bailey's argument, we now see cracks in their defense of the rights of the abstract individual. It is no longer self-evident that the individual's choices should be protected above other considerations. Instead, one could argue that the history of discrimination and misrecognition of those who define their identities as gay or lesbian requires that it is our protection that should be prioritized. In addition, the fairness of allowing the choices Greenberg and Bailey advocate needs to be evaluated within the social conditions in which those choices are in fact made: a social and political context where equality for same-sex sexual orientation does not exist.

The Private and the Public

In Greenberg and Bailey's negative articulation of rights, it is assumed that there is a space where the individual exists, where the state has no right (or limited right) to interfere; this is the private sphere of family. The private sphere is where the individual can exist without surveillance and judgment by others. It is the haven from the hardships and toil of the public sphere. From classic to contemporary liberal political thinking, the significance of the nuclear family as that haven and the gendering of that space are inescapable. Writers such as Pateman (1989) and Moore (1999) argue that liberalism's celebration of impartiality and reason in the public sphere is based on the gendered separation of particularity and emotion into the feminized private sphere of the nuclear family. The private sphere has been the site where all the things that make the individual not autonomous—dependency, need, emotion, connection—are contained and dealt with by women (Kittay 1995).

Brown (1992) argues that the private/public separation is based on classic liberalism's assumption of male patriarchal right, which contemporary liberalism is yet to relinquish. Due to the gendered separation of spheres, liberalism has lacked a concern with the forms of oppression that take place in the private sphere. In the words of Moore (1999), "Although liberal theory was invested in protecting every citizen's right to privacy, it was wholly unconcerned with the content of the decisions, judgements, and preferences exercised in that realm" (37). Various problems have been allowed to occur in the private sphere because the state has no right to be there: domestic violence and child abuse were ignored for years because of a gendered presumption that the private space was beyond the scope of law and justice. In reality, the state, via the mechanisms of welfare and law (for example, the criminalization of homosexuality in many Western countries), has always been present in the private sphere. The liberal response has been to see such entries of the state into the private realm as, at best, a necessary evil; where possible instead the state should avoid meddling with private matters, whether internal family dynamics or issues of private morality. This is insufficient for feminists, who see the boundary between the private and public as a device that justifies state refusal to respond to the problems that occur in what is framed as the private, including the social implications of the choices made there (McLaughlin 2003). Once the state is seen as playing a role in the operation of the family, then concepts of justice themselves need to address both the public and private, as Abbey (2007) asserts, in a feminist defense of a form of "comprehensive liberalism": "Once the family becomes the subject of justice, at least some of 'the virtues of private life' become part of a theory of justice" (7).

It is significant that Greenberg and Bailey focus on the right to choose to be similar to one's family members, to share the same values. The model of family and parents they wish to protect from the curtailment of rights is not a family of difference, of blurred boundaries, of chosen relationships and connections (Richardson 2005). It is a private unit made up two parents who wish to enclose their family in the bonds of similarity. The model of family being constructed is unforgiving of difference and the reality that neither families nor individuals can be predetermined. This version of family life is an illusion, created through a false belief that individuality is about determining, controlling, the relations one chooses to be part of. What kind of intimate family life develops from a dream of predeterminacy? The dark side of the celebration of parental liberty is that liberty can become surveillance as families then feel an obligation to construct their intimate relations in a way that generates the "best" genetic outcome (Murray 2002).

We know that there are different forms of family living, not all of which are based on constructions of privacy; some are instead embedded in social relationships (Jamieson 1998). In the contemporary period in Western countries, we have seen greater visibility, and at times greater legal recognition, of different patterns of family relationship and intimacy that are not always centered on heterosexual co-residence of a couple with their children (Roseneil 2006). It is increasingly difficult to draw a clear line between the private and the public once what is presumed to lie within the private—the nuclear family—is repositioned as only one version of family life, rooted not in biology but instead in a historical and structural gender inequality.

Choice Is a Private Matter of No Social Significance

What has been laid out so far is a disclosure of problematic exclusions and denials within the prioritization of individual choice. The individual is a social construct, embedded with gendered values, which can be critiqued and should not necessarily sit at the center of rights and justice. The individual can operate autonomously only if there is a private sphere positioned as separate from the public and made up of distinct nuclear families. If the boundaries of the private and public are instead the product of a particular social arrangement, then it is illegitimate to say that the state has no right to interfere with the operation of the private sphere. There is no logic to saying that choices made there are private and of no social significance, because the social is embedded in what is thought of as the private.

Choices made in the private sphere help constitute the values and norms of the public. For example, Rapp (1998, 1999) has shown how "private choices" about undergoing screening for congenital conditions and how to respond to any diagnosis are embedded in and informed by social and cultural values, which means that this not about an individual making a private choice but about a community actor making a choice that makes sense and can be defined within that broader context. The choices being made around screening cannot be examined without that social and cultural understanding. At the same time, the choices people make are informed by the societal values they share or resist, and their choices either support or challenge those societal values. This is the important argument made by disability activists who challenge liberal defenses of prenatal screening for congenital conditions (Hubbard 1997; Shakespeare 1998; Asch 2000; Jennings 2000; Press 2000). The private choices of individuals are drawn from and embedded in societal disapproval of disability, and this disapproval is reinforced through the continued articulation of those choices and state support of them (Jennings 2000; Press 2000).

Liberal writers argue that they are not interested in what the content of the good life should be; instead, they just want to ensure that the individual has the space to develop their private version of it. Nevertheless, in any liberal construction of the rights of the individual, there is an implied version of what the good life is. In Greenberg and Bailey, the good life is about shaping one's family life according to one's own choices, their assumption being that parents would make the child as similar to them as possible by choosing heterosexuality. One could argue that this, like the varied versions of family life emerging through new patterns of living, is unproblematic. However, the problem is, what version of the good life is offered by this form of family shaping, and does it come into conflict with other versions of the good life?

Cornell (1998) argues that the space within which individuals define their version of the good life is the *imaginary domain*. The development of our own sense of our sexuality—our conception of ourselves as "sexuate beings"—and how we live our intimate sexual lives is fundamentally important to our personal well-being. An unfair society is one in which individuals are not free to develop, express, and live according to their self-representation and self-definition of their sexuate being—a process vital to a complete sense of self. If the state protects the imaginary domain, this gives it the right to enter the private sphere. When the state does not protect the imaginary domain, as part of the processes through which rights are realized for the individual, some groups' definitions of the good life are privileged over others.

A fair and just society is one in which different versions of the good life are acknowledged and given the space to exist. The choices Greenberg and Bailey wish to allow parents as their private rights are in conflict with an expansive version of society that provides an equal space for lesbian and gay men to make our choices and live our lives. If choices are not fully private but instead emerge out of cultural values, and in their articulation either support or challenge such values, then the choice to avoid same-sex sexual orientation is supportive of discriminatory cultural norms. Unlike other forms of family life emerging, this kind of family shaping makes a claim to be a better, more socially legitimate, form. For this reason, the state does have a right, even within a liberal formulation, to intervene, because the scope to imagine a good life, which involves same-sex sexual orientation, is made more difficult by other versions of the good life that deny that orientation's legitimacy.

The Defense against Private Choice

Now that feminist liberal arguments have opened up space for us not to presume that the rights of the individual trump other issues and concerns, we have greater scope to identify the broader social and ethical costs of allowing choice in certain matters.

Both feminist (Strathern 1996) and disability theorists (Hubbard 1997; Jennings 2000) examining reproductive technologies used to aid conception or enable preselection link the increase in the language of choice to the emergence of these technologies. Celebrations of technological advances that offer new techniques for conceiving or diagnosing conditions in a fetus focus on how such technologies provide for existing desires to have a child or to know what problems a child may face. However, the more technologies enable such options and choices, the more prospective parents, in particular women, are supposed to wish to exercise them and the more abnormal it becomes to remain childless or deliberately unaware of the future for the fetus. Technologies are presented as providing for pre-existing desires to have a choice (to be a mother, to be a mother of a "normal" child). By opening up the possibility of particular choices, technology helps generate the value of choice. The practice constructs the choices it serves, it generates the "liberty" it seeks to enable, and in doing so, it encourages a notion that family relations are predictable and manageable.

If we take forward the argument that particular technologies and practices construct the choices they appear to help resolve, and that notions of normality are altered by the operation of those technologies and practices, we can propose some important forms of indirect harm that could result from preselection of sexual orientation. In a world of sexual hierarchies and dreams of the nuclear family wrapped in sameness, preselection of sexual orientation encourages the notion that same-sex sexual orientation is different and open to question, constructing lesbian and gay sexuality as outside the norm. In debates in which same-sex sexual orientation is treated as a separate category of human condition, the social production of "othering" is taking place. To preselect to avoid the future harm that being gay is assumed to involve helps construct the world as a place where that harm takes place. Just as having an impairment due to a congenital condition appears less "comprehensible" to those encouraged to remove this presence from society, being lesbian or gay, or worse still, being someone whose sexuality cannot be explained or defined via genetics, also becomes less comprehensible (Stein 2002).

Preselection encourages discrimination because it is influenced by and shapes notions that bonds, family or otherwise, are based on similarity and that sexual orientation is something one wishes to control and correct. As Parens and Asch (2000, 8) indicate, "discrimination results when people in one group fail to imagine that people in some 'other' group lead lives as rich and complex as their own." The preselection being defended by Greenberg and Bailey is a form of indirect harm because it represents such a failure of imagination. The harm occurs through the opportunity lost to engage properly with questions of discrimination in important policy and provision debates, within which a libertarian variety of bioethics has an insider position. Preselection to avoid same-sex sexual orientation does not need to occur in practice for the kind of indirect harm indicated here to take place.

Conclusion

Greenberg and Bailey's piece is a useful example of a particular, but prevalent, form of liberal bioethics. The danger in their approach is that the unquestioned centrality of the individual and the assertion that choice and liberty are fundamental values that lie at the heart of society lead to high demands for proof before anything can be put in the way of the exercise of those rights and choices. Drawing from feminist critiques of liberal thinking, this chapter has highlighted how Greenberg and Bailey's argument is a form of speech and ethical thinking that emerges in a particular political and institutional culture. If the individual is a product of a particular/dominant ethical style rather than a (or *the*) source of legitimacy, we obtain a space within which to question the superiority of individual rights arguments, which force the burden of proof onto those who propose a restriction of rights.

There is a wider problem that emerges from the recourse to genetics being made in contemporary debates about the causes of different human conditions.

Through the promise of the gay gene, in everyday debates sexual orientation is being framed as an essential trait; the gene does not need to be found for the assumption to be made. Therefore, harm exists when sexuality is narrowed to being a genetic trait, even without genetic technologies and knowledge available that could remove the gene. Genetic imaginaries (Rose 2000, 2006), alongside other social processes and patterns of regulation, are shaping the boundaries of acceptable sexuality; the danger is that much of this framing of sexual orientation as genetic is happening supposedly for the benefit of gay and lesbian people. The right to be free (from discrimination and difference) is being offered to those individuals who can prove they are genetically gay or lesbian. Those who argue for the benefits of genetic explanations participate in the construction of the sexual and intimate hierarchies of the twenty-first century (Brookey 2002; Jasanoff 2003).

Choices here are in tension. Liberty to be gay also apparently means that someone else should have the liberty to try to ensure they do not have a gay child. The choice to predetermine one's child's sexuality or the choice to legitimate oneself as gay through the gay gene takes away social and individual choice to express sexuality, family, and intimacy in varied ways that owe nothing to DNA. Even if we support choice as an important political value, we need to consider what individual choice does not provide and how it appears as a political value apparently able to "trump" other possible versions of rights, which might go against the primacy of individual choice. Is choice a good in itself that cancels out all others? Are there choices that as a society we wish to decide we would rather not exercise? Are there choices I would rather not have to make? As we explore those questions, it appears that there is far more to consider in the ethics of choice than simply letting people make their own.

A liberal framework is incapable of conceptualizing the processes put in motion by the exercise of choice. Without a vision able to capture the competition over choices and the full scope of what it is to be human in relations with others, the possible harm that generating (not just allowing, but generating) choices could create will stay hidden. Individuality remains a valuable political concept and tool, still needed in feminist, lesbian and gay, and disability politics, but it requires a different, more humane and connected context. There is a need for moral and ethical debates about many of the areas covered here, including genetics, sexual practice, intimacy, and family forms. Ethics needs to be explored as a social question open to capturing the contingencies in its formulations and its standpoint. The insider position that liberal articulations of bioethical issues have obtained is a significant barrier in both the United States and the United Kingdom to achieving a broader conception of the issues at stake in genetic and reproductive technologies. Without the acknowledgment that ethical concerns can be constructed and debated from different positions, this barrier will not be removed. Therefore, liberal bioethics needs to share its space more willingly and openly with alternative ethical approaches to considering bioethical problems—in particular, approaches more able and willing to place individuals in contexts and to understand the social conditioning and production of choices, values, and implications.

REFERENCES

Abbey, R. 2007. Back toward a comprehensive liberalism? Justice as fairness, gender, and families. *Political Theory* 35:5–28.

Asch, A. 2000. Why I haven't changed my mind about prenatal testing: Reflections and refinements. In *Prenatal testing and disability rights*, ed. E. Parens and A. Asch. Washington, D.C.: Georgetown University Press.

Bauman, Z. 1993. *Postmodern ethics*. Oxford: Blackwell.

———. 2001. Postmodern ethics. In *The new social theory reader*, ed. S. Seidman and J. C. Alexander. London: Routledge.

Benhabib, S. 1992. The generalized and the concrete other. In *Ethics: A feminist reader*, ed. J. Hornsby, and S. Lovibond. Oxford: Blackwell.

Braidotti, R. 2002. *Metamorphoses: Towards a materialist theory of becoming*. Cambridge: Polity.

Brookey, R. A. 2002. *Reinventing the male homosexual: The rhetoric and power of the gay gene*. Bloomington: Indiana University Press.

Brown, W. 1992. Finding the man in the state. *Feminist Studies* 18:7–13.

———. 1993. Wounded attachments. *Political Theory* 21:390–410.

Butler, J. 1990. *Gender trouble: Feminism and the subversion of identity*. London: Routledge.

Cavarero, A. 1992. Equality and sexual difference: Amnesia in political thought. In *Beyond equality and difference*, ed. G. Block and S. James. London: Routledge.

Cornell, D. 1998. *At the heart of freedom: Feminism, sex, and equality*. Princeton, N.J.: Princeton University Press.

Fox, R. 1990. The evolution of American bioethics. In *Social science perspectives on medical ethics*, ed. G. Weisz. Boston: Kluwer Academic Publishers.

Fraser, N. 2001. Recognition without ethics? *Theory Culture and Society* 18:21–42.

Gilligan, C. 1993. *In a different voice*. Cambridge, Mass.: Harvard University Press.

Greenberg, A. S., and J. M. Bailey. 2001. Parental selection of children's sexual orientation. *Archives of Sexual Behavior* 30:423–37.

Haimes, E. 2002. What can the social sciences contribute to the study of ethics? Theoretical, empirical and substantive considerations. *Bioethics* 16:89–113.

Hamer, D. H., and P. Copeland. 1994. *The science of desire*. New York: Simon & Schuster.

Haraway, D. J. 1991. *Simians, cyborgs, and women: The reinvention of nature.* New York: Routledge.

Harding, S. 1993. Rethinking standpoint epistemology: What is "strong objectivity?" In *Feminist epistemologies,* ed. L. Alcoff and E. Potter. London: Routledge.

Hubbard, R. 1997. Abortion and disability: Who should and who should not inhabit the world? In *The disability studies reader,* ed. L. J. Davis. London: Routledge.

Jamieson, L. 1998. *Intimacy: Personal relationships in modern societies.* Cambridge: Polity Press.

Jasanoff, S. 2003. Just evidence: The limits of science in the legal process. *Journal of Law, Medicine and Ethics* 34:328–41.

Jennings, B. 2000. Technology and the genetic imaginary. In *Prenatal testing and disability rights,* ed. E. Parens and A. Asch. Washington, D.C.: Georgetown University Press.

Kittay, E. F. 1995. Taking dependency seriously: The Family and Medical Leave Act considered in light of the social organization of dependency, work and gender equity. *Hypatia* 10:8–29.

LeVay, S. 1993. *The sexual brain.* Cambridge, Mass.: MIT Press.

Lister, R. 1997. *Citizenship: Feminist perspectives.* Basingstoke, U.K.: Macmillan.

McLaughlin, J. 2003. *Feminist social and political theory: Contemporary debates and dialogues.* Basingstoke, U.K.: Palgrave.

McMillan, J. 2002. Sex selection in the United Kingdom. *Hastings Center Report* 32:28–31.

Moore, M. 1999. The ethics of care and justice. *Women and Politics* 20:1–16.

Murphy, T. F. 1990. Reproductive controls and sexual destiny. *Bioethics* 4:121–42.

———. 1995. Abortion and the ethics of genetic sexual orientation research. *Cambridge Quarterly of Healthcare Ethics* 4:340–50.

Murray, T. H. 2002. What are families for? *Hastings Center Report* 32:41–45.

Mustanski, B. S., M. G. Dupree, C. M. Nievergelt, S. Bocklandt, N. J. Schork, and D. H. Hamer. 2005. A genomewide scan of male sexual orientation. *Human Genetics* 116:272–78.

Myser, C. 2003. Differences from somewhere: The normativity of whiteness in bioethics in the United States. *American Journal of Bioethics* 3:1–11.

Nussbaum, M. C. 1999. *Sex and Justice.* New York: Oxford University Press.

———. 2003. *Frontiers of justice: Disability, nationality, species membership (The Tanner lectures).* Cambridge, Mass.: Belknap Press of Harvard University Press.

Okin, S. M. 1994. Gender inequality and cultural differences. *Political Theory* 22:5–24.

Osborne, T. 1994. Power and persons: On ethical stylisation and person-centered medicine. *Sociology of Health and Illness* 16:515–35.

Parens, E., and A. Asch. 2000. Reflections and recommendations. In *Prenatal testing and disability rights,* ed. E. Parens and A. Asch. Washington, D.C.: Georgetown University Press.

Pateman, C. 1988. *The sexual contract.* Cambridge: Polity Press.

———. 1989. *The disorder of women: Democracy, feminism, and political theory.* Cambridge: Polity Press.

Paul, D. B. 2001. Where libertarian premises lead. *American Journal of Bioethics* 1:26–27.

Phillips, A. 1993. *Democracy and difference.* Cambridge: Polity Press.

Press, N. 2000. Assessing the expressive character of prenatal testing: The choices made or the choices made available? In *Prenatal testing and disability rights,* ed. E. Parens and A. Asch. Washington, D.C.: Georgetown University Press.

Rapp, R. 1998. Refusing prenatal diagnosis: The meanings of bioscience in a multicultural world. *Science, Technology and Human Values* 23:45–70.

———. 1999. *Testing women, testing the fetus: The social impact of amniocentesis in America.* London: Routledge.

Rawls, J. 1972. *A theory of justice.* Oxford: Clarendon Press.

Richardson, D. 2005. Desiring sameness? The rise of a neoliberal politics of normalisation. *Antipode* 37:515–35.

Robertson, J. A. 2001. Preconception gender selection. *American Journal of Bioethics* 1:2–9.

———. 2003. Extending preimplantation genetic diagnosis: Medical and non-medical uses. *Journal of Medical Ethics* 29:213–16.

Rorty, R. 1989. *Contingency, irony, and solidarity.* Cambridge: Cambridge University Press.

Rose, H. 2000. Risk, trust and scepticism in the age of the new genetics. In *The risk society and beyond,* ed. B. Adam, U. Beck, and J. Van Loon. London: Sage.

Rose, N. 2006. *The politics of life itself: Biomedicine, power, and subjectivity in the twenty-first century.* Princeton, N.J.: Princeton University Press.

Roseneil, S. 2006. On not living with a partner: Unpicking coupledom and cohabitation. *Sociological Research Online* 11.

Rudy, K. 1999. Liberal theory and feminist politics. *Women and Politics* 20:33–57.

Savulescu, J. 2001. Procreative beneficence: Why we should select the best children. *Bioethics* 15:413–26.

Sevenhuijsen, S. 1998. *Citizenship and the ethics of care.* London: Routledge.

Shakespeare, T. 1998. Choices and rights: Eugenics, genetics and disability equality. *Disability and Society* 13:665–81.

Stein, E. 2002. Precis of the mismeasure of desire: The science, theory and ethics of sexual orientation. *Law and Philosophy* 21:305–16.

Steinbock, B. 2002. Sex selection: Not obviously wrong. *Hastings Center Report* 32:23–28.

Strathern, M. 1996. Enabling identity? Biology, choice and the new reproductive technologies. In *Questions of cultural identity,* ed. S. Hall and P. du Gay. London: Sage.

Tong, R. 2007. Feminist thought in transition: Never a dull moment. *Social Science Journal* 44:23–39.

CHAPTER TEN

Toward a Methodology for Technocratic Transformation

Feminist Bioethics, Midwifery, and Women's Health in the Twenty-first Century

AL-YASHA ILHAAM, PH.D., AND
INA MAY GASKIN, M.A., C.P.M.

As a collaboration between a philosopher and a midwife who are both women's health activists, this chapter takes Rosemarie Tong's view that feminist bioethicists should seek not just consciousness-raising in theory but in a conclusive "*program of action* aimed at overcoming gender inequities in the realms of medicine and science," without which our discourse is "morally incomplete" (Tong 1997, 75). Our purpose here is to strengthen the bond and base of knowledge between bioethics discourse and the women's health movement, and more specifically, to analyze the perspectives of midwifery and obstetrics in light of some of the public health issues associated with childbearing, including infant mortality, premature birth, lack of insurance or prenatal care, maternal mortality and morbidity, and, as indicated by the World Health Organization and the Centers for Disease Control and Prevention, the recent rise in cesarean sections (Simkin 2003).

We begin with a discussion of collaborative methodologies in bioethics and then turn to a consideration of midwifery's critique of technological intervention in childbirth. This critique should be of great interest to bioethicists, as its challenges reflect commensurate technological changes in medicine, concerns raised by the civil rights movement, and critical theories that connect definitions of the body to power and social institutions, all proclaimed to be integral to the foundations of the discipline (Engelhard 2003). But to the contrary, we generally find, as Helen Bequaert Holmes writes, that "bioethics nestles happily inside its little cocoon. It seems almost unaware of social movements such as the women's movement, especially the women's health movement and the midwifery debate"

(Holmes 1999, 54). To address this issue, we note that feminist theorists have challenged the methodological and epistemological limitations of bioethics discourse and emphasized that women's health activism informs and is informed by feminist ideologies.

Below, we aim to show that midwifery in the United States has presented a similar feminist critique through its persistent challenge to patriarchy in medical practice and to some of the epistemological, epidemiological, and theoretical claims of obstetrics that reduce the agency of childbearing women. We offer a consideration of women's health advocacy that combines feminist bioethics and midwifery research to critique the findings of ethics boards and medical editorials on the relationship between technology and reproductive choice. We then propose a way that feminist bioethics and midwifery can work together toward defining a feminist reproductive rights agenda.

Bioethics, Collaboration, and Cognitive Authority

In the early years of the discipline, bioethics urged links between philosophers and physicians as an opportunity to provide useful reflection for medical practitioners, for finding valuable case studies for bioethics research, and for insight into the functioning of ethics boards. William Ruddick's assessment of medical ethics notes that "physician-philosopher collaboration ... has posed meta-ethical questions about the role of professional codes, religious principles, ethical theories and principles, committee consensus, clinical experience, and moral intuitions in the analysis and decision of clinical cases" (Ruddick 1998). Collaboration between philosophers and physicians had benefits for both professions and was central to the casuist strain of bioethical theory. However, feminist theorists observed that philosopher-physician collaboration as a teaching and research methodology could mutually reinforce patriarchal tendencies in philosophy and medicine by privileging the perspectives of M.D.s over nurses and female health care workers in other fields and by resting moral questions on the responsibility of the physician as opposed to (or as primary over) the concerns of the patient (Pinkus 1986; Mahowald 1999).

Gwen Anderson et al. note that collaborative work generally follows one of three major models: multidisciplinary, interdisciplinary, or transdisciplinary. In the multidisciplinary model, "each person works from within his or her own disciplinary philosophy," and final decision making often "lies with one discipline and often with only one person on the team (Anderson, Monsen, and Rorty 2000, 44). In the interdisciplinary model, three or more disciplines are represented, and a more collaborative approach is suggested, yet this model still reinforces "hierarchical relationships" in actual practice. The transdisciplinary model "considers each member of the team an equal partner" (Anderson, Monsen, and Rorty 2000, 45) and has the greatest potential to transform the tendencies of structured power relationships through a "shared philosophical perspective." On the basis of the existing literature, one can argue that most of the philosopher-clinician collaboration in bioethics takes the multidisciplinary approach with the physician as the final authority, while ethics committees often vacillate between the multidisciplinary and interdisciplinary models, with transdisciplinarity being a rarely achieved goal (Anderson, Monsen, and Rorty 2000, 46).

In these early collaborations, the philosopher's contribution often centered on identifying guiding principles of medical ethics derived from traditional ethical theory and applying them to specific practitioner-patient situations as case studies. This emphasis may have limited alternative approaches to medical (and ethical) decision making. Renee Fox's early survey (1976) provides a consideration of ethical issues in advanced medical technology from the view of social science and public health, two fields she found marginalized from the bioethics discourse. She describes how and to what effect bioethics is divided between practitioners, theorists, and policy analysts and the subsequent methodological issues that arise in bioethics research from professional situatedness and the complexities of interprofessional collaboration. Her categorization of bioethicists into philosopher-theologians, physician-biologists, and lawyers demonstrates the divisions of intellectual labor and forms of collaboration and inclusion in the field (Fox 1976, 240). Fox notes that normative ethics was a field in crisis in the 1950s and that philosophers who recognized the lack of explicated moral grounds for medical decision making in the era of scientific reason also identified a more general crisis in ethical theory, commensurate with important and increasing technological changes in medical practice (Fox 1976). She cautions that theoretical methods derived from existing practices and politics could reinforce disturbing trends in health care technology, including aspects of access and research agendas (Fox 1976).

The role of philosophers in medical ethics has usually been perceived as limited and subordinate to the authority of physicians. As part of a collection of five respondent articles from the *Hastings Center Report*, Cheryl Noble writes that philosophers seeking to claim technical expertise on social problems risk becoming defenders of a conventional morality already supported by structures of social and epistemic power (Noble 1982). This caution is considered by Tom Beauchamp in the collection in light of the feminist and multicultural critiques of the principlist approach (Beauchamp 1982). Beauchamp's account of writing *The Belmont Report* and the first edition of *Principles of Biomedical Ethics* reveals that he faced consistent conflict between an approach that was "as philosophical as possible" and a combatant view from doctors and lawyers looking for "a minimalist statement relatively free of the style of academic philosophy" (Beauchamp 2003, 21). Reflecting the desires of a collaborative process, *The Belmont Report* took the road less jargon encumbered, and the *Principles* text then went on to provide the theoretical groundwork for the fledgling field of bioethics (Beauchamp 2003).

Feminist theorists such as Holmes have noted with concern that biomedical ethics risks becoming a consultation field for doctors who regulate the entry of other researchers. The forging of relationships between philosophers and clinical practitioners has created legitimacy around analytical processes in keeping with the existing paradigms of knowledge: the "cognitive authority" of medicine, as Holmes (1999) describes. This cognitive authority renders the truth claims of medicine as valid, while its concurrent social authority demonstrates the pervasiveness of the medical model in social institutions. The collaborative bridge between philosophers and medical practitioners provides the humanities with access to scientific knowledge and its epistemological credibility. "Who can be called a 'bioethicist?' Any M.D. who wants to be. But attorneys, clergy, persons with master's degrees in bioethics, and philosophy doctorates—they must have connections" (Holmes 1999, 47). Further, while bioethics has been critical of the power relations in medicine and has sustained some gender analysis, similar structures within academe complicate the ability for women in bioethics to obtain a critical distance. Holmes notes that within the field of bioethics, as in medicine, "a kind of subtle brutality conditions female practicing bioethicists to revere authority figures in medicine and to dampen critical views of the assumptions underlying mainstream bioethics discourse and standard medical practice" (Holmes 1999, 49).

Theories about the doctor-patient relationship illustrate some of these methodological concerns. As a physician whose early writings on the inadequacies of the Hippocratic Oath threw down the gauntlet to philosophers to reconsider longstanding attachments to normative ethics, Edmund Pellegrino argues that philosophers look for "principled arguments for the resolution of professional and clinical ethical dilemmas" and can provide insight into theoretical tendencies within the physician's moral reasoning (Pellegrino 2003, 5). Pellegrino's emphasis on the "clinical encounter" in bioethics claims the doctor-patient relationship as the locus of ethical decision making: "My thesis was, and remains, that the obligations specific to physicians arise from the special features of the personal relationship between the person who is ill and the person the ill person seeks for help. The resulting relationship has certain features that give it a special character that generates special mutual moral duties" (Pellegrino 2003, 5).

Pellegrino's (2003) doctor-patient relationship model emphasizes particular asymmetrical structures of power and ability, reflecting differentials of control related to the impairment of the patient: "I argued that illness wounded our humanity, challenged our self-image, limited our freedom in special ways, and made us vulnerable ontologically and existentially" (7). With this characterization, the clinical encounter also structures the conditions of agency, where the "vulnerable, dependent and anxious human beings" who are patients look for the moral characteristics of "fidelity, trust, benevolence, truth-telling, intellectual honesty, humility, courage, suppression of self-interest at a minimum" in their physicians.

The emphasis on the physician's inherent morality and structural power in the doctor-patient relationship model has been critiqued through the interdisciplinarity of bioethics discourse and the intervention of feminist thought. Ruddick (1998) notes that "although still supported by religious texts and medical tradition, this ideal physician is increasingly criticized as 'paternalistic,' too willing to act on judgments of a patient's best interests without the patient's knowledge or consent." The doctor-patient relationship as the central dynamic of moral decision making has also been called into question by several changing conditions in medicine resulting from the shift from ameliorative care to technological medicine; from private practice to HMO/insurance managed care; and from the primacy of the physician-patient dyad to a larger range of influential people and factors, including family, friends, and cultural contexts and to emphases on language and dialogue rather than the doctor's emotions and empathy (Koop 1990). Susan Foley Pierce (1997) argued that managed care calls for including nurse's perspectives in collaborative models with the aim of creating a new model for moral dynamics that decentralizes the doctor-patient relationship and physicians' authority. The feminist perspective particularly recognizes the shift in power from physicians to corporations as an economic transaction with related power dynamics; Holmes writes, "Our society reveres doctors; we consider their advice more enlightened than anyone else's. But now managed care administrators 'manage' doctors: physicians must toe the line, the bottom line" (Holmes 1999, 46).

In the past few decades, bioethicists and their approaches have become an essential component of medical review boards, research institutions, and professional ethics associations. But their near absence from health advocacy programs, managed care policy reform, and/or legal challenges to the increasing health disparities between privileged and marginalized ethnic and economic sectors suggests that the field has sided strongly with existing institutions of power and knowledge and has not created or supported counterstructures or critiques of the prevailing system. Holmes notes again that "bioethics has become an essential part of western medicine even though it doesn't improve health" (Holmes 1999, 46). Suggesting that this might be related to reinforcing dominant ideologies through the collaborative model, Dan Brock (2000) proclaimed the need for bioethics to forge links with public health in the way that it has with clinicians. It is likely, however, that the same issues that have resulted in the marginalization of health professionals who are not M.D.s will continue to thwart the efforts to include public health perspectives in the bioethics literature, especially if the views and research of nurses, midwives, childbirth educators, and women's health activists aren't routinely incorporated.

Midwifery, Obstetrics, and the Shaky Middle Ground

The discussion of collaborative models and professional perspectives brings us to the contrasting ideas of childbirth that frame the midwifery/obstetrics debate. The issues include whether the shift from midwifery to obstetric care has produced better birth outcomes and whether midwifery can maintain its professional stance in an increasingly technology-driven medical field. The epistemic issue is the question of whether birth generally requires a high level of medical intervention to secure the health and safety of the mother and child.

The concept of birth as necessitating technology is debated by research in midwifery and through analyses of holistic or natural versus technological birth and has been argued against by both of us in prior works (Gaskin 2003; Ilhaam 2005). Robbie Davis-Floyd (1992) points to the technocratic model of birth as the dominant episteme in obstetric care. The technocratic model emphasizes technology as lifesaving, both vesting technology with a moral quality, the ability to save lives, and affirming the need for interventions with the perspective that birth is always a possibly perilous act requiring medical management. In contrast, the holistic model counters the technocratic with the view of birth as a life occurrence, which ought not to be threatening, and with the perspective that technology may hinder rather than help the experience. Davis-Floyd (1992) details the extent to which the "technocratic" model of birth contrasts with the "holistic" model of birth and now predominates in hospitals worldwide. Davis-

Floyd also remarks that the middle ground, described as the "natural" birth movement, is a tenuous compromise in which intentions toward the holistic model are often thwarted by the dominance of the technocratic model. She argues that the dominant form of obstetrical practice is fetus-centered rather than woman-centered. This focus on the fetus encourages the use of invasive technology to gather fetal information. This technology, in turn, further erodes the autonomy of pregnant and birthing women by making them appear more and more superfluous to the birthing process.

In *Women, Power, and Childbirth* (1995), Kathleen Doherty Turkel provides a survey of the feminist analyses of modern childbirth technologies in light of the efforts to create and sustain a freestanding birth center staffed by midwives. Turkel compares the ideologies of midwifery and obstetrics around the issues identified as "technology, patriarchy and capitalism" (cf. Rothman 1989). She also notes that the issue of whether birth is medical or not determines its position vis-à-vis the discourses of science, nature, and the professional authority of medicine.

> First and foremost, pregnant women are seen as "patients." Pregnancy is viewed as a "condition" requiring treatment from physicians, technicians, and nurses who make use of a variety of procedures, tests, and high-tech diagnostic tools to assess the health of the pregnant woman and of the developing fetus and the overall progress of the pregnancy. Birth itself takes place in a hospital setting under the direction of a physician and the assistance of nurses and technicians who rely upon an array of technologies to assess the progress of the event. (cf. Rothman 1989; Davis-Floyd 1992)

Turkel describes the technocratic model in general as "1) a belief that technological development is neutral with regard to social interests and synonymous with progress, 2) a belief that technical information and expertise should provide the grounds for decision making, and 3) a belief that efficiency, productivity, rationality and control should serve as the standards by which we judge not only machines and organizations, but human beings as well" (Turkel 1995). She also notes that sexism leads childbirth dynamics to replicate existing imbalances of power women experience in the society at large. "In the case of medical practice, when women are the patients, the physician-patient relationship embodies the basic dualism between masculine and feminine. There is no shortage of evidence that women experience treatment by the medical profession which cannot be explained by the basic split between layperson and expert which characterizes medical practice in this society" (Turkel 1995, 24). Turkel notes with concern that young women are increasingly inclined toward the technocratic model of child-birth and are largely unaware of the critiques offered by midwifery and the women's health movement:

> I discuss childbirth frequently in the university courses which I teach. While some of the students are critical of dominant birth practices, most belong to the "what if something goes wrong" school of thought. They might agree with some of the criticisms of hospital practices and procedures and they might like the idea of birth outside the hospital, but they believe that birth needs to take place in a hospital, "in case something goes wrong." Hospitals have all the high-technology equipment that an emergency might require. It is the technology that is important. (Turkel 1995, 8)

This confirms Davis-Floyd's view about the internalization of the technocratic model (Davis-Floyd 1992), of concern in part because of its subordination of women's power to the power of machines, which Rothman also considers. "Rothman, specifically, talks about the ideology of technology as a way of thinking about the world in mechanical-industrial terms" (Turkel 1995, 17). These ideological terms include the values of productivity, time management, cost-benefit analysis, and control. As Rothman describes, "In technological society we apply ideas about machines to people, asking them, too, to become more efficient, productive, rational, and controlled" (Rothman 1989, 53).

Given that the technocratic model predominates in most hospitals, perhaps one problem is that one has to look at out-of-hospital practice outcomes to have any idea about what women are capable of and to see how seldom complications occur in healthy pregnant women who receive good maternity care. Birth statistics from the Farm Midwifery Center in Summertown, Tennessee (the basis of Gaskin's midwifery practice and research), represent more than 2,000 births and document that 95.1 percent of the births were completed at home (Gaskin 2003). The statistics at the Farm represent not just different birthing techniques but different ideologies about women's power and the ability of the body to respond to the experience of labor when guided by support, encouragement, and the prediction of positive outcomes as opposed to fear, alienation, and the prediction of negative outcomes. At the Farm, many of the clients have been grand multips (had five babies or more over their lifetimes) or had breech births or twins, but still the cesarean rate has remained below 2 percent, with good neonatal outcomes and with little need for medical intervention or medication.

Paula Treichler's (1990) analysis of feminism and the meaning of childbirth highlights the development of a contemporary midwifery movement and notes that its main successes are in the liminal space provided by insurers for (cheaper) nonmedicalized forms of care. Ideologically, midwifery directly challenges the cognitive and social authority of medicine, yet in actual practice, complex negotiations result from the attempts to fuse the two forms of labor and delivery support. Treichler notes that the ideological differences that distinguish obstetrics and midwifery have their roots in structures of power that benefit from the primacy of the medical paradigm: "The problem of traditional childbirth for women is rooted not in 'medicalization' per se but in monopoly: monopoly of professional authority, of material resources and of what may be called linguistic capital—the power to establish and enforce a particular definition of childbirth" (Treichler 1990, 3).

Both Treichler and Turkel note that birth centers represent a tenuous compromise in the midwifery/obstetrics debate and are extremely vulnerable in this regard. Turkel writes that "the birth center exists within a structural context which supports the medical model. On the one hand, they challenge the assumptions and practices of the medical model. On the other hand they require the recognition and support of the legal and financial institutions which support the medical model" (Turkel 1995, 150). While Wolf claims the freestanding birth center as the possible best of both worlds, the balance of power that favors the technocratic model can affect the operation of such institutions. Birth centers are often the first targets of insurance adjustments, and some have only been able to survive by being incorporated into hospitals. Institutional protocol designed to reduce liability and reinforce the technocratic paradigm often becomes the order of the day. As Davis-Floyd (1992) notes, even when women wish to have intervention-free births, they are often convinced or even required by hospital protocols to have enemas, shaving, episiotomies, IVs, monitoring, and medications they might not want or even need. The Farm Midwifery Center serves an example of how working outside the dominant model may produce better birth outcomes and prove more empowering than finding a niche within it.

Feminist Bioethics and the Public Health Sector: Technology as Reproductive Choice

Feminist bioethicists have taken notice of the women's health advocates who have been critical of the increasing role of surgery and medications in women's health, especially in the management of pregnancy, childbirth, and menopause. Women's health activists have recently protested the national rise in cesarean sections, have raised concerns about increased and underreported maternal deaths resulting from cesarean surgery, and have critiqued the influential public opinions on elective cesareans issued by ethics committees and leading members of the American College of Obstetrics and Gynecology (ACOG). The case for and against elective cesarean section has gained some attention in obstetric journals and popular debates about health care options. From the standpoint of feminist bioethics, to what extent can requests for elective cesarean surgery be thought to represent the patient's rights, and in what way can these be called feminist rights?

The use of reproductive rights language in reference to elective cesareans raises some initial questions. The March/April 2000 issue of *ACOG Clinical Review* included an editorial by W. Benson Harer Jr., then ACOG's president, entitled "Patient Choice Cesarean." Harer (2000) cites comparable outcomes in cesarean and vaginal deliveries, and noting that the change is coming from women, the reproductive rights language used seems appropriate: "Traditional paternalistic medicine held that therapeutic choice is dictated by the 'doctor knows best' theory, and therefore paternalistic choice prevailed. The time is coming—if not already here—for 'maternal-choice cesarean.'"

While doctors and patients use terms like "paternalism" and "choice," which invoke reproductive rights and suggest that elective cesarean might qualify as one, many women's health advocates regard cesarean section as a necessary and lifesaving procedure in some instances and view unnecessary cesareans as a violation of women's bodily integrity and a further medical complication of the birthing process (Rothman 1991; Davis-Floyd 1992; Goer 2001). Yet many women's health professionals in obstetric medicine and midwifery can attest to patients who have requested—even demanded—cesarean birth, with problematic results in medical and ethical terms. One such woman, whose baby was recently born in Franklin, Tennessee, demanded that her baby (her first) be born by cesarean. Her obstetrician, reluctant at first, went ahead and scheduled the surgery. As the doctor made the incision, she cut into the placenta, which was lying directly under the lower segment of the uterus (it usually lies higher in the uterus). The hemorrhage that followed nearly killed the mother and did permanently injure the baby.

Such stories happen more often than women know. They are never mentioned on television programs about birth, which only show good outcomes. These same programs show close details of cesarean surgery but must obscure the view of the vagina during a vaginal birth (Gaskin 2003). And while Naomi Wolf (2001), Robbie Davis-Floyd (1992), and Barbara Katz Rothman (1999) have all written clearly about the capacities and representations of women's bodies and their effect on surgery, birth, and the creation of the technologically dependent body, images and practices persist in making the technologically mediated birth the standard of medical care.

An analogy might be drawn between the high rate and public views of cesarean section as a birth option and surgical sterilization as a contraceptive method. Jurema Werneck et al. (2001) write on the surgical sterilization of black women in Brazil, where the cesarean rate and maternal death rate are also high. In Brazil, tubal ligation is now the primary method of contraception available to women ages 15–49 (Werneck et al. 2001, 116). Werneck argues that while sterilization can be seen as "a pure expression of a woman's power" based on a notion of "liberal feminism" from Euro–North American feminists, she believes that in Brazil this statistic instead represents the limited range of effective options for women where "delivering babies is not an easy process. On the contrary, we face neglect, disrespect and danger, with high rates of maternal mortality." She claims that surgical sterilization represents the extreme of technological rationality as "a choice for those without choices" (Werneck 2001, 117).

Werneck's analysis also considers the role of economic factors for childbearing women, particularly in developing nations or in minority populations in developed countries. Wendy Savage (2002) draws our attention to the socioeconomic factors in elective cesarean section:

> The rising CSR [cesarean section rate] is not just about medical or woman power, advances in medical technology or changing societal expectation, it is about the organization of services and money. The highest rates are found in countries in which the medical system is dominated by private practice, as for example in the US and Australia. In South America the even higher rates are said to be due to social factors, while Chile, with a rate of 37 per cent nationally, is thought to have the highest rate in the world. The recent steep rise followed a change in the organization of payment for health care.

The Ethics Committee of ACOG submitted an opinion on the elective cesarean ("Surgery and Patient Choice: The Ethics of Decision Making"). ACOG considers the "right of patients to have a surgical procedure when the scientific evidence supporting it is incomplete" (American College of Obstetrics and Gynecology 2003). The major proposition of "Surgery and Patient Choice" is that increasing numbers of childbearing women are requesting cesarean sections as a birthing option, yet the lack of empirical knowledge on which to make a decision about risks and benefits creates ambiguity for doctors and patients alike. The opinion affirms the patient's right to choose a cesarean birth when corroborated by her physician's assessment of the medical benefits of the procedure over those of a vaginal birth. Speaking to a critique of the process and decision that alleged a mere corroboration of prevailing medical directives, committee member Michael Zinberg (2004) says, "The group reached its conclusions after more than a year of difficult deliberations that applied the highest of ethical principles: in the absence of data on the long-term risks and benefits of elective cesarean versus vaginal delivery in healthy women, no single, correct response exists for a physician confronting such a patient request."

For some women, the fear of childbirth is itself substantial enough to consider the experience of labor and delivery more frightening than the prospect of surgery. A Scandinavian obstetrics journal reports that "severe fear of childbirth complicates between 6 and 10 percent of parturients. Often, fear of childbirth leads to request for an elective cesarean section (CS). In Finland, Sweden and the United Kingdom, fear of childbirth or maternal request is the reason for about 7% to 22% of CS births" (Saisto 2003). The response of women's health activists to this concern might acknowledge psychological and social factors but might also underestimate or minimize their influence toward a valid patient choice. Goer's (2001) assertion that fear is just "not a good enough reason for major abdominal surgery" seems to dismiss the psychological condition of fear on feminist grounds, without any further consideration of the possibility that fear might actually be a relevant reason to consider a cesarean section, even while cesarean section may not be the only or even best solution. It seems clear from labor-support professionals that psychological factors play a role in the physical abilities of women in childbirth and that fear in first stage labor can produce "increased heart rate and blood pressure, blood sugar and decreased contractions" in the laboring woman and the fetal production of catecholamines, which may reduce the fetal heart rate and inhibit the progression of labor (Simkin 2003). In this case, the biological condition that might warrant a cesarean section is precipitated by psychological conditions but is managed as a set of physical symptoms. This biological response, however descriptive and causal, does not completely describe the conditions of labor that produce the social context for the emotions and tension, as "fear of childbirth is not an isolated problem but associated with the woman's personal characteristics, mainly general anxiety, low self-esteem and depression, and dissatisfaction with their partnership, and lack of support" (Saisto 2003).

Wolf (2001) notes that elective cesarean "would seem to be a version of the feminist 'your body, your right'—except that women are not often given the whole picture of what is at stake." When construed in terms of rights, a "right" to a cesarean section on grounds of autonomy might consider Werneck's analysis as part of a broader feminist critique of autonomy that raises concerns about a potentially dangerous reinforcement of Western individualism that avoids the interdependent or dialogical notions of self (vis-à-vis others) for the (Western/masculine fantasy of) self without attachment or dependence (Tong 1997). Tong notes that feminist approaches to bioethics are characterized by looking at choice in terms of social networks and membership in groups that confer support. This correlates to the issue of labor support, which is proven to reduce the cesarean section rate. Physicians who argue for patient autonomy also argue that national and individual practitioner statistics are irrelevant when determining the appropriateness of cesarean section in any given case and (despite public health opinions) may not even see rising cesarean section rates as a problem. "No one knows what the best cesarean rate should be—or even what is a good range. Obstetricians are obligated to recommend cesarean delivery in any given case based on the best available evidence of the balance of risk and benefits for mother and child. If the mother agrees, a cesarean is performed. The statistics shouldn't matter" (Harer 2000).

Yet, for midwives, women's health activists and in the public health sphere, these statistics can matter. For one thing, if women become so frightened of childbirth that 80–90 percent choose cesarean, the skills that obstetricians are supposed to have mastered will atrophy, and these doctors will be helpless to perform the hand maneuvers that are sometimes necessary when women give birth too rapidly for surgery to be a safe option. There have been instances of babies being lost because of physician ignorance of the normal process of vaginal breech birth. The limited range of options in childbirth stems in part from medical practitioners, who, according to Holmes, "tend to vacillate between two poles: an unthinking voluntarism that offers patients (such as pregnant women) an undiscriminating 'choice' among the assorted techniques in their armamentaria, with little attention to individualizing risks and benefits to the particular patient under treatment, or a rigid paternalism that silences those experiencing the symptoms and imposes on them a statistical norm that may have no bearing on their particular situation" (Holmes 1999, 11).

Conclusion

We are concerned with the documented rise in maternal mortality from elective cesarean sections as well as emergency cesarean sections. We assert that the ambiguity about the safety of cesarean section that seems to confound the ACOG's Ethics Committee comes from the dominant model of childbirth, which reveres technological intervention in contrast with the feminist health model and epidemiological facts, as well as from consistent underreporting of surgical complications (Gaskin 2003). Further, if women today are socially adjusted to the technocratic model of childbirth, this is not proof of its efficacy but rather attests to the effectiveness of an ideology that has support from the existing conditions of sexism and disempowerment. Patriarchal cultures can reinscribe notions of inadequacy and inferior status on the bodies and minds of women. Women from cultures where their power is denied will sometimes agree that the unequal status they endure is justified and even to their benefit (Hellsten 2002). In societies where female genital surgery is performed on girls, women may defend the practice on the grounds that their marital fidelity is increased as their sexual pleasure is reduced (Althus 1997). Similarly, we live in a culture in the United States where for most women the need for technological medical assistance during childbirth is considered the rule rather than the exception. It is commonly believed that women cannot give birth without technology, and most women would be afraid to consider childbirth without the aid of an obstetrician. For first-time mothers, terms such as "unproven pelvis" or "failure to progress" proclaim that a woman must have demonstrated her prior ability to have a baby rather than assuming this ability as a natural matter of course (Wolf 2001). If elective cesarean is a choice motivated by fear and commerce rather than empowerment, it is hard to argue that cesarean section increases a woman's power or self-possession in the birthing process. As Goer (2001) notes: "The contention that there is a groundswell of consumer demand for elective cesarean that should be honored is not sustained, although ongoing efforts to convince women that cesarean section is preferable may yet succeed in making the imaginary groundswell a reality."

Our plan of action, therefore, is to make this analysis a contribution toward a praxis for educating women about childbirth and for developing transdisciplinary, nonhierarchical, collaborative models in the production of knowledge about ethics and childbearing. Midwifery in the United States has presented a persistent challenge to patriarchal medical knowledge through the assertion of epistemological, epidemiological, and theoretical claims that counter those of obstetrics. Feminist bioethics and midwifery research can work together to critique the findings of ethics boards and medical editorials on the relationship between technology and reproductive choice and to raise connected questions about science, nature, race, gender, class, and power in the current approach to feminist reproductive rights.

REFERENCES

Althus, F. 1997. Female circumcision: Rite of passage or violation of rights? *International Family Planning Perspectives* 23 (3): 130–33.

American College of Obstetrics and Gynecology. 2003. News release: Surgery and patient choice: The ethics of decision making. October 31.

Anderson, G. W., R. B. Monsen, and M. V. Rorty. 2000. Feminism and genetic nursing: Globalizing transdisciplinary teams. In *Globalizing feminist bioethics*, ed. R. Tong, G. Anderson, and A. Santos-Maranan. Boulder, Colo.: Westview.

Beauchamp, T. L. 1982. What philosophers can offer. *Hastings Center Report* 12:13–14.

———. 2003. The origins, goals and core commitments of *The Belmont Report* and *Principles of Biomedical Ethics*. In *The story of bioethics: From seminal works to contemporary explorations*, ed. J. Walter and E. Klein. Washington, D.C.: Georgetown University Press.

Brock, D. 2000. Broadening the bioethics agenda. *Kennedy Institute of Ethics Journal* 10 (1): 21–38.

Davis-Floyd, R. 1992. *Birth as an American rite of passage*. Berkeley: University of California Press.

Engelhardt, H. T. 2003. The foundations of bioethics: Rethinking the meaning of morality. In *The story of bioethics: From seminal works to contemporary explorations*, ed. J. Walter and E. Klein. Washington D.C.: Georgetown University Press.

Fox, R. 1976. Advanced medical technology: Social and ethical implications. *Annual Review of Sociology* 2:231–68.

Gaskin, I. M. 2003. *Ina May's guide to childbirth*. New York: Bantam Bell.

Goer, H. 1999. *The thinking woman's guide to a better birth*. New York: Perigee Books.

———. 2001. The case against elective cesarean section. *Journal of Perinatal and Neonatal Nursing* 15 (3): 23–6.

Harer, W. B. 2000. Editorial: Patient choice cesarean. *ACOG Clinical Review* March/April.

Hellsten, S. K. 2002. Multicultural issues in maternal-fetal medicine. In *Ethical Issues in Maternal-Fetal Medicine*, ed. D. Dickerson. Cambridge: Cambridge University Press.

Holmes, H. B. 1999. Closing the gaps: An imperative for feminist bioethics. In *Embodying bioethics: Recent feminist advances*, ed. A. Donchin and L. Purdy. Lanham, Md.: Rowman & Littlefield.

Ilhaam, Al-Yasha. 2005. Women deserve holistic birth options. *ICTC Newsletter* (Spring): 10–12.

Koop, C. E. 1990. Health care in the US: The social issues. *Second Opinion* 13 (3): 12–20.

Mahowald, M. B. 1999. Collaboration and casuistry. In *Pragmatic bioethics*, ed. G. McGee. Nashville: Vanderbilt University Press.

Noble, C. 1982. Ethics and experts. *Hastings Center Report* 12 (3): 7–9.

Pellegrino, E. 2003. From medical ethics to a moral philosophy. In *The story of bioeth-*

ics: From seminal works to contemporary explorations, ed. J. Walter and E. Klein. Washington, D.C.: Georgetown University Press.

Pierce, S. F. 1997. A model for conceptualizing the moral dynamic in health care. *Nursing Ethics* 4 (6): 483–95.

Pinkus, R. L. 1986. Superman meets Don Quixote: Stereotypes in clinical medicine. *Journal of Medical Humanities and Bioethics* 7:17–32.

Rothman, B. K. 1999. *Recreating motherhood.* New York: W. W. Norton.

Ruddick, W. 1998. Medical ethics. In *Encyclopedia of ethics,* 2nd ed., ed. L. Becker and C. Becker. New York: Garland/Routledge.

Saisto, T. 2001. *Obstetric, psychosocial and pain-related background and treatment of fear of childbirth.* PhD diss., Department of Obstetrics and Gynecology, University of Finland, Helsinki.

Savage, W. 2002. Cesarean section: Who chooses—the woman or her doctor? In *Ethical issues in maternal-fetal medicine,* ed. D. Dickerson. Cambridge: Cambridge University Press.

Simkin, P. 2003. Cesareans on the rise again. Conference presentation at Childbirth and Postpartum Professionals Association meeting, May 3.

Tong, R. 1997. *Feminist approaches to bioethics.* Boulder, Colo.: Westview.

Treichler, P. 1990. Feminism, medicine, and the meaning of childbirth. In *Body/politics: Women and the discourses of science,* ed. M. Jacobus, E. F. Keller, and S. Shuttleworth. New York: Routledge.

Turkel, K. D. 1995. *Women, power and childbirth: A case study of a free-standing birth center.* Westport, Conn.: Greenwood.

Werneck, J., F. Carneiro, and A. A. Rotania, with H. B. Holmes and M. R. Rorty. 2001. Autonomy and procreation: Brazilian feminist analyses. In *Globalizing feminist bioethics,* ed. R. Tong, G. Anderson, and A. Santos-Maranan, 114–34. Boulder, Colo.: Westview.

Wolf, N. 2001. *Misconceptions: Truth, lies, and the unexpected on the journey to motherhood.* New York: Random House.

Zinberg, S. 2004. Letter to the Editor. *Washington Post,* February 14.

PART FOUR

Understanding Difference

*Making and Breaking Connections
within and between the Margins*

LAUREL BALDWIN-RAGAVEN, M.D.C.M., AND
JACKIE LEACH SCULLY, PH.D.

The authors in this section grapple with issues that have not traditionally been central to the agendas of either mainstream or feminist bioethicists. The next four chapters invoke some of the most ethically troubling and morally unresolved dynamics of the twenty-first century: those involving rich and poor; "white" and "black"; the global North and South; the colonizer and the First Nation; those producing nation-building policy and those subject to these plans; the "normal" and the "disabled." Whether we choose to admit it or not, these are issues of great importance from a critical perspective; they deeply inform existing power relationships and are key to the health and well-being of majority populations the world over and to those living in marginal spaces everywhere.

In this brief commentary, we situate the chapters in this section within some of the most important arguments raised by scholars and activists about difference and suggest ways forward toward meaningful engagement for feminist bioethicists. Inherent in this critique is the frequently problematic role that academics—in their roles as professionals as well as global citizens—play in constructing knowledge, especially if that entails accepting as immutable the unequal burdens of health and illness and contributing (both wittingly and otherwise) to the "structural violence" that many see as the root cause of the suffering pervading the daily lives of the world's most vulnerable people—exacerbating their "difference" (Farmer 2003; Ho 2007). The relative absence of scholarly work in these areas is related to the way in which the purview of bioethics has been largely to explore the impact of biomedical technology on *individual* patients. Feminist bioethics has challenged the narrowness of this view, arguing for an enlargement of the scope of the bioethics project. Yet this move may still retain a focus on "crises" within medicine to the neglect of "housekeeping" issues, effectively shutting out legitimate areas of bioethics concern, including the relationship between poverty and health, and inequities grounded in race, class, geographic location (Holmes 2001), and disability. Staking out what "counts" as bioethical inquiry has had the twin effects of (de)limiting parameters and sanctioning relevance.

In addition to content, there are methodological and theoretical limitations to how bioethics has approached problems of difference and marginalization. Mainstream bioethics for the most part retains an individualistic over a collective perspective. Yet the canonical approach to identifying and analyzing bioethical problems, through the lens of personal autonomy, has limited applicability in a global context. To address *racial and ethnic differences* in bioethics, one needs to see these issues as dominated by power relationships of a structural kind that mainstream bioethics is less used to examining than the individualized, relatively flat power differential within doctor–(paying) patient relations. An important exception is the recent interest in public health or population-based bioethics (Mann 1997; Brock 2000; Rogers and Brock 2004; Daniels 2006). Yet even here, bioethics' engagement with issues of global health inequalities, neoliberal economic policies, and health care marketization is colored by strong trends toward ideals of behavioralism and personal responsibility. All of this is in keeping with Catherine Myser's (2003) critique of the domination of North American bioethics by "whiteness," which, she says, if left unexamined, "risk(s) reproducing white privilege and white supremacy in its theory, method and practice." Myser traces the cultural construction of bioethics in the United States in parallel with those norms and values of "WASP whiteness," arguing that the discipline is unlikely to decenter itself enough to engage in the real work of dismantling the "dominance and normativity of whiteness."

The categories of gender, race, global location, ethnicity, class, religion, sexual preference, and age are becoming increasingly familiar lenses through which to analyze relations of hierarchy and power; the consideration of physical, cognitive, and affective variations from the norm that we call *disability*, however, continues to be neglected by mainstream bioethics. But it is important to recognize that the process through which disabled people have been marginalized in bioethics is radically different from that of other social/ontological categories mentioned above. The viewpoints of women and other "minorities" have mostly been excluded because mainstream bioethics has not seen the particularities arising from their social positioning as analytically relevant. In contrast, bioethics has always found the difference represented by physical or mental variation to be *highly* relevant (see discussion in Vehmas 2003; Scully 2008). The biomedical model depicts disability as a morphological or physiological deviation from the established norm. It is precisely these measured deviations from the statistical norm, and their eventual normalization, that are biomedicine's business. Moreover, developments in medicine over the last three or four decades have greatly extended the repertoire of ways in which disability can be medically "managed" and such deviations normalized. Among the most ethically contentious of medical interventions to "correct" or altogether avert disability are the sophisticated techniques developed for prenatal screening and genetic diagnosis, preimplantation genetic diagnosis, and fetal therapy. There are other less high profile but ethically troubling areas, for example, the surgical normalization of conjoined twins or intersex individuals (Dreger 2004; Parens 2006). Most often, these medical interventions are presented in bioethical discussion as means to increase parental choice and to reduce potential suffering. But their responsible use also demands some form of public consensus on the moral meaning (or lack of it) of various impairments, which by and large does not yet exist. Further, it requires that the meaning of concepts such as "moral good," "choice," and "suffering" in this context be subject to critical scrutiny.

Positioning and Voice

Some scholars argue that the specific concrete and complex realities of social margins are beyond their ability to disentangle due to the great (physical as well as cultural) gulf between themselves and those experiencing these problems. Given the limitations of our sources of knowledge beyond our own experience, it is plausible that we really don't know much about the lives of others, whether they live on the other side of the world or across the proverbial railroad tracks.

Can the relative lack of firsthand knowledge ever be surmounted sufficiently to portray an unfamiliar experience with accuracy or even comment on it in intellectually authentic and nonpatronizing ways? As one feminist philosopher suggests, to speak on behalf of people living at the margins "may not only mute the voices of other[s] but even suggest that they are incapable of speaking for themselves. Regardless of the speaker's motivations, the structure and context of their discursive interventions may have the consequence of positioning the subjects of their discourse as less than equal" (Jaggar 1998, 11). From this perspective, no matter how good the intentions, it may be impossible to overcome the power differential between those who are speaking and those who are being represented.

More than women and some other marginalized groups, people with long-term disability are underrepresented within the mainstream of the discipline (Scully 2008). Bioethicists are not exempt from the normal accrual of impairments as they age, but this alone does not give them special insight into disability, and certainly not into the experiences and perspectives of those whose sense of self has developed over the long term in the context of an impairment. Feminist bioethicists are acutely aware of the extent to which bioethical issues that feature prominently in many women's lives—primarily those concerning reproduction and its control—continue to be discussed in their absence. Equally, bioethical issues that concern people with disabilities, especially those involving third-party evaluations of quality of life, such as prenatal screening and some end-of-life decisions, have been extensively debated in bioethics with virtually no input from people with firsthand knowledge of them.

In part as a result of this exclusion, much of the early writing on bioethical issues to emerge from within the disability community was vociferously critical of biomedical interventions aimed at preventing impairment (see Rock 1996; Asch 1999), often claiming that these techniques devalue the lives of people with disabilities and legitimate their eradication on eugenic grounds (Bailey 1996). Mainstream bioethics in its turn has countered that this claim confuses *disability* (or impairment) with *people with disabilities*, that is, that attempting to eradicate impairments that drastically reduce an individual's quality of life does not imply any judgment on the value of that individual's life. Going further, some bioethicists have argued for a general moral obligation to have the "best children possible" (Harris 2007; Savulescu 2007). In general, the disability countercritique has focused on bioethics' neglect of the social nature of disability and has problematized the use mainstream bioethics makes of such concepts such as "quality of life" and "best child" (Parens and Asch 2002; Wasserman, Bickenbach, and Wachbroit, 2005).

The Philosophy and Politics of Difference

Notwithstanding the tendencies to trivialize or essentialize variation or to sidestep it altogether, there have been important attempts within medicine, philosophy, ethics, disability studies, and feminism to develop deeper understandings of what difference means and how best to intervene around ensuing power differentials. Bioethics is therefore confronted with the task of considering the meaning of difference from the multiple disciplinary points of view it draws upon. For example, is there any connection between the 0.1 percent variation in our human DNA and the discrimination, domination, and oppression we witness on the basis of race, ethnicity, gender, inherited disease, or even class? Should we view disability as a biological hurdle to be diagnosed and repaired or as the result of a society erecting barriers through its narrow construal of what is normal? How much of the racial and ethnic disparities in health outcomes are due to health care providers' internalization of the idea that social stratification is more biologically determined than politically constructed? By examining some key themes within the discourse of difference, we attempt here to make sense of where feminist bioethics is now and where those on the margins may seek to engage with or disassociate from areas of potential common concern.

Appeals to either negate or transcend difference in favor of universal goals are embedded in Enlightenment doctrine, secularism, Marxism, and feminism as well as anticolonial and global human rights movements. These approaches may acknowledge difference but stress that such difference is insignificant compared with the universality of human suffering and human flourishing that forges a common bond across seemingly disparate divides. Taken to its extreme, we could come to believe therefore that there is no *real* difference between any of us.

Yet the stock we place in overarching solidarity becomes problematic when it seeks to camouflage the tough work that needs to be done to combat racism, sexism or other -isms. As Patricia J. Williams states so poignantly: "We must be careful not to allow our intentions to verge into outright projection by substituting a fantasy of global seamlessness" (Williams 1997, 3–4). To ignore that there *is* difference, or to believe that difference does not matter, is to negate the painful reality of our interconnected lives. It gives us the privilege of relegating other people's suffering to an advent of misfortune (Shklar 1990) rather than facing our complicity in the devastating injustice that determines for the most part where we live, where we go to school, the occupations we enter, the people with whom we are intimate, the children we bear (or don't), and how and when we die.

Feminist bioethics began to articulate its objectives at a time when views about difference and identity were becoming well-worked notions in many related disciplines, including feminist philosophy. Feminist bioethicists were able to respond to voices that criticized mainly Western white female privilege for not only limiting the scope of feminist concerns but also sabotaging systemic or structural social change that would disrupt racially or globally entrenched hegemonies. Among these were North American black and Latina feminist scholars (see *inter alia:* hooks 1989; Hurtado 1997; Collins 2000) who had charged late-twentieth-century feminism with ignoring/homogenizing their concerns and pursuing instead a political and intellectual agenda that reinforced existing power relations, preventing the elimination of racial injustice. Similarly, some Asian,

African, and Latin American women intellectuals sought to disrupt categories that did not serve their interests; in particular Eurocentric constructions of theory and representation of "Third World" women as victims (Weedon 1998, 83). Their critiques problematized the condemnation by many Western feminists of cultural practices that seemed clearly to oppress women—such as female genital cutting, bride burning, dowry payment, and some inheritance patterns—accusing them of misunderstanding (or downright disparaging) the inherent complexities of moral judgments of these longstanding practices (Brems 1997). By pointing out many examples of falsely shared assumptions, "subaltern" writers have successfully challenged Western feminism's idealized solidarity across a global sisterhood (Mohanty 1984; Spivak 1993; Narayan 1998; Swartz 2005).

From its inception, then, feminist bioethics has addressed these tensions by clearly establishing, at least theoretically, its own identity as one of plurality, as well as its supportive relationship with other marginalized groups. The International Network on Feminist Approaches to Bioethics (FAB) has posted a foundational document on its website, stating goals that recognize intersecting forms of oppression:

> [FAB] aims to develop a more inclusive theory of bioethics encompassing the standpoints and experiences of women and other marginalized social groups. It examines presuppositions embedded in the dominant bioethical discourse and creates new methodologies responsive to the disparate conditions of women's lives across the globe. FAB is committed to a non-hierarchical model of organization and seeks to include all who share its goals. Academics, professionals, grassroots activists, and concerned persons from all fields are welcome. (International Network on Feminist Approaches to Bioethics, 2007)

Central to this mission is overcoming divisions across vulnerable groups and "recognizing the need for a cross-cultural perspective on bioethical issues that is responsive to non-dominant social groups" (Donchin 2000, 107). Susan Sherwin similarly states that we need a "broadened moral perspective... (that) encourages us to pay particular attention to... the disadvantaged and oppressed and not to automatically assume the standpoint of the privileged" (Sherwin 2001, 187).

Disability and Feminist Bioethics

We have included a contribution on disability to draw attention to the distinctive nature of feminist bioethics' emerging engagement with this form of difference. First, the concept of *disability* as an overarching social category (as opposed to individual *impairments*) has only recently entered the literature (Braddock and Parish 2001, 11–60; Borsay 2005). Second, disability poses distinct problems of definition, reflecting both the heterogeneity of impairments and the lack of consensus within various disciplines about whether disability is best understood as a biological phenomenon, a social construct, or something constructed through the mutual interaction of biology and society (Shakespeare 2006; Thomas 2007; Scully 2008). Only recently have some feminists started to think and write about disability as a form of social exclusion in itself, and one that might intersect or synergize with gender. Feminist bioethicists who have published in this area include Fine and Asch (1988); Kittay (1999); Silvers, Wasserman, and Mahowald (1999); and Wendell (1996).

Feminism in its turn has had a visible impact on disability scholarship. Within disability studies, disability is now increasingly recognized as a phenomenon or experience that is *gendered* (Morris 1993; Meekosha 1998; Thomas 1999; Garland-Thomson 2005). But because it is an embodied experience, and also because it involves bodies that exist in particular social settings, it is not gendered straightforwardly. Feminist perspectives on disability therefore highlight the acquisition of empirical data about disability and gender. They also draw on subjective accounts of living with disability in a way that many nonfeminist disability studies fail to do.

Moreover, feminism and disability intersect on a theoretical level. Responding to what many see as the narrowness of an exclusively medical understanding of impairment, in the 1970s the disability movement in Britain put forward a "social model" of disability. Among the characteristics of this model is the sharp distinction it draws between *impairment* (as the "biological substrate," the measurable bodily variation) and *disability*, which the social model argues results directly from social exclusion (Oliver 1990). This finds a parallel in the sex/gender distinction developed within feminist theory, where sex is understood as biologically determined and gender as a social and/or culturally constructed category (see Gatens 1995). But just as the sex/gender dichotomy has come under renewed scrutiny within feminism, with the "naturalness" of biological sex no longer seeming so secure (for example, in debates around intersexuality and transsexuality: Fausto-Sterling 2000; Butler 2001), so disability theory is also reexamining the relegation of impairment to the biological domain. And just as feminist theory has treated gender, disability theory is formulating an understanding of impairment as socially and discursively constructed. Further, following feminism's questioning of the sex/gender dichotomy (and posing the question of whether this is a meaningful dichotomy at all) disability scholars, especially advocates of the social model, have begun to reflect on the theoretical consequences of drawing a sharp line between impairment and disability.

Both the British strong social model, with its materialist view of disability as the result of societal forces that act to prevent people with impairments from participating in paid work, and the civil rights model that predominates in the United States, in which disabled people are a minority group with legitimate claims to have their civil rights protected, have political advantages. However, the critiques they offer of complex *bioethical* questions about disability are limited. Neither model directly confronts our cultural assumptions about the ontological or ethical meaning of impaired bodies or cognitive function; yet it is precisely these meanings that are at stake in the bioethical justification offered for normalization. In contrast, feminist bioethics' engagement with disability is able to draw on the parallel in which feminist theory challenges normalizing assumptions about gendered bodies, thereby reframing disability as "a socially constructed identity and a representational system similar to gender" (Garland-Thomson 2005, 1559).

In addition to theoretical arguments, disability bioethics may also find feminist methodologies useful. Feminist bioethical analysis situates ethical issues, such as prenatal testing decisions, within the societal and political contexts in which they are made. Doing so necessarily highlights how those contexts constrain our thinking not only about what constitutes disability, but also about what interventions are appropriate, and even about which factors are relevant to ethical analysis. Without disregarding the physical reality of bodily variance, it is nevertheless true that the disabling impact of an impairment is significantly influenced by social expectations, economic structures, technological developments, and so on. A close analysis of the relevant social and political contexts enables us to separate out more clearly the disability-associated disadvantages that are the direct result of an impairment and those that are mainly the consequence of social arrangements or attitudes that have the potential to be altered. This distinction is generally ignored or elided in mainstream bioethical analyses, which focus predominantly on anomalous bodies as problematic biomedical deviations.

A feminist analysis of power relations in disability also offers what we might call a therapeutic as well as a diagnostic aspect. As well as identifying who participates in and who is excluded from decision making and parameter setting in bioethical dilemmas, a feminist analysis highlights the practices through which power inequalities are maintained and examines how such relations may be made more equitable. This scrutiny ideally includes examining power relations *between* women, as well as the ones that feminists are generally more comfortable looking at, between women and men. Here we begin to see how the relationship between disability and feminism within bioethics can be mutually beneficial. Like many non-white, non-Western, non-straight, and/or non-middle-class women, disabled feminists claim that they were tacitly excluded from much of the feminist movement of the late twentieth century. For black, lesbian, and/or working-class women, these exclusions operate primarily through the barriers of money, employment, and education—the familiar forms of economic, social, and cultural capital (Fowler 1997). But for women with disabilities, exclusion entails additional types of barriers. Remedying the exclusion requires not simply the political recognition that the voices of disabled women and men have been absent from the debate, but tangible, sometimes costly measures—like ramps, lifts, Braille note takers, and sign language interpreters—to ensure access to the sites where the political and theoretical discussion takes place.

Disability therefore acts as a reminder to feminist bioethicists to think hard and to notice where lines are unwittingly being drawn that determine which women (and men) contribute to the bioethical conversation and which don't. But disability expands feminist bioethics' thinking in more fundamental ways too. As Rosemarie Garland-Thomson (2005) writes, "Feminism challenges the belief that femaleness is a natural form of physical and mental deficiency or constitutional unruliness. Feminist disability studies similarly questions our assumptions that disability is a flaw, lack or excess." A feminist bioethics of disability therefore is not just about applying feminist theory to prenatal selection, assisted suicide, or other issues that concern people with disabilities. Nor is it a matter of expanding bioethical debate to include empirical data about the views of disabled women or the impact of particular practices on them. Disability should serve to remind feminist bioethicists that the roots of feminist challenge lie in women's recognition of the ethical, social, and political significance of the deviant body: put bluntly, women are marked as different (in complex and culturally specific ways) because their *embodiment* is classified as different from men's. This does not mean that women's lives are biologically determined but rather that gender and its consequences are embodied as well as social phenomena. Likewise, disability theory points up the ethical, social, and political significance of bodies that are "deviant" for other reasons and offers a view of disability that is embodied, material, cultural, and social.

The following chapters challenge some of our well-honed assumptions about feminism's ability to traverse methodological, ideological, and positional subjectivities with ease. Ruth Groenhout reviews how notions of difference inherently assume deviation from an ideal norm (usually white and male), and how race-based categories have been exploited in research that affects public, not just individual, health. She cites the example of BiDil, approved by the U.S. Food and Drug Administration for the treatment of heart failure exclusively in African Americans, the first racially customized drug in the world. Extending a feminist critique of principle-based ethics to its treatment of race and ethnicity, Groen-hout proposes applying care theory to research and policy decisions because it moves policy makers and researchers beyond the individual focus to recognize "the many ways that all of us are socially connected, constituted and dependent" so that we will "have some sense of how social factors, rather than individual genetic heritage, may have an impact on people's lives and decisions." Practically, she emphasizes the need to reconnect theory with action, calling for research that ideally begins and ends in the community and putting forward the model of community based participatory research.

The next chapter addresses the contentious matter of whether feminist bio-ethics brings any added value to attempts by Indigenous scholars and activists to reform how medical research is conducted and disseminated. While arguing that there may be strategic benefits to be gained from an "informal alliance" between feminist bioethicists and the Indigenous peoples of Australia, authors Jennifer Baker, Terry Dunbar, and Margaret Scrimgeour are realistic about the limitations of any such relationship. Documenting how the problematic behavior of some non-Indigenous feminists has thwarted Indigenous goals to date, this chapter makes clear the potential for misunderstanding and breach of trust and the frequently expropriated rights of representation.

Jing-Bao Nie then explores the often-contradictory analyses of Western feminists addressing China's one-child policy that began nearly a quarter-century ago. Nie is both a scholar of feminism and a researcher of China's birth-control program. He presents a nuanced view of how feminism has both influenced and been influenced by this massive demographic project. He is hopeful that although bioethics and feminism have to date largely ignored "population control and world poverty," he sees China as a potentially rich area for ethical engagement.

Together, these three contributions challenge feminist bioethics to look again at its response to radical critiques as well as its engagement with "other" forms of difference. The final chapter in this section is an example of how the phenomenon of disability can push bioethicists and feminists to think harder about the complexity and strangeness of bodies. While there are many ways of doing this, Mary B. Mahowald applies feminist standpoint theory (the claim that experiences connected with specific, usually marginal, social positions offer an alternative and sometimes privileged insight into social phenomena: see Hartsock 1987; Harding 2004) in a systematic fashion to examine the discrimination surrounding disability. Focusing on cognitive impairment, Mahowald makes a case for an account of normality based on the concept of flourishing rather than on function. From an egalitarian feminist position she argues that standpoint theory is one way in which "the inevitable nearsightedness of the dominant group" in policy making can be made to take account of otherwise excluded marginalities, like disability.

These contributions return us to the question of feminist bioethics' willingness both to attend to and to act on such radical critiques. How ready are feminist bioethicists to do what is necessary for genuine collaborative work, for example, altering language and frameworks and embracing different epistemologies? As we have seen, embedded in efforts to incorporate diversity are tendencies to (re)create scholars in our own image. Chadwick and Schuklenk (2004) echo this caution when they say: "The current assumption seems to be that the developing world needs our training and needs to be subjected to significant doses of our ethical views and ideologies, instead of funding allowing it to develop its own capacities based on its own thinking." It remains to be seen if feminist bioethics has reached the maturity to truly engage in open self-criticism and to foster a more transparent dialogue with those (similarly or not) situated on the margins of mainstream bioethical discourse. Still, the intention within feminist bioethics to desire a plurality of perspectives (Tong 2001) and the enrichment this can bring is an excellent starting point from which to find common ground and to illuminate divergences.

REFERENCES

Asch, A. 1999. Prenatal diagnosis and selective abortion: A challenge to practice and policy. *American Journal of Public Health* 89 (11): 1649–57.

Bailey, R. 1996. Prenatal testing and the prevention of impairment: A woman's right to choose? In *Encounters with strangers,* ed. J. Morris, 143–67. London: Women's Press.

Borsay, A. 2005. *Disability and social policy in Britain since 1750: A history of exclusion.* Basingstoke, U.K.: Palgrave.

Braddock, D. L., and S. L. Parish. 2001. An institutional history of disability. In *The disability studies handbook,* ed. G. Albrecht, K. Seelman, and M. Bury, 11–60. London: Sage.

Brems, E. 1997. Enemies or allies? Feminism and cultural relativism as dissident voices in human rights discourse. *Human Rights Quarterly* 19 (1): 136–64.

Brock, D. W. 2000. Broadening the bioethics agenda. *Kennedy Institute of Ethics Journal* 10 (1): 21–38.

Butler, J. 2001. Doing justice to someone: Sex reassignment and allegories of transsexuality. *GLQ* 7:621–36.

Chadwick, R., and U. Schuklenk. 2004. Bioethical colonialism? *Bioethics* 18 (5): iii–iv.

Collins, P. H. 2000. *Black feminist thought: Knowledge, consciousness, and the politics of empowerment*, 2nd ed. New York: Routledge.

Daniels, N. 2006. Equity and population health: Toward a broader bioethics agenda. *Hastings Center Report* 36 (4): 22–35.

Donchin, A. 2000. Bioethics: Feminist. In *Routledge international encyclopedia of women: Global women's issues and knowledge*, ed. C. Kramarae and D. Spender, 105–7. New York: Routledge.

Dreger, A. D. 2004. *One of us: Conjoined twins and the future of normal*. Cambridge, Mass.: Harvard University Press.

Farmer, P. 2003. *Pathologies of power: Health, human rights, and the new war on the poor*. Berkeley: University of California Press.

Fausto-Sterling, A. 2000. *Sexing the body: Gender politics and the construction of sexuality*. New York: Basic Books.

Fine, M., and A. Asch. 1988. *Women with disabilities: Essays in psychology, culture, and politics*. Philadelphia: Temple University Press.

Fowler, B. 1997. *Pierre Bourdieu and cultural theory: Critical investigations*. London: Sage.

Garland-Thomson, R. 2005. Feminist disability studies. *Signs: Journal of Women in Culture and Society* 30:1557–87.

Gatens, M. 1995. *Imaginary bodies: Ethics, power and corporeality*. London: Routledge.

Harding, S. 2004. A socially relevant philosophy of science? Resources from standpoint theory's controversiality. *Hypatia* 19:25–47.

Harris, J. 2007. *Enhancing evolution: The ethical case for making better people*. Princeton, N.J.: Princeton University Press.

Hartsock, N. 1987. The feminist standpoint: Developing the ground for a specifically feminist historical materialism. In *Feminism and methodology: Social science issues*, ed. S. Harding, 157–80. Bloomington: Indiana University Press.

Ho, K. 2007. Structural violence as a human rights violation. *Essex Human Rights Review* 4 (2): 1–17.

Holmes, H. B. 2001. When health means wealth, can bioethicists respond? *Health Care Analysis* 9:213–28.

hooks, b. 1989. *Feminist theory: From margin to center*. Boston: South End Press.

Hurtado, A. 1997. *The color of privilege: Three blasphemies on race and feminism*. Ann Arbor: University of Michigan Press.

International Network on Feminist Approaches to Bioethics. 2007. www.pdcnet.org/member-fab.html.

Jaggar, A. M. 1998. Globalizing feminist ethics. *Hypatia* 13 (2): 7–31.

Kittay, E. F. 1999. *Love's labor: Essays on women, equality, and dependency*. New York: Routledge.

Mann, J. M. 1997. Medicine and public health, ethics and human rights. *Hastings Center Report* 27 (3): 6–13.

Meekosha, H. 1998. Body battles: Bodies, gender, and disability. In *Disability studies reader: Social science perspectives*, ed. T. Shakespeare, 163–80. London: Cassell.

Mohanty, C. T. 1984. Under Western eyes: Feminist scholarship and colonial discourses. *Boundary* 212 (3): 338–58.

———. 2003. *Feminism without borders: Decolonizing theory, practicing solidarity*. Durham, N.C.: Duke University Press.

Morris, J. 1993. Feminism and disability. *Feminist Review* 43:57–70.

Myser, C. 2003. Differences from somewhere: The normativity of whiteness in bioethics in the United States. *American Journal of Bioethics* 3 (2): 1–11.

Narayan, U. 1998. Essence of culture and a sense of history: A feminist critique of cultural essentialism. *Hypatia* 13 (2): 86–106.

Okin, S. M. 1998. Feminism, women's rights and cultural differences. *Hypatia* 13 (2): 32–52.

Oliver, M. 1990. *The politics of disablement*. Basingstoke, U.K.: Macmillan.

Parens, E. 2006. *Surgically shaping children: Technology, ethics, and the pursuit of normality*. Baltimore: Johns Hopkins University Press.

Parens, E., and A. Asch, eds. 2002. *Prenatal testing and disability rights*. Washington, D.C.: Georgetown University Press.

Rock, P. J. 1996. Eugenics and euthanasia: A cause for concern for disabled people, particularly disabled women. *Disability and Society* 11:121–8.

Rogers, W., and D. Brock. 2004. Public health ethics. *Bioethics* 18 (6): iii–vi.

Savulescu, J. 2007. In defense of procreative beneficence. *Journal of Medical Ethics* 33:284–88.

Scully, J. L. 2008. *Disability bioethics*. Lanham, Md.: Rowman & Littlefield.

Shakespeare, T. 2006. *Disability rights and wrongs*. London: Routledge.

Sherwin, S. 2001. Moral perception and global visions. *Bioethics* 15 (3): 175–88.

Shklar, J. N. 1990. *The faces of injustice*. New Haven, Conn.: Yale University Press.

Silvers, A., D. Wasserman, and M. B. Mahowald. 1999. *Disability, difference, discrimination: Perspectives on justice in bioethics and public policy*. Lanham, Md.: Rowman & Littlefield.

Spivak, G. 1993. Can the subaltern speak? In *Colonial discourse and post-colonial theory*, ed. P. Williams and L. Crisman, 66–111. New York: Harvester Wheatsheaf.

Swartz, S. 2005. Can the clinical subject speak? Some thoughts on subaltern psychology. *Theory and Psychology* 15 (4): 505–25.

Thomas, C. 1999. *Female forms: Experiencing and understanding disability*. Buckingham, U.K.: Open University Press.

———. 2007. *Sociologies of disability and illness*. Basingstoke, U.K.: Palgrave Macmillan.

Tong, R. 2001. Towards a feminist global bioethics: Addressing women's health concerns worldwide. *Health Care Analysis* 9:229–46.

Vehmas, S. 2003. Live and let die? Disability in bioethics. *New Review of Bioethics* 1:145–57.

Wasserman, D., J. Bickenbach, and R. Wachbroit. 2005. *Quality of life and human difference: Genetic testing, health care, and disability*. New York: Cambridge University Press.

Weedon, C. 1998. Postmodernism. In *A companion to feminist philosophy,* ed. A. M. Jaggar and I. M. Young, chap. 8. Malden, Mass.: Blackwell.

Wendell, S. 1996. *The rejected body: Feminist philosophical reflections on disability*. New York: Routledge.

Williams, P. J. 1997. *Seeing a colour-blind future: The paradox of race*. London: Virago Press.

CHAPTER ELEVEN

The Difference Difference Makes

Public Health and the Complexities of Racial and Ethnic Differences

RUTH GROENHOUT, PH.D.

Conceptions of Health and Public Policy: An Introduction to the Problem

Public health research and public health practices represent a context within which central theoretical problems of difference become issues of application. Practice and theory cannot be kept separate here because of the nature of public health, and theoretical flaws become magnified in important ways. The history of research on public health matters indicates the ways that theoretical models of difference have been harmful to people. Think, for example, of the assumptions on the part of most researchers during the early years of modern medicine about what good research should look like, namely, that good research was defined by being relevant to, conducted on, and exclusive in its focus on one particular model of human existence, namely, a homogeneous group of Anglo men, middle-aged, able-bodied, and middle class. Some research focused only on this group; other research, such as the infamous Tuskegee study that specifically focused on differences from this group, did so with a clear assumption that difference indicated less than fully human status (Waltraud and Harris 1999; Reverby 2000; Pence 2004). By and large, population groups who differed from the "standard model" were considered exceptions to the general rule even when, as in the case of women, they made up slightly more than half of the population. Even now, although U.S. research supported by the National Institutes of Health is required to include both ethnic minorities and women, it is still common to find studies that make no mention of whether the research applies to either group, whether they were included in the study, or whether there are significant differences in how they react to any given treatment protocol.

Difference inevitably poses this problem in the context of public health re-search because we do not have good paradigms for incorporating pluralism into our models of research. The models we have assume either a unified single model of health, one that in turn inevitably assumes a single model of human being (the Western European middle-class male model), or subjective "definitions" of health determined by the whims of the individual. As soon as a single determinative model is given up, there is a tendency to assume that we are left with nothing but ungrounded subjectivism. The assumption that these are our only two options follows, in part, from the theoretical framework most contemporary health care ethics adopts, namely, a principles-based, consensus-oriented model (DuBose, Hammel, and O'Connell, 1994; Beauchamp and Childress 2001). Principles-based reasoning espouses an unrealistically individualistic account of human existence in conjunction with a noncontextual account of reasoning and autonomy; these fea-tures set up a context within which we do not have any good theoretical way to think about pluralism other than by framing it as complete subjectivism.

A completely subjectivist account of health is no standard at all, particularly in the context of public health policy, where we are making collective decisions about collective resources, benefits, and burdens. Public policy cannot be based on completely subjective standards, because it involves decisions about public expenditures of tax dollars, laws that set parameters for children's health, and limitations on what can count as a treatment for various conditions (Coughlin, Soskoline, and Goodman 1997). None of these is possible without an account of what actually counts as "health," whether for a particular subsection of the popu-lation, such as children, or for considerations of treating particular conditions such as mental illness. In all such cases, a background conception of health is necessary for making policy decisions, and considering health to be a completely individual, subjective concept is neither practically workable nor beneficial to the individuals who are covered by the policy.

In public health studies, we need a paradigm for thinking about multiple ways of being human while maintaining a commitment to the full flourishing of all. I focus on public health in this chapter because by definition, public health is sup-posed to focus on the health of all included in the public. In that context, an eth-ics of care offers the best resources for thinking about what it means to concep-tualize a model of public health research that does not begin with a single model of human health but a pluralistic model, and yet nonetheless allows us to strive for health for all concerned.

An ethics-of-care framework has been developed by a number of thinkers, both within and without bioethics, out of a concern that contemporary models of ethics are designed to fit the lives of disembodied rational beings rather than the embedded, enmeshed, physical, and relational lives that humans actually live out (see *inter alia:* Gilligan 1982; Noddings 1984, 2002; Ruddick 1989; Held 1993, 2006; Groenhout 2004). Care ethics recognizes the situated, particularistic nature of human lives, the relational matrices within which decisions are made, and the social dimensions of autonomy, identity, and authority (Kittay 1999; Kittay and Feder 2000; Hamington and Miller 2006). This recognition allows care ethics to discern and address issues of difference in health research and policy in ways that are more appropriate to lived experience.

Mapping the Terrain

Already in this chapter I have used a number of terms that are used with regularity in discussions of health care, all of which are contentious and difficult to define. I'd like to briefly review these concepts, discuss why their definitions are so controversial, and suggest alternative definitions.

The first, and probably most amorphous term, is health. Many writers on the topic of public health adopt the definition offered by the World Health Organization: health is a "state of complete physical, mental, and social well-being, not merely the absence of disease or infirmity" (World Health Organization 1948). Although this definition is undoubtedly the most commonly cited in the literature, it is also the most contentious. Some of those who reject it do so on the grounds that it requires far too much for health. For example, everyone in a society that is badly structured turns out to be unhealthy within this definition because they lack *complete* social health. If we also think that many societies have had unhealthy structures, it turns out that perhaps no one, anywhere, has ever been healthy. Others reject the WHO definition because it precludes a notion of health that recognizes the compatibility of health with physical or mental disabilities. They point out that a diabetic who carefully manages her condition, for example, can presumably live a healthy life with a chronic disease; a similar case can be made for someone with controlled depression.

For the moment I'd like to offer another, provisional definition of health. Health is better understood as a state of being that permits the individual to flourish to the greatest extent possible as a human, given the limitations that arise from the physical condition and capacities of the individual, but only such limitations that arise in a social and cultural context that does not itself pose intractable hurdles to achieving flourishing. When limitations are a direct result of social and cultural impediments, full health may be impossible to achieve, though a reasonable level of health may still be possible with a variety of coping mechanisms. On this view, health is in large part an instrumental good—one that we value in human life because without health, accomplishing any of our life goals and values becomes much more difficult, sometimes impossible (for an elaboration, see, for example the *Ottawa Charter for Health Promotion* [World Health Organization 1986], which defines health as a "resource for everyday life, not the objective of living"). As well, we need not be in a state of physical perfection to be healthy. We can consider ourselves healthy, and be correct in so doing, when we recognize that we have physical limitations but can still act to make our own lives as good as possible within those limitations, given that they are not caused by social conditions that are in direct conflict with human flourishing. Social structures that deny people's basic rights, that permit violence against ethnic or racial minorities, that allow for widespread poisoning of the environment, do make it impossible to achieve a healthy life for many, and this definition tries to separate such issues from physical conditions that may not be avoidable or curable, that need to be accommodated rather than fought.

Public health, like health itself, is also more difficult to define than one might expect. While health is defined in terms of the state of well-being (or lack thereof) of individuals, public health, in at least one standard discussion, is defined as "what we as a society do collectively to ensure the conditions in which people can be healthy" (Mann et al. 1999, 29). So, this definition presumes, health is a condition of individuals. Public health, however, rather than being the collective health of a public group, refers to the collective activities of a social group that aim at producing the conditions of health, a definition that appears to be two steps removed from health itself, that is, it refers to collective action (one step) aimed at producing conditions (two steps) that are necessary for health. Public health, then, presumes the existence of a "we"—those who are responsible, presumably, for the collective action, as well as a collective sense of the nature of health, itself a contested concept.

Both "health" and "public health," then, are concepts that are hard to define exactly, and their definitions involve a variety of controversial assumptions about group membership, collective responsibility, and the existence of standards for defining well-being. When we add to this the difficulty of theoretically accommodating deep differences between individuals and social groups in a pluralist social system, we add another layer of complexity to the whole picture.

Difference has generally been taken to be an inherently hierarchical notion in Western philosophy. It takes on this valence when it is assumed to be difference from a particular norm or standard, so those who are not of Western European

(WE) heritage, for example, are considered to be the groups who instantiate "difference," while those who are WE are not different but the norm. When this model is adopted, the group or positions taken as the norm benefit from unspoken and often untheorized assumptions of "the right way to be" while groups identified with difference are assumed to be problematic, or inferior, or in need of justification (Mills 1998; Spelman 1988; Alcoff 2006).

While it is easy to note that difference can carry automatic connotations of inferiority, however, it is much more difficult to develop a theoretical perspective from within which to think about difference in ways that do not automatically establish an illegitimate hierarchy. And certain types of reasoning, I want to argue, operate with an internal logic that makes nonhierarchical difference particularly difficult to think. Principles-based reasoning, in particular, with its automatic and (often) unnuanced assumption that autonomy is (a) a central value; (b) easy to recognize; and (c) easily identified in its absence, offers an example of such a theory. Care theory, a more recent feminist addition to discussions of bioethics, offers an alternative conceptual structure that makes difference easier to incorporate into ethical discussions.

To see this, however, it is necessary to step back a bit and think about how difference and normativity play out in the context of public health, particularly public health concerns in the arena of research on primary and secondary health prevention (Berg and Mol 1998), to gain some perspective on why and how we find ourselves where we are today. Although I will be focusing on issues of research for reasons of convenience, much of this analysis would also apply to non-research concerns about public health, issues that involve the funding of various treatments, for example, provision of public health services.

Including Racial and Ethnic Data

Researchers are now required by law to include women in studies of new treatments and techniques, at least for new treatments requiring U.S. Food and Drug Administration regulatory approval. But that does not mean that medical data are collected in ways that include both men and women regularly in studies. As I write, the *New York Times* carries an article reporting on a study that found significant differences between two different types of statins, medications used to lower blood cholesterol (Kolata 2003). The article notes that the research subjects were predominantly men, but the percentage is not provided. The reporter throughout speaks in terms of statins preventing heart disease in people (not men) and makes no mention of tracking racial or ethnic diversity in the study.

The study involved 502 patients, and it may not have included a sufficiently large number of non-Anglo patients to provide any statistically relevant data for non-white ethnic groups, but we are not given that information in this public presentation of medical data.

Both race and sex raise problems of difference. In the case of biological sex, although there is a relatively clear correlation between genetic factors and biological components of sexual development and nature, researchers sometimes show little awareness of the socially constructed nature of many aspects of gender. In the case of racial and ethnic difference, the situation is even more complex. Researchers have found that there are some statistical correlations between continent of origin and certain genetic variations, but also that these variations are slight and that only a small proportion of variations separate continental populations (Jorde and Wooding 2004). In the public mind, however, race and racial differences are not a matter of general geographical points of origin but distinct categories of human existence, and these are the categories used when making research and treatment decisions.

The *New England Journal of Medicine* reported that a combination of two older drugs, isosorbide dinitrate and hydrazaline, commercially known at BiDil, provides a significant benefit in African Americans with heart failure (Taylor et al. 2004). The combination had not been found to be effective in white populations. This is, of course, good news for those individuals for whom this protocol can be beneficial. But at the same time, the research and the reporting expose a set of worries that need to be addressed. Not all African Americans share the same genetic makeup. Africans arrived in North America from different geographic locations within Africa and most have extensively mixed genetic inheritances that include a large portion of European or Native American genes. Likewise, many U.S. citizens are placed in the category "white" because of phenotypic characteristics yet have genetic inheritances that reveal their origins in African geographic regions. While geographic inheritances may correlate in significant ways with certain genetic variations, phenotypic categories are not nearly so exact. The social construction of racial categories, however, works against researchers' awareness of these distinctions, making skin color and facial features (seemingly obvious phenotypic "markers") the only identifying characteristics for research.

Racially disaggregated data do have the potential to improve public health services and need to be recognized as important. But having said that, we also need to be aware that racially and sexually indexed data can do harm to the very groups who should benefit. We need a clear view of the double-edged nature of the data before we simply begin collecting and disseminating information. The racial beliefs that usually shape research protocols are often problematic. All African Americans do not share the same genotype. Presumably those with sub-Saharan backgrounds differ in important ways from those from Northern Africa, to pick one obvious example, but these possibilities are obscured by American racial stereotypes. On the basis of these stereotypes, one is (or isn't) black, and medicines can now be administered following a quick visual observation (and racial assignation) of someone's phenotypic characteristics.

The idea that racial categories are absolute, easily apparent, and homogeneous should be known to be false by anyone who thinks about it for more than a few moments. But the recognition that racial categories have a large grain of social fiction about them does not always trickle down to concrete medical practices. Rather than investigate how possible differences in metabolic pathways affect the actions of various drugs, practitioners observe that a drug does or does not work in some individuals who are socially categorized as black. That this may result in some who statistically benefit from it being excluded from treatment without comment goes unrecognized. That this may also result in using the treatment in others inappropriately, namely, those who may look stereotypically black but who may not share the geographically based genetic heritage that makes the treatment appropriate, may also go unrecognized.

When we talk about collecting racial, ethnic, or gender data, then, we must avoid the naïve assumption that collecting data will result in better treatment options and better health. Sometimes it does. I do not want to be misunderstood as a critic of those who want better treatment for heart disease in African Americans, and I think that research of this sort is essential for developing better medicine generally. But it is not only the case that racial categories, inappropriately applied, can improperly include or exclude people from important treatment protocols. The history of medical research indicates the more worrisome possibility that research that takes difference into account can be used in ways that are harmful to the groups identified as different.

Both gender and racial or ethnic differences affect the caregiver's perception of the patient. It has been common in the past for caregivers to tell women that their health concerns were unreasonable for a variety of reasons. Either women were assumed to be naturally physiologically defective, or they were particularly prone to psychological problems, or they were disposed to treat minor problems as if they were serious. In the case of osteoporosis, it was female physiology that was defective. Recent studies of the treatment of heart disease in women and men highlights the extent to which men's reporting of symptoms is taken seriously while women's is often treated as whining, with the result that particular conditions in women are more likely to be fatal than similar conditions would be in men. (I am not advocating an opposite reaction—that of overtreatment. We have seen the problems that can arise from treating menopause, for example, as if it were a medical condition to be fixed.) Similar cases can be cited for racial biases in treatment, particularly pain control. There is a fairly widespread assumption among health care workers that African Americans are complainers: that they don't really feel much pain but complain sooner at more modest discomfort, and that therefore their requests for pain control can be dismissed, treated as less severe, or discounted (Smedley, Stith, and Nelson 2003).

In the case of racial and ethnic minorities, the situation is exacerbated by disparities in access to insurance and primary care providers. Racial and ethnic minorities use teaching hospitals, clinics, and emergency rooms for their usual source of care in far higher numbers than whites (Smedley, Stith, and Nelson 2003, 102–11). Those sites, in turn, are staffed by non-U.S.-trained physicians to a great degree. The interactions between minority patients and international medical graduates are far more challenging in terms of cultural insensitivity and miscommunication than are those between almost any other group (Smedley, Stith, and Nelson 2003, 116–20). When research on racial and ethnic differences is carried out or disseminated in this context, it may not always be used to provide better care but can instead contribute to an atmosphere of second-class treatment for those identified by the research as "different."

Some theorists have argued that collecting more data on the specificities of disease etiology in ethnic subpopulations will result in a tendency among caregivers to dismiss the concerns of individuals from specific ethnic groups on the grounds that the condition is not something that can be fixed, it's just "how those folks are." And it is worth noting that how this dismissal works generally plays out to the detriment of those in "marked" categories. That is, stereotypes about Western European men result in their testimony being given attention and credence, caregivers wanting to provide care, research on medications providing adequate information for treatment, and the like. For women, on the other hand, stereotypes can work to diminish perceptions of accuracy in testimony, caregivers tend to assume that they need or deserve less attention, and research that provides inadequate data for their treatment is not automatically considered faulty.

While noting that this is a real and worrisome danger, I should also note that the collection of data in all of these cases has been precisely the way that the problem has been addressed. If it were not for data collection that did focus on racial and gender specifics, the problems would not be widely known. Acquiring data is a double-edged sword. It is not enough to accumulate the data; one also has to be sure that they are properly used.

We can summarize part of the problem here by noting that we continue to fall back into the trap of treating difference as difference-from-a-norm, that the norm is one of a particular ethnic group, sex, and class, and that difference is still, in each of these problematic ways, a matter of deviance and inferiority. Presumably this should be a point at which we can bring in philosophical theorizing to resolve some of these difficulties, to suggest ways in which we can think about differences without equating them with deviance or simply to provide a framework that allows us to distinguish differences that are problems from differences that are simply differences. But the main model of reasoning in contemporary bioethics is ill suited for this job.

Principles-based Reasoning and the Problem of Difference

Principles-based (PB) reasoning is the model of ethical theorizing most widely used and taught in the contemporary health care context (Fox 1994; Beauchamp and Childress 2001). It is an account of ethical theorizing that we can almost always assume many others will share. Whether discussing issues in the context of a hospital ethics committee, talking policy concerns with lawmakers, or reviewing a research protocol for tests involving human subjects, the use of principles-based reasoning allows one to speak in terms that are widely shared, generally accepted, and handy for conducting ethical debates. I teach it in my own classes, in part so that my students can share in what has become the lingua franca of contemporary bioethical debates, particularly in the United States.

Although we can acknowledge that PB reasoning is the dominant language of contemporary bioethics, we should also be aware of the ways in which it skews our reasoning by the form it imposes on our discussions. In particular, PB reasoning requires us to make three moves that can be problematic and that lead to difficulties in dealing with the sorts of racial and gender differences this chapter is concerned with. The first involves the abstract individualism that is at the heart of PB reasoning, the second is the privileging of a particular notion of autonomy that fits with abstract individualism, and the third is the compartmentalized reasoning that principles tend to force on us. All of these structural biases are strengths as well as weaknesses. They have provided some of the features that make PB reasoning so powerful and popular in bioethics, but they also lead to serious problems when we are trying to deal with the sorts of differences and complexities that arise when discussing ethnicity, race, gender, and class.

I'll begin with abstract individualism. PB reasoning assumes the notion of the individual as an isolated, autonomous being. This is an enormously powerful way of initiating one's reasoning in health care ethics, and its strengths should not be overlooked. Racial and ethnic minorities, and women of all heritages, recognize that their acknowledgement as individuals in their own right is an enormous advance over social systems that assigned ownership of all such groups to Western European males. But while individualism is an important moral advance, it is not without its own problematic baggage.

Treating people as isolated individuals obscures the extent to which their situation in society, the options they have open to them, and the authority and power available to them are constructed by social structures rather than being matters of individual choice or achievement. It also obscures the extent to which an individual's assimilation of information may be affected by ethnic heritage or class, so that individual decision making may be influenced by features of a situation that are quite separate from the information an individual may be assumed to be using to make her decision. For example, women are often socialized to be "nice," that is, eager to please and to meet the expectations of those around them. An individual woman, making decisions about end-stage cancer treatment, may be strongly influenced by the force of personality of the caregiver who discusses treatment options with her and may need to be accompanied by family or community members in order to gain the psychological power she needs to make a decision that does not accord with the caregiver's opinion. Too strong an emphasis on individualism, however, coupled with the caregiver's natural tendency to see agreement as rational, can lead to the caregiver missing the individual's need for social support.

In the context of public health research, particularly when the research is conducted in non-Western countries, this individualist focus can lead the researchers to lose sight of the many ways that all of us are socially connected, constituted, and dependent. Recent controversies over a number of research protocols in Third World countries, including studies of zidovudine (or AZT) to prevent mother-to-child transmission of HIV that used placebos in the control group, suggest that researchers need to be constantly reminded that researchers and subjects, though both individuals, do not stand in equal relationships of power or social status (Angell 1997). Research into health-related effects of race in the United States substantiates this: it is not difficult to find published research that describes the category of "black race" as an unfavorable biologic parameter because it correlates with higher rates of mortality and morbidity in many contexts. But treating the category as if it (alone) were the source of these problematic statistics allows researchers to assume that something about the individual, perhaps genetic inheritance or behavior patterns, creates the increased risk. It then becomes easy for researchers to ignore the contributions of historical racism and economic disenfranchisement to these statistics (Roach 2000). In situations in which race and ethnicity are the focus of a study, it is particularly important that researchers have some sense of how social factors, rather than individual factors, may have an impact on people's lives and decisions.

The ideal of individualism that lies close to the heart of PB reasoning is embodied in standard research protocols that treat the subjects of research as individuals. Whether we are concerned with signatures on consent forms or the selection of one treatment protocol rather than another, the subjects are largely assumed to be complete in and of themselves. This has led to problems in obtaining informed consent in the developing world. The Western notion of the individual who signs a form taking on the responsibility for knowing what the form signifies may not apply. In communities with strongly hierarchical structures, those signing the form may be doing so at the command of a superior and may have no clear sense that they could refuse if they wanted to.

Individualism in PB reasoning is closely connected to the notion of autonomy. Respect for individuals is usually translated into protection of the individual's autonomy. And, in a manner similar to my discussion of individualism, though I will be somewhat critical of the notion of autonomy as it currently functions in this context, I also want to note that I have no desire to return to the days of unbridled paternalism. The moral and legal protection of autonomy is vital to an ethical health care system; at the same time, the protection of autonomy can become problematic when it produces social structures that have the effect of undermining the very values they are meant to protect.

These dilemmas are largely waved out the back door of PB reasoning by the method of assuming that they represent glitches in the application of principles but no real problem for PB reasoning itself. I would argue, on the contrary, that they represent intractable problems for PB reasoning altogether, precisely because it is a system that denies real differences of perspective, value systems, and knowledge bases in the groups that are subject to the applications of the principles. So, when autonomy is held up as a central value of PB reasoning, those advocating it are not encouraged to ask whose autonomy is in question and what that means—the assumption is that autonomy is the same for all people pretty much all of the time and that it is a concept that does not need to be specified or given substantive content.

This assumption is simply not true. In practice, autonomy generally ends up meaning "whatever would be chosen by the average middle-aged, middle-class individual," so whenever decisions depart from that model, their autonomy is questioned. But if that unspoken norm were rejected, there seems nothing within PB reasoning itself to replace it. In the context of PB reasoning, autonomy is intended to be a minimalist concept without specified connections to social context, caregiver's perspectives on different social classes, or ingrained patterns of self-worth and respect for authority. These aspects of the caregiver-patient interaction determine what autonomy can mean for any given individual. Without such a contentful account of what autonomy is, there can be no real standard of autonomy. If we acknowledged that the concept was vacuous, this would make PB reasoning itself vacuous. (I take it that vacuity is a transitive property.) To avoid the loss of any principled basis for ethical decisions, we revert to declaring some people and decisions autonomous, and the ones we so baptize are those that fit with one particular, class-bound, limited picture of how things ought to be (MacKenzie and Stoljar 2000; Young 2002).

Again, when we think about standard models of public health research, we find that the implicit standard of autonomy is largely determined by assumptions about what the "reasonable person" would do or believe, and those standards assume a relatively isolated individual. In discussing the case of a healthy man who volunteers to undergo a moderately disabling operation to aid in a research project investigating a disease from which the man's wife suffers, Douglas Lackey notes that most institutional review boards would not approve such a protocol. "There is a tendency," he writes, "among researchers and many IRB members to regard people with medical problems as morally ideal subjects for research on those problems, even when the prospect that the research will produce therapy for these subjects is nil... On the other hand, the participation of normal subjects... is viewed as altruism verging on the irrational" (Lackey 1993, 178). In both cases, however, the individual volunteering for research faces exactly the same level of disabling potential, and both volunteer out of a concern for others, because the research offers no short-term potential for treatment of the condition.

That volunteering in this case is seen as rational and autonomous on the part of the woman with an illness but not on the part of her healthy husband suggests that judgments about autonomy are not based on a neutral standard of (say) harm and rational capacity. Lackey argues that other-directed concerns should not be automatically dubbed irrational; that they are suggests a particular set of assumptions about rationality that may be problematic. I would agree with him. But I would also note that it is not just the nature of rationality that this example throws into question. It also reflects differing assumptions about what can count as an autonomous decision when one is healthy or has a disease.

Autonomy and rationality, as this case might suggest, are closely connected, and PB reasoning faces problems in this area as well. Because of the tendency to separate analyses into considerations of each particular principle in isolation, PB encourages compartmentalized reasoning. If we are concerned with autonomy we focus on individual rights, autonomy, and competency. If we are concerned about beneficence we use a utilitarian calculus to measure costs and benefits. When we speak of justice, we tend to adopt a (roughly) contract model of reasoning; could all concerned rationally accept this outcome? And when these various principles come into conflict, we "weigh" them, though what criteria we use for weighting is not specified.

This description does capture a certain amount of moral reflection. As I have noted, I teach PB reasoning to my students because it is a valuable skill to have. But if we stop there, we will have missed significant features of moral reasoning, precisely because this style of reasoning lends itself too easily to compartmentalized thinking. When the question is one of an individual, whether patient or research subject, our reasoning automatically moves to the autonomy track, then notes whether the person is (or appears to be) competent, and the need for reflection ends when we conclude that the person is competent and that he or she has given consent. But, as mentioned earlier, consent means different things in different contexts, particularly when the power and authority differential between researcher and subject is great.

Again, to pick an example: one aspect of contemporary medicine that produces great frustration in both researchers and health care workers is "noncompliant" patients or subjects. Researchers, physicians, and nurses find it aggravating that subjects can sign up for a project, apparently giving full and informed consent. Their caregivers then arrange for appropriate medications or treatment protocols, or engage in education about the health effects of, say, an unhealthy diet, and follow up, only to find that the patient is not taking the medication or has not made appropriate dietary changes. Obviously, this causes enormous headaches for those trying to acquire data about those medications or dietary changes. Issues of noncompliance are generally slotted under the heading of autonomy. The individual has the information or the medication she or he needs but refuses to comply. And studies of noncompliance often focus on whether the information is too complex, or the regimen of medications too difficult to understand, or whether there are ways of controlling subject behavior to enforce compliance. But treating the problem as purely a matter of autonomy may itself be part of the problem.

Human behavior is affected by factors far beyond the simple issue of whether someone simply chooses to act responsibly or not. One interesting consideration that rarely finds its way into our thinking about autonomous decisions has been raised by some recent studies on violence. In particular, exposure to violence in one's home and neighborhood has a negative impact on health promotion and may increase risky behaviors (Saunders-Phillips 2000). This is important information, because it suggests that there are social and environmental factors that have an impact on people's (apparently) autonomous choices. Women dealing with abusive spouses, for example, may find it hard to follow a medically prescribed diet carefully. Other factors, such as survival, may seem far more central to their day-to-day existence. Or their concern to avoid angering their partner may make following a prescribed diet difficult. Noting social features of individual's lives can alert us to the ways in which simply providing medications or information may not be experienced by a patient or client as help but as an additional duty or burden in the context of a life already too full of struggle. But seeing this requires us to enlarge our field of vision beyond the constraints of autonomy reasoning and to locate individuals in their social and community context.

Care Theory as an Alternative Theoretical Model

What sort of alternative to this abstract, compartmentalized account of bioethical reasoning can we then turn to? One option is care theory, an account of ethics that has been developed in a wide array of contexts but has proven particularly appropriate for deliberation in the health care context (see *inter alia* Tong 1997; MacKenzie and Stoljar 2000; Cates and Lauritzen 2001; and Kittay and Feder 2002).

Care ethics does not offer a set of principles with which to perform calculations about the moral wrongness and rightness of various policies or procedures. Instead, it offers a set of considerations to guide our practical reasoning on particular issues. It begins by noting that ethics cannot be a matter of disinterested reasoning about issues. Ethical reflection begins with care, with an attitude of emotional involvement directed at the good of those affected by the particular issue at hand. Two aspects of care are worth noting here. The first is that care theorists point out that we are always motivationally or emotionally committed in any set of actions or deliberations. Care theory does not require us to add something new to our moral reasoning in this sense. But care theory does require a level of motivational displacement. For deliberation to be done right, it must issue from a commitment to the good of the other. This need not conflict with one's own good, though it sometimes may, nor is it a sentimentalized projection of one's own feeling onto another, though people sometimes confuse this with care.

Care theorists and other philosophers working in the context of moral epistemology have argued convincingly (and some psychologists have offered corroborating evidence) that reasoning, particularly reasoning that involves moral and social issues, is inherently affective (see, for example, Polanyi 1962; Taylor 1985; Code 1991). Without emotional connections one cannot reason accurately, and perhaps one cannot reason at all (Nussbaum 2003; Damasio 2005). (Nothing said here implies, of course, that emotions alone make reasoning good.)

But those of us trained in Western philosophy rarely think of ourselves as emotionally involved when we deliberate about ethical matters. We conceive of ourselves, instead, as impartial, unconnected, logical machines. This self-image provides an effective cover, however, for the emotional commitments that we do have, but to which we can remain blind as long as we portray our reasoning as "impartial reason." What we offer seems to be just the deliverances of some impartial reason, the same conclusion any good thinker would come to if considering this particular issue. This also lets us dismiss anyone who reaches another conclusion—the fact that they differ from us indicates that they failed in logic or reason at some point, because we, impartial reasoners that we are, reached another conclusion.

When, however, we begin with a recognition that all moral reasoning involves emotions and assumed sets of values, it becomes more difficult to represent our own reasoning as pure logic. If we know we start from a particular standpoint, with a particular set of emotional commitments, then those commitments themselves become part of the reasoning process. Insofar as they are foregrounded, then, we are also able (though not guaranteed) to put them under a certain level of critical scrutiny, asking, in particular, to what extent our reasoning assumes the values of our own perspective, to what extent it can adopt a perspective of concern for those who are affected by our reasoning.

As feminist theorists and others have repeatedly pointed out, this is not an easy task. The historical particularity of various groups produces deep areas of disagreement and misunderstanding between them, so that when one (usually privileged) group reasons about another (frequently less privileged), the reasoning assumes all sorts of values, baptizes any number of beliefs as "irrational," and generally produces a one-sided, simplistic, and sometimes unfair result. Further, the recognition that my own reasoning is limited and partisan cannot, by itself, correct the myopia. If my reasoning as a bioethicist is to have any relevance to the values and beliefs of another group, I need to begin with an admission of ignorance. I don't know how the world looks to others, I don't know what sorts of reasoning makes sense to them, and to dictate from my "superior" position how they should understand their ethical situation and options is unbearably patronizing.

But admitting ignorance should push theorists in the direction of trying to learn. If we are concerned to think through issues of public health and difference, then we cannot do this apart from a shared public conversation with the various groups whose difference is at issue. However, this is not the way bioethics is traditionally done. Bioethics, like many other philosophical disciplines, takes place in the privacy of one's office, in the company of a few well-loved books, and to the gentle hum of a computer, the quiet tapping of a keyboard. It is almost shocking to think of conducting philosophical and ethical discussions in public, perhaps in a town meeting or in a community center, with people who do not always follow the ground rules of academic discourse, even more shocking to find out that one's own reasoning may not even seem to have much relevance to other groups. Challenging the dominant view, Cheryl Sanders (1994) points out: "Clearly African-Americans are engaging in biomedical ethical discourse on a daily basis, but not necessarily in ways that that European-Americans would regard as scholarly or even noteworthy. Further, it may be that African-Americans have thoughtfully concluded that Western biomedical ethics is not useful or applicable to their dilemmas precisely because their data and input have not been taken into account."

If we are committed to the notion that bioethics must involve the true incorporation of multiple perspectives, and if we are committed to speaking with others instead of for them, then the isolation that has so often been the status quo in bioethics needs to end. We need to resist any policy development that allows only one perspective to be voiced; we need to think about the ways in which the structures of authority and power in the contemporary world make it hard for multiple perspectives to be heard at the higher levels of policy construction; and we need to begin to learn to hear what is already being discussed in locations far removed from academic conferences and professional journals.

When we return to the issue of research on racial and ethnic differences in various treatment protocols, for example, this model of reason emphasizes the need that researchers and caregivers both have to discuss with subjects or patients their own identification in terms of ethnic and racial background and the reasons why certain protocols might or might not be appropriate for particular groups. While it may seem like an obvious thing for caregivers or researchers to do, the simple step of discussing ethnic background with subjects rather than assigning them, perhaps without their knowledge, to certain categories, would be a significant change from current practices. It is a change, moreover, that signifies a move away from the image of researcher as rational, all-knowing authority and toward an understanding of the research-subject relationship as one to which both parties bring important knowledge.

Acknowledging the value-laden-ness of the search for knowledge also pushes us toward a different standard for the construction of research protocols. The knowledge gained from research on a particular population may not align with the values of the population being studied, and that lack of alignment may be the source of some of the "noncompliance" that causes so many headaches for researchers. A model of incorporating subjects into the planning stages of research when that is possible, including them in the shaping of the values that structure the research as well as the values that structure the outcomes of the research, can sometimes result in subjects who care more about the research and so are committed to following protocols more carefully. This requires a shift in the way we think about research, however, from a model of a powerful, controlling researcher who is the guarantor of the behavior of the subjects studied to a model that assumes that researcher and subjects are both "owners" in some sense of the research and the outcomes.

This brings us to another difference between care theory and a principles-based approach to bioethics. Principles approaches do not automatically generate a recognition for the ways that the power dynamics of a situation can affect both what is admitted into the reasoning process as evidence and how the logic of the situation moves toward a particular conclusion. When, for example, scientists or physicians speak, they are accorded authority, and we rarely stop to question whether they are speaking on a topic on which they have genuine expertise (the rates at which airborne viruses spread) or on a topic on which they are no more expert than the next person (the difficulty of providing care for the homeless). Authority tends to be transitive, and those who are experts in one field often find that the rest of their reasoning is accepted by others as authoritative as well. The opposite is also true; those who are not accorded expertise on the basis of education are often assumed to be incompetent generally, even when they are quite proficient at any number of real-world tasks.

Care theory is sometimes criticized for relying on models of relationships in which the power dynamics are unequal: the parent-child relationship, for example. But as a number of care theorists have pointed out in response to this criticism, relationships in the real world are unequal, and there are always power dynamics at play in social interactions, especially between differently situated ethnic and racial groups. If our ethical theories are to be appropriate to the lives people actually live, they cannot begin with the fiction of absolute equality, nor should they automatically assume that in every case equality is the correct ideal to strive for.

If we begin our moral reasoning with the recognition that power relationships are rarely equal, we can approach disparities without denying them. Care theory offers a way of thinking about the proper uses and misuses of power in various relationships, an analysis that has come from thinking through unequal relationships such as the parent/child relationship, or the caregiver/client relationship in health care. In such a context, care theorists note, power is improperly used when it serves to advance the interests of the powerful at the expense of the vulnerable. (The qualifier is important. It is not the case that any use of power in one's own interests is necessarily bad. It can be morally good. But when it is used at the expense of the weaker partner in a relationship, it is used wrongly.) A similar picture of the proper use of power can be found in Howard Brody's (1992) discussion in *The Healer's Power*, where he argues that those who have power need to begin by owning their power, aim it at appropriate ends, and share it, using it to generate power in the other. When we fail to do this, we are likely to avoid responsibility by denying the power we wield, while simultaneously using it to undermine the other or consolidate our own advantage.

Public policy research, then, requires just this sort of analysis of the structures of decision making. Current systems of public health rely heavily on top-down bureaucratic approaches to decisions about what research will be funded, how it will be disseminated, and what the policy implications will be. Care theory would argue for a more situated structure for decision making, involving community members in decisions about funding allocation, research priorities, and how the research will be used.

Conclusion

But what of the issue with which I began, the problem of how to understand health in a pluralistic way without falling into an unworkable subjectivism? One of the important features of the care theory approach I have been developing here is that it does offer a partial answer to that problem, though not a complete answer. The part of the answer it provides is a move away from isolated individualism as our predominant model of human interaction. PB theories tend to assume a picture of the individual, isolated from everyone and everything in society, confronting the health care system. In that model, of course, the only two loci for a definition of health would be the institution (using a generalized, impersonal measure of health) and the individual (who, isolated and disconnected, can offer only an idiosyncratic or subjective notion to counter the generalized one).

Care theory, on the other hand, offers a picture of deliberation about health that situates people in the context of their families, communities, and social groups. In this model we don't start with a universal statement about abstract individuals; we start with real people who face specific health issues, with limited budgets that can only be used for a finite number of research protocols. In that context of situated reasoning, the notion of health is not free-floating and subjective, but it is also not a bland universal. It can be contested and modified, but it does not start from a vacuum in the way that a completely subjectivist view does.

Community-based (or participatory) research offers a paradigm of how this might work. Community-based research is conducted in partnership with a given community rather than being conducted *on* a community by others unconnected with it (Minkler and Wallerstein 2002; Blumenthal and DiClemente 2003; Heffner, Zandee, and Schwander 2003; Israel et al. 2005). It requires a relationship of partnership and trust between researchers and subjects, and it blurs the boundaries between them as well. It requires more time and more contextualized understanding of the study by both researchers and subjects. Community members are involved at a number of different levels in such research; they help define the questions to be investigated, participate in discussions about methodology, are engaged in regular feedback about the progress of the research, and are one of the target audiences for the resulting reports of research findings.

In this context, community members are able to contribute to the conception of health adopted in particular cases of research, in conversation with those conducting the research. If health is in many ways an instrumental value, then the aims of people in the community are rightly taken into account in determining what health means. At the same time, the specialized knowledge that researchers have, their understanding of disease processes or environmental risks, provides valuable information for the community as it deliberates about which health goals should be of highest priority. The process of deliberation about these issues, while time consuming and sometimes frustrating, is crucial for the production of public health research that meets the needs of the communities in which it is undertaken.

These heavier investments in relationships and time pay off in a number of ways for both communities and researchers. They provide for a higher commitment on the part of the community participants to the research; they make the researchers accountable to the community, and they produce studies that are less likely to overlook significant variables or ignore the contextual nuances of the protocol being studied. Further, the structure of such research prevents an easy assumption on the part of researchers that their own understanding of the situation is correct or complete. Community-based participatory research begins with listening to others, not with telling them how things are.

Care theory offers a better account of moral reasoning in the context of health care than principle-based theory, particularly when we come to issues of public health with their important historical situated-ness, applications to diverse and disagreeing populations, and concerns about the fairness of distributing public funds and benefits, as well as burdens and taxes. But it should be noted that while the theory offers a more nuanced, less cookie-cutter approach to ethics, it cannot, as no theory can, fix the situations we find in the world by itself. Theory cannot change the world. It can open our eyes to changes that could be made, but the actions it recommends remain mere recommendations until and unless we choose to act.

REFERENCES

Alcoff, L. M. 2006. *Visible identities: Race, gender, and the self.* New York: Oxford University Press.

Angell, M. 1997. The ethics of clinical research in the Third World. *New England Journal of Medicine* 337 (Sept. 18): 847–49.

Beauchamp, T. L., and J. F. Childress, eds. 2001. *Principles of biomedical ethics,* 5th ed. New York: Oxford University Press.

Berg, M., and A. Mol, eds. 1998. *Differences in medicine: Unraveling practices, techniques, and bodies.* Durham, N.C.: Duke University Press.

Blumenthal, D., and R. DiClemente, eds. 2003. *Community-based health research: Issues and methods.* New York: Springer.

Brody, H. 1992. *The healer's power.* New Haven, Conn.: Yale University Press.

Cates, D. F., and P. Lauritzen, eds. 2001. *Medicine and the ethics of care.* Washington, D.C.: Georgetown University Press.

Code, L. 1991. *What can she know? Feminist theory and the construction of knowledge.* Ithaca, N.Y.: Cornell University Press.

Coughlin, S. S., C. Soskoline, and K. Goodman. 1997. *Case studies in public health.* Washington, D.C.: American Public Health Association.

Damasio, A. 2005. *Descartes' error: Emotion, reason, and the human brain.* New York: Penguin.

DuBose, E., R. Hammel, and L. O'Connell, eds. 1994. *A matter of principles? Ferment in U.S. bioethics.* Valley Forge, Penn.: Trinity Press International.

Fox, R. 1994. The entry of U.S. bioethics into the 1990s. In *A matter of principles? Ferment in U.S. bioethics,* ed. E. R. DuBose, R. Hamel, and L. O'Connell. Valley Forge, Penn.: Trinity Press International.

Gilligan, C. 1982. *In a different voice: Psychological theory and women's development.* Cambridge, Mass.: Harvard University Press.

Groenhout, R. 2004. *Connected lives: Human nature and an ethics of care.* Lanham, Md.: Rowman & Littlefield.

Hamington, M., and D. Miller, eds. 2006. *Socializing care: Feminist ethics and public policy issues.* Lanham, Md.: Rowman & Littlefield.

Heffner, G. G., G. L. Zandee, and L. Schwander. 2003. Listening to community voices: Community-based research, a first step in partnership and outreach. *Journal of Higher Education Outreach and Engagement* 8 (1): 127–39.

Held, V. 1993. *Feminist morality: Transforming culture, society, and politics.* Chicago: University of Chicago Press.

———. 2006. *The ethics of care: Personal, political, global.* Oxford: Oxford University Press.

Israel, B., E. Eng, A. Schulz, and E. Parker, eds. 2005. *Methods in community-based participatory research for health.* San Francisco: Jossey-Bass.

Jones, J. 1993. *Bad blood: The Tuskegee Syphilis Study.* New York: Free Press.

Jorde, L. B., and S. P. Wooding. 2004. Genetic variation, classification, and "race." *Nature Genetics Supplement* 36 (11): s28–33.

Kittay, E. F. 1999. *Love's labor: Essays on women, equality, and dependency.* New York: Routledge.

Kittay, E. F., and E. K. Feder, eds. 2002. *The subject of care: Feminist perspectives on dependency.* Lanham, Md.: Rowman & Littlefield.

Kolata, G. 2003. Study of two cholesterol drugs finds one halts heart disease. *New York Times,* September 13.

Lackey, D. P. 1993. Commentary on the case study Can a healthy subject volunteer to be injured in research? In *Cases in bioethics: Selections from the Hasting Center Report,* 2nd ed., ed. B.-J. Crigger. New York: St. Martin's Press.

MacKenzie, C., and N. Stoljar. 2000. *Relational autonomy: Feminist perspectives on autonomy, agency, and the social self.* New York: Oxford University Press.

Mann, J., S. Gruskin, M. Grodin, and G. Annas. 1999. *Health and human rights.* New York: Routledge.

Mills, C. W. 1998. *Blackness visible: Essays on philosophy and race.* Ithaca, N.Y.: Cornell University Press.

Minkler, M., and N. Wallerstein, eds. 2002. *Community-based participatory research for health.* San Francisco: Jossey-Bass.

Noddings, N. 1984. *Caring: A feminine approach to ethics and moral education.* Berkeley: University of California Press.

———. 2002. *Starting at home: Caring and social policy.* Berkeley: University of California Press.

Nussbaum, M. 2003. *Upheavals of thought: The intelligence of emotions.* Cambridge: Cambridge University Press.

Pence, G. 2004. *Classic cases in medical ethics,* 4th ed. Boston: McGraw Hill.

Polanyi, M. 1962. *Personal knowledge: Towards a post-critical philosophy.* New York: Harper & Row.

Reverby, S. 2000. *Tuskegee's truths: Rethinking the Tuskegee Syphilis Study.* Chapel Hill: University of North Carolina Press.

Roach, M. III. 2000. Race and health: Implications for health care delivery and promotion. In *Promoting human wellness: New frontiers for research, practice, and policy,* ed. M. S. Jamner and D. Stokols. Berkeley: University of California Press.

Ruddick, S. 1989. *Maternal thinking: Toward a politics of peace.* Boston: Beacon Press.

Sanders, C. J. 1994. European-American ethos and principlism. In *A matter of principles? Ferment in U.S. bioethics,* ed. E. R. DuBose, R. Hamel, and L. O'Connell. Valley Forge, Penn.: Trinity Press International.

Saunders-Phillips, K. 2000. Health promotion in ethnic minority families: The impact of exposure to violence. In *Promoting human wellness: New frontiers for research, practice and policy,* ed. M. S. Jamner and D. Stokols. Berkeley: University of California Press.

Smedley, B. D., A. Y. Stith, and A. R. Nelson, eds. 2003. *Unequal treatment: Confronting racial and ethnic disparities in health care.* Washington, D.C.: National Academies Press.

Spelman, E. V. 1988. *Inessential women: Problems of exclusion in feminist thought.* Boston: Beacon Press.

Taylor, A. L., S. Ziesche, C. Yancy, P. Carson, R. D'Agostino Jr., K. Ferdinand, M. Taylor, et al. for the African-American Heart Failure Trial Investigators. 2004. Combination of isosorbide dinitrate and hydrazaline in blacks with heart failure. *New England Journal of Medicine* 351 (20): 2049–57.

Taylor, C. 1985. Rationality. *Philosophy and the human sciences: Philosophical papers* 2. Cambridge: Cambridge University Press: 134–51.

Tong, R. 1997. *Feminist approaches to bioethics.* Boulder, Colo.: Westview Press.

Waltraud, E., and B. Harris, eds. 1999. *Race, science, and medicine, 1700–1960.* New York: Routledge.

World Health Organization. 1948. *Constitution of the World Health Organization.* www.who.int/governance/eb/who_constitution_en.pdf.

———. 1986. *The Ottawa Charter for Health Promotion.* www.who.int/healthpromotion/conferences/previous/ottawa/en/.

Young, I. M. 2002. Autonomy, welfare reform, and meaningful work. In *The subject of care: Feminist perspectives on dependency,* ed. E. F. Kittay and E. K. Feder. Lanham, Md.: Rowman & Littlefield.

CHAPTER TWELVE

Feminist Bioethics and Indigenous Research Reform in Australia

Is an Alliance across Gender, Racial, and Cultural Borders a Useful Strategy for Promoting Change?

JENNIFER BAKER, PH.D., TERRY DUNBAR, B.B.B.S., M.P.E.&T., AND MARGARET SCRIMGEOUR, ED.D.

This chapter explores the potential of applying feminist bioethics scholarship to support the cross-disciplinary agenda for Indigenous research reform in Australia. Feminist bioethics is a well-established branch of bioethics concerned generally with inequities and the distribution of power in public health processes (Rogers 2006) and, more specifically, the relationship between gender, sex, and ethics in medicine and health care. Similarly, the Indigenous Research Reform Agenda in Australia is concerned with addressing unequal power distribution within the construction of research and the inequitable flow of benefits to Indigenous peoples from health and other research activity.

An alliance between Indigenous peoples in Australia and feminist bioethicists could open up new ways of disclosing the marginalizing influence that mainstream research institutions and their representatives continue to have on the interests of Indigenous peoples. The bioethical center in Australia (represented principally by the National Health and Medical Research Council and associated higher education institutions) must somehow be convinced that research that positions Indigenous peoples as "objects" of inquiry should be regarded as exploitative and unlikely to lead to sustainable and positive change.

The absence of a shared language or framework for considering fundamental differences between Indigenous and mainstream concepts of research and bioethics is one of the most immediate and challenging issues to be addressed. Those involved in the development of feminist bioethics have argued for many years that the rights of minority and marginalized groups must be upheld through public health and institutional reform and to this end have developed theoretical frameworks to support their case for change. It might prove useful, therefore, for Indigenous peoples to draw on the experience of those involved in the international field of feminist bioethics to convince members of the mainstream research establishment in Australia of the need for fundamental changes to the way Indigenous research is ethically assessed and conducted.

We begin our discussion by outlining key elements of the Indigenous Research Reform Agenda and then draw on the history of engagement between Indigenous peoples and feminist movements in Australia to indicate some possible barriers to the development of alliances between these groups into the future. We then identify some connections between Indigenous conceptions of bioethics and feminist bioethical theories that may provide the basis for mutually beneficial future collaborations.

The Indigenous Research Reform Agenda

Historically, mainstream research institutions and their representatives have taken a leading role in identifying and determining the cause of a wide range of Indigenous "problems" in Australia. This situation has resulted in the positioning of Indigenous peoples as objects of inquiry and recipients of Western philanthropy. Over the past thirty years, Indigenous representatives have advocated fundamental reform of health research involving Indigenous interests. This advocacy for change has hinged on the argument that the mainstream research community lacks the necessary commitment and capacity to deliver on the promise of improved health and social outcomes for Indigenous peoples in exchange for their cooperation as research stakeholders and subjects.

In recent years, the research reform agenda has extended from the health field to include a range of social science disciplines. This evolving and cross-disciplinary reform agenda is underpinned by a commitment to the principles of Indigenous self-determination and an argument for due recognition of Indigenous cultural authority, knowledge, diverse cultural protocols, priorities, and values within the construction of research (Humphery 2000; Anderson, Griew, and McAullay 2003; Henry et al. 2004). Promoting Indigenous participation in all aspects of research, including deliberations over proposals for research, represents a cornerstone of the reform agenda.

Despite sustained advocacy and the intervention of structural support in some fields, progress toward improving the flow of benefits from research to Indigenous peoples remains slow. Institutional support for the advancement of Indigenous priorities and ways of doing research remain inadequate, and reform proposals do not seem to be gaining significant traction within the mainstream research community. In the health research field for example, Indigenous peoples continue to question the value of research with limited potential for delivering tangible benefits to Indigenous participants. Indigenous health research activity in Australia has been described by various commentators as seriously damaging, insensitive, intrusive, and exploitative (Dodson 2000; Thomas 2004).

Michael Dodson (2000), a former Aboriginal and Torres Strait Islander Social Justice Commissioner in Australia, warned against the complacency of considering exploitative research practices a thing of the past. Commenting on human genome research in Australia, he pointed out that the human rights and cultural values of Indigenous peoples were potentially compromised by the conduct of the International Human Genome Diversity Project (HGDP). Dodson argued that the HGDP is little more than another example of the colonialism and exploitation that characterizes the clash between Indigenous and non-Indigenous people for centuries. According to Dodson, throughout the HGDP, the dominant discourse of Western science asserted its authority over marginalized knowledge such as that of Indigenous peoples.

Uneven progress toward the achievement of research reform in Australia is attributed by some commentators to the maintenance of unsupportive institutional processes for the governance and ethical assessment of proposals for Indigenous research. It has been argued, for example, that local Indigenous priorities and values are underrepresented within the ethical assessment of Indigenous research. This situation contributes significantly to the ongoing marginalization of Indigenous interests within the research process (Anderson, Griew, and McAullay 2003; Gillam and Pyett 2003).

Investigator-driven research that proceeds with scant reference to Indigenous priorities and Indigenous values remains the main paradigm for research across a range of academic disciplines in Australia. The question of who should initiate research in Indigenous community contexts is central to the resolution of tensions between Indigenous advocates for research reform and the so-called research establishment. Reform proponents argue strongly that the establishment of Indigenous health research priorities should be located within the control of the community-based Indigenous health sector (Anderson 1996). This approach is supported to help achieve a closer alignment between the interests of researchers and the interests of Indigenous peoples (Henry et al. 2004).

Although not commonly disclosed, researcher resistance to increased levels of Indigenous involvement in research activity is cited as a possible reason for the persistent marginalization of Indigenous interests (Dunbar and Scrimgeour 2006). In this regard, some commentators do not accept that the research reform process has gone far enough to protect the interests of Indigenous peoples. Commenting on the situation in New Zealand, Tuhiwai Smith, a Maori academic, points out that "clearly, there have been some shifts in the way non-Indigenous researchers and academics have positioned themselves and their work in relation to the people for whom the research still counts. It is also clear, however, that there are powerful groups of researchers who resent Indigenous people asking questions about their research and whose research paradigms constantly permit them to exploit Indigenous peoples and their knowledges" (Tuhiwai Smith 1999, 17).

Indigenous research reform advocates argue that the expertise of outsider researchers should be positioned as complementary to the cultural authority and knowledge of local Indigenous peoples and that the development of Indigenous research capability should be a central aspect of collaborative efforts. In summary, the current positioning of Indigenous research reform advocates in Australia includes commitments to

- reject institutionalized research approaches that have historically marginalized the knowledge, perspectives, and values of Indigenous peoples;
- adopt research approaches that have a capacity for sustainable community development;
- adopt research approaches that are more respectful of Indigenous values and inclusive of Indigenous knowledge and worldviews; and
- support the development of Indigenous research capacity and the development of systems to ensure that the management of research is under Indigenous community control. (Humphery 2000; Henry et al., 2004)

Although the level of Indigenous representation within the organization of the National Health and Medical Research Council (NHMRC) has increased in Australia over recent years, and new guidelines for Indigenous health research have been developed and implemented, commentators still argue that current institutional structures inadequately provide for representation of local Indigenous community interests in the ethical assessment of research (Gillam and Pyett, 2003; Dunbar and Scrimgeour 2006). In addition, there is continuing concern that mainstream investigator-driven research agendas still dominate in the health research field (Henry et al. 2004a). This situation continues despite the existence of nominated Indigenous health research priority areas within both the National Aboriginal and Torres Strait Islander Health Council Health Strategy (National Aboriginal and Torres Strait Islander Health Council 2002) and the RAWG Road Map, a strategic framework for the development of a health research agenda (National Health and Medical Research Council 2002).

An NHMRC publication, *Keeping Research on Track: A Guide for Aboriginal and Torres Strait Islander Peoples about Health Research* (National Health and Medical Research Council 2005) aims to provide guidance to Indigenous community members engaging with outsider health researchers. The stated aim of the document is to "help people to become familiar with the stages in the research journey. It helps us to understand the steps that we need to follow in order to make research work for us" (National Health and Medical Research Council 2005).

Mounting pressures from the forces of globalization and the past eleven years of aggressive assimilation policy under the previous Federal Liberal government are just two possible reasons why an Indigenous position on the reform of research practice and ethical assessment of research has been slow to gain traction in Australia. Clearly, Indigenous reform objectives based on the promotion of Indigenous self-determination and the recognition of cultural diversity between and within Indigenous communities are not compatible with a mainstreaming policy approach and the associated homogenizing influence of globalization.

In an interview entitled "Finding a Moral Compass—The Notion of Core Values in the Face of Pluralism and Globalisation," Hogan (2005), a feminist commentator, pointed out that within the most unfettered forms of globalization, Western practices are advanced endlessly, which in turn leads to "the creation of homogenised systems of thought that can wipe out local cultures, local languages, local social structures, and often livelihoods as well" (5). Hogan's observation is a sobering reminder to Indigenous peoples and other minority and marginalized groups in society, of the urgency associated with the project to assert their authority over research dominated by mainstream community and global corporate interests.

If the agenda for research reform is to be successfully advanced in Australia, mainstream institutions, funding providers, and those responsible for the ethical assessment of research must somehow be convinced of the need to change long-standing approaches to the funding, brokerage, ethical assessment, and conduct of Indigenous research. In particular, there is a pressing need to disclose the way collective and individual Indigenous interests are routinely marginalized through research processes that deny the reality of individual and community Indigenous agency.

The History of Engagement between Indigenous Peoples in Australia and Feminist Movements

Formal engagement between Indigenous women in Australia and feminist movements has been minimal (Bergman 1984). In the 1980s, Bergman attributed this situation to the widespread belief among Indigenous women that the concentration by feminists on women's rights was irrelevant and that the oppressive forces of racism was a more pressing issue in their lives. During this time, Pat O'Shane (an Indigenous lawyer) reportedly referred to the existence of a tremendous spirit of sisterhood among Aboriginal women. Bergman (1984) suggested that this "collective solidarity" amounted almost to "hostility against outsiders" (35).

The emergence of an agenda for reform of Indigenous research in Australia coincides with a small but significantly increased representation of Indigenous peoples in upper levels of the academic hierarchy. Critical analysis conducted by this group of academics continues to challenge dominant assumptions about the nature of Indigenous disadvantage and has led to proposals for new frameworks of engagement between the academy, government agencies, and key service providers to the broader Indigenous community. Within this context, the potential represented by feminist theoretical frameworks for advancing the sociopolitical reform agendas of Indigenous peoples has also come under scrutiny.

Indigenous women in Australia have argued that feminist movements remain dominated by the interests of Western women and that feminist theoretical frameworks provide an inadequate basis for the advancement of Indigenous positions on key social, health, and well-being issues (Moreton-Robinson 2000, 2003; Smallacombe 2004). This positioning is also common among representatives of minority group interests internationally. It is argued, for example, that many "feminisms" promote the notion of a generic woman who is white and middle class and that historically women of color have not been engaged as full participants in white feminist organizations (Collins 2000).

A debate in Australia during the late 1980s over the right of a non-Aboriginal self-described feminist researcher to publicly disclose a sensitive cultural issue involving abuse of Aboriginal women in a remote Northern Territory community marked a significant turning point in relations between Aboriginal women and Western feminists in Australia. An already strained relationship became openly hostile. This debate (commonly referred to as the Bell-Huggins debate) led to contestation over representation rights and contained reference to the application of racially blind frameworks for analyzing complex social and cultural issues, the adoption by outsider researchers of exclusionary and unrepresentative agendas, contravention of Indigenous cultural integrity and privacy, and insufficient regard for the primacy of Indigenous knowledge (Moreton-Robinson 2003).

In a book entitled *Talkin' Up to the White Woman: Indigenous Women and Feminism* (2000), Moreton-Robinson (an Indigenous academic) argued that white Australian feminist theory has traditionally centered on notions of whiteness. She also suggested that white middle-class feminists use race privilege to write about their gendered oppression, while whiteness remains "invisible, unnamed and unmarked in their work" (2000, 42). More recently, Moreton-Robinson (2003) argued against engagement between Indigenous women and white feminists in Australia on the following basis: "If we enter feminism and its debates, it is not on our own terms, but on the terms of White feminists whose race confers dominance and privilege. What sort of sisterhood can be constructed when we begin from such unequal positions within a politics that defines our racial difference yet masks its own?" (77).

In an article entitled "Speaking Positions on Indigenous Violence," Indigenous academic Sonia Smallacombe (2004, 54) points out that she regards herself as "Indigenous first and as a woman second." In her view, this difference in perspective and priorities for action sets many Indigenous women apart from their Western feminist counterparts. She explains that while Indigenous women must continue to fight within their own communities for gender equality, the primary focus right now has to be on "healing the dignity of our people and our communities" (54). Further, Smallacombe argues for the right of Indigenous women to make choices and decisions in ways that "heal ourselves and our cultural identity" (54).

The charge by minority group members that some feminists actively promote forms of "cultural essentialism" is an important issue underlying tensions between Indigenous women and their non-Indigenous counterparts in Australia. The practice of homogenizing Indigenous experience supports the broader mainstreaming agenda of government and reflects a poor understanding of the substantial differences between and within Indigenous cultural groups. Internationally, commentators such as Narayan (1998) have also argued that feminist efforts to avoid gender essentialism have led to a cultural essentialism that effectively denies the heterogeneous nature of some cultural groups.

Connections between Indigenous Conceptions of Bioethics and Feminist Bioethical Theorizing

Contemporary feminist bioethics has emerged as an international movement over the last decade and is distinguished by concerns about the representation of feminist perspectives in research (Beauchamp and Childress 2001). Feminists working in bioethics share significant commonalities, both in their criticisms of dominant structures and in their efforts to build a more adequate framework that is responsive to the disparate situations of women and other groups whose health needs are underrepresented (Donchin 2004). According to Donchin, the development of a distinctively feminist approach to bioethics integrates insights of the women's health movement with cross-disciplinary analysis of structural relationships that divide and marginalize people.

Until now, feminist bioethics has focused mainly upon theoretical analyses and the identification and description of gender-related issues in health and connected fields, and there has been little examination of the ways that feminist bioethics scholarship can influence policy and practice (Rogers 2006). The development of alliances between feminists and other minority and marginalized groups, such as Indigenous peoples, might open the way for feminist bioethical theories to be usefully applied as the basis for challenging mainstream institutional research policies and practices.

The initiative to incorporate the concerns of Indigenous peoples and other minority groups into feminist bioethical theorizing signals an important shift in focus. Holmes (1999) explains the necessity for this shift as follows: "The practice of bioethics has been defined by its context (hospitals) and practitioners (essentially, doctors and their friends). Women in the field have done little to provide a unique shape to bioethics and... the field could change if the needs and concerns of those commonly left out of the ethics committee room: the sick, lower-echelon health care workers, women, and other marginalized groups were taken seriously" (47).

Before we can chart a course for Indigenous peoples and feminists to work together over bioethical issues, it is necessary to identify some points of similarity and difference in approach. As feminists we need to ask how this important groundwork can be carried out. Of central importance is the thorny question of representation rights. As discussed in the previous section, the relationship between Indigenous women and feminists in Australia seems to have stalled over unresolved tensions involving representation rights and alleged breaches of trust.

The positioning of feminist researchers in relation to those who are marginalized is raised by Sharpe and Spivak (2002), who suggest that it is important to earn the trust of research participants. They also warn that fieldwork involving outsider feminists and minority and marginalized peoples is not just about creating and sharing discourse with academic peers. Instead, they remind researchers that "you are a person who is clearly not a subaltern person, who has moved into a group which clearly is subaltern with no kind of mobility. And you are earning trust so that you can do whatever it is that you are there to do" (Sharpe and Spivak 2002, 612).

Further, they remind feminists that doing "whatever it is you are there to do" (usually in the service of the state or a research institution) requires a mindfulness about community that for most Indigenous academics and researchers in Australia is part of the politics of their identity, arising from a shared history of colonial oppression. It is not necessarily an experience easily understood by most non-Indigenous researchers. For Indigenous researchers, the interests of community are high on the agenda, and community perspectives are given priority. Such a close connection to community may be unfamiliar to many Western-trained researchers, and when they do not accept that community interests are central to research practice, an invisible form of silencing or marginalizing is taking place.

The wariness and thoughtfulness demonstrated by Indigenous researchers may be misinterpreted by their non-Indigenous colleagues (who are often positioned as outsiders to the world of Indigenous affairs) as a lack of confidence and authority. This attitude, however, is evidence of an approach that is not individualistic and that places primary emphasis on protecting and respecting wider Indigenous community interests. As Collins (1997) reminds us, "Individualism continues as a taproot in Western theorizing, including feminist versions" (375).

A problem to be negotiated when considering alliances across racial, cultural, and gender borders over bioethical issues is one of definition. It is apparent, for example, that when feminists and Indigenous peoples in Australia talk about bioethics, they do not always mean the same thing. Garvey et al. (2004) disclose the potential for misunderstanding by suggesting that "the terms 'ethics' and 'bioethics' are not evident within Aboriginal cultures because the ethical convictions that form these cultures cannot be dissociated from them" (571). Instead, Garvey and colleagues argue that Indigenous values are woven through the very fabric of Aboriginal cultures and that "Aboriginal societies do not differentiate bioethics or the process of healthcare decision making from the values, narratives, and contexts that define and structure all dimensions of living" (571).

There are some points of connection between an "ethics of care" described within feminist bioethics theory and the notion of "accountability to others" referred to by Indigenous commentators in Australia. Accountability in this context is considered in terms of relationship, reciprocity, and community responsibility, which are identified as being fundamental to Indigenous cultural life (National Health and Medical Research Council 2003; Garvey et al. 2004; Henry, Houston, and Mooney 2004). The concept of an "Aboriginal ethic of accountability to others" relates closely to the pivotal role of "community" in Indigenous cultural life. Communitarianism in Aboriginal society contributes to the care and nurture of others with whom they are related, and within Indigenous societies, commitment to communitarianism is a mechanism for ensuring that personal behavior remains socially grounded (Henry, Houston, and Mooney 2004). This is a point that seems to be lost on those who represent the bioethical center of research in Australia. There is a persistent lack of regard for the central importance of involving Indigenous community representatives in decisions about research that involves Indigenous interests.

Feminist accounts of care ethics derive from the philosophical tradition of virtue ethics, which incorporates virtues that it is claimed are exemplified by women, such as those necessary for taking care of others, including patience, ability to nurture, and self-sacrifice (Donchin and Purdy 1999). Commenting on the implications of care ethics for colonized peoples internationally, Narayan (1995) warns that the concept of "care" may alienate some minority group members who associate it with the paternalistic "caring" practiced by colonizers.

In Australia, the failure by successive Australian governments to "care" for Indigenous peoples has had devastating consequences. The forced removal of Indigenous children from their families (which occurred until the 1960s), and the continuing level of Indigenous poverty, leading to drastically shortened life expectancy, provide justification for Indigenous community suspicion about the colonial notion of "care." There is also a danger that a focus on the role of women in "caring" may draw attention away from the oppressive nature of neoliberalcolonial state rule for Indigenous peoples and the politically driven advancement of mainstreaming policy agendas.

An awareness of histories of oppression that have in fact privileged the development of Western notions of science in a range of global contexts suggests the need to focus on an ethics of justice as well as an ethics of care (Lange 1998). Narayan (1995) argues for the development of this dual focus in the following way: "I point to a colonial care discourse that enabled colonizers to define themselves in relation to 'inferior' colonized subjects. The colonized however had very different accounts of this relationship. While contemporary care discourse correctly insists on acknowledging human needs and relationships, it needs to worry about who defines these often contested terms. I conclude that improvements along dimensions of care and justice often provide 'enabling' conditions for each other" (133).

The potential effectiveness of an ethics of care, relative to an ethics of justice, as the basis for theorizing the positioning of marginalized and minority groups over bioethical issues is a source of debate (Narayan 1995; McClure 1999; Hogan 2005). Hogan (2005), for example, argues that an ethics of care draws attention to the values of interconnectedness and relatedness, whereas the language of human rights can provide excessive focus on the individual as the center of rights and responsibilities. Hogan does not propose the concept of care as an alternative to justice considerations but more as "a corrective to the disinterested and abstract concerns that the rhetoric of justice might contain" (2005, 13). These collaborations require acts of "border crossing" by Indigenous peoples and feminists across cultural, racial, and gender boundaries. This process is recognized as being complex, contradictory, and sometimes stressful for individuals (Anzaldua and Moraga 1983; Anzaldua 1987; Gaard 2001; Crawford 2003). Commenting on the experience of Indigenous women in Australia, Crawford (2003) warns that "constant border-crossings can cause subjects to feel so fragmented that a despairing immobility can take hold. Indigenous women in Australia must juggle the priorities of their survival in the personal and public sense, taking risks for land, for histories, families, feminisms, sexualities and cultures" (172). The problem remains that minority group members engaged in acts of border crossing can be marginalized and negatively affected in inadvertent ways by feminists with good intentions, and mainstream feminists can be demoralized when their good intentions are not met with trust.

We anticipate that those individuals currently engaged in the project to improve the responsiveness of the bioethical center in Australia to the diverse concerns of Indigenous peoples may support an informal alliance with feminist bioethics. There is a pressing need to identify a bioethical framework capable of disclosing the intersecting oppressions of race, gender, and globalization and then to apply this framework as the basis for promoting Indigenous community involvement in all stages of the research process.

Conclusion

In this chapter we have touched on some points of similarity and difference between Indigenous and feminist concerns over bioethics. For example, more detailed analysis of convergences between feminist conceptions of a "care ethics" and an Indigenous notion of "accountability to others" is required. The potential effectiveness of an ethics of care relative to an ethics of justice as a vehicle for promoting Indigenous concerns about bioethics must be debated as well. It is also important that ongoing Indigenous concerns regarding representation rights are addressed. After all, a commitment to the appropriate representation of Indigenous interests is at the heart of Indigenous calls for reform of research practice in Australia.

In their efforts to challenge the bioethical "center" over the way minority group interests are considered within the ethical assessment of research, feminists and Indigenous peoples in Australia share a common purpose. A proposed alliance between these two broad groups comes at a time when Indigenous advocates are struggling to challenge the mainstream research establishment on a number of fronts. In the Indigenous health research field, intervention by advocates from within the NHMRC establishment, from representatives of Indigenous community-controlled organizations, and from Indigenous academics has resulted in Indigenous concerns about research ethics and research methodology gaining a higher profile. There is no question, however, that there is still a long way to go before Indigenous peoples in Australia are positioned as the main beneficiaries of research in which they participate.

An informal alliance between the International Network for Feminist Approaches to Bioethics and Indigenous peoples could provide access to international forums in which the representation of minority and marginalized group interests in research is given serious consideration. The development of an alliance across difference is a complex undertaking, and the proposed alliance between feminists and Indigenous peoples over bioethical issues is likely to generate contestation in Australia. However, an alliance with feminist bioethics represents a valuable opportunity for advancing a reform agenda based on the premise that the mainstream research establishment must change the way it deals with Indigenous concerns if the promised benefits from research are to flow to Indigenous peoples.

REFERENCES

Anderson, I. 1996. Ethics and health research in Aboriginal communities. In *Ethical intersections: Health research, methods and researcher responsibility*, ed. J. Daly, 153–65. Sydney: Allen & Unwin.
Anderson, I., R. Griew, and D. McAullay. 2003. Ethics guidelines, health research and Indigenous Australians. *New Zealand Bioethics Journal* 4:20–27.
Anzaldua, G. 1987. *Borderlands la frontera: The new mestiza*. San Francisco: Aunt Lute.
Anzaldua, G., and C. Moraga. 1983. *This bridge called my back: Writings by radical women of color*. New York: Kitchen Table: Women of Color Press (first published in 1981).
Beauchamp, T. L., and J. F. Childress, eds. 2001. *Principles of biomedical ethics,* 5th ed. New York: Oxford University Press.
Bergman, M. 1984. Black sisterhood: The situation of urban Aboriginal women and their relationship to the white women's movement. In *Australian women and the political system,* ed. M. Simms, 20–47. Melbourne: Longman Cheshire. 1984.
Collins, P. H. 1997. Comments on Hekman's *Truth and Method*: Feminist standpoint theory revisited: Where's the power? *Signs* 22 (2): 375–81.

————. 2000. *Black feminist thought: Knowledge, consciousness, and the politics of empowerment.* New York: Routledge.

Crawford, J. 2003. *Culture, risk and belonging: Black women write Australia.* Ph.D. thesis, Department of English and Cultural Studies, University of Melbourne.

Dodson, M. 2000. Human genetics: Control of research and sharing of benefits, *Australian Aboriginal Studies* (Spring-Fall): 56–71.

Donchin, A. 2004. Feminist bioethics. In *The Stanford encyclopedia of philosophy,* ed. E. N. Zalta.

Donchin, A., and L. Purdy, eds. 1999. *Embodying bioethics: Recent feminist advances.* New York: Rowman & Littlefield.

Dunbar, T., and M. Scrimgeour. 2006. Ethics in Indigenous research—Connecting with community. *Journal of Bioethical Enquiry* 3 (3): 179–85.

Gaard, G. 2001. Tools for a cross-cultural feminist ethics: Exploring ethical contexts and contents in the Makah whale hunt. *Hypatia* 16 (1): 1–26.

Garvey, G., P. Towney, J. McPhee, M. Little, and I. Kerridge. 2004. Is there an Aboriginal bioethic? *Journal of Medical Ethics* 30:570–75.

Gillam, L., and P. Pyett. 2003. A commentary on the NH&MRC draft values and ethics in Aboriginal and Torres Strait Islander health research. *Monash Bioethics Review* 22 (4): 8–19.

Grossman, M., ed. 2003. *Blacklines: Contemporary critical writing by Indigenous Australians.* Carlton, Victoria: Melbourne University Press.

Henry, B., S. Houston, and G. Mooney. 2004. Institutional racism in Australian healthcare: A plea for decency. *Medical Journal of Australia* 180 (10): 517–20.

Henry, J., T. Dunbar, A. Arnott, M. Scrimgeour, and L. Murakami Gold. 2004. Links Monograph 5: *Indigenous Research Reform Agenda—A review of the literature.* Darwin: CRC for Aboriginal Health.

Hogan, L. 2005. *Finding a moral compass—The notion of core values in the face of pluralism and globalisation.* Transcript, Radio National Encounter, March 20. www.abc.net.au/rn/relig/enc/stories/s1323408.htm.

Holmes, H. B. 1999. Closing the gaps: An imperative for feminist bioethics. In *Embodying bioethics: Recent feminist advances,* ed. A. Donchin, and L. Purdy, 45–64. New York: Rowman & Littlefield.

Humphery, K. 2000. *Indigenous health and Western research.* Vic Health Koori Health Research and Community Development Unit Discussion Paper 2.

Lange, E. A. 1998. Fragmented ethics of justice: Freire, liberation theology and pedagogies for the non-poor. *Convergence: International Journal for Adult Education* (Invitation by Peter Mayo to special tribute issue for Paulo Freire): 31 (1–2): 81–94.

McClure, M. A. 1999. Responding to difference: Engaging multicultural/postcolonial concerns and revisiting an ethic of care. *APA Newsletter* 98 (2).

Moreton-Robinson, A. 2000. *Talkin' up to the white woman: Indigenous women and feminism.* St. Lucia: University of Queensland Press.

————. 2003. Tiddas talkin' up to the white woman: When Huggins et al. took on Bell. In *Blacklines: Contemporary critical writing by Indigenous Australians,* ed. M. Grossman, 66–77. Carlton, Victoria: Melbourne University Press.

Narayan, U. 1995. Colonialism and its other: Considerations on rights and care discourses. *Hypatia* 10 (2): 133–40.

———. 1998. Essence of culture and a sense of history: A feminist critique of cultural essentialism. *Hypatia* 13 (2): 86–106.

National Aboriginal and Torres Strait Islander Health Council. 2002. *National Aboriginal and Torres Strait Islander health strategy.* Canberra: NATSIHC.

National Health and Medical Research Council. 1999a. *National statement on the ethical conduct of research involving humans and supplementary notes.* Canberra: NHMRC.

———. 1999b. *Human research ethics handbook.* Canberra: NHMRC.

———. 2001. *Human research ethics handbook: Commentary on the National statement on ethical conduct in research involving humans.* Canberra: NHMRC.

———. 2002. Aboriginal and Torres Strait Islander Research Agenda Working Group (RAWG). *The NHMRC road map: A strategic framework for improving Aboriginal and Torres Strait Islander health through research.* Canberra: NHMRC.

———. 2003. *Values and ethics: Guidelines for ethical conduct in Aboriginal and Torres Strait Islander health research.* Canberra: NHMRC.

———. 2005. *Keeping research on track: A guide for Aboriginal and Torres Strait Islander peoples about health research ethics.* Canberra: NHMRC.

Rogers, W. 2006. Feminism and public health ethics. *Journal of Medical Ethics* 32:351–54.

Sharpe, J., and G. Spivak. 2002. A conversation with Gayatri Chakravorty Spivak: Politics and the imagination. *Signs* 28 (2): 609–24.

Simms, M., ed. 1984. *Australian women and the political system.* Melbourne: Longman Cheshire.

Smallacombe, S. 2004. Speaking positions on Indigenous violence. *Hecate* 30 (1): 47–55.

Thomas, D. 2004. *Reading doctors' writing: Race, politics and power in Indigenous health research, 1870–1969.* Canberra: Aboriginal Studies Press.

Tuhiwai Smith, L. 1999. *Decolonizing methodologies: Research and Indigenous peoples.* London: Zed Books.

CHAPTER THIRTEEN

China's Birth Control Program through Feminist Lenses

JING-BAO NIE, PH.D.

A Massive Project of Social Engineering

Two human miracles have occurred China in the past three decades—one economic and the other demographic. The historic economic takeoff and the sharp fertility decline have transformed Chinese society to a far greater extent than Mao's total revolution and left the world in wonder, even shock. They have various international impacts as well, evidently and potentially.

In the very period of withered planned economy and relaxed state control over society, the Chinese Party–government has been forcefully promoting state-planned reproduction, *jihua shengyu* (literally, "planned reproduction," officially translated as "family planning"). Along with the reintroduction of a laissez-faire market economy systematically abolished in Mao's era, the establishment of a wholesale population program constitutes the centerpiece of a far-reaching reform agenda initiated in the late 1970s. While it is commonly known as *dusheng zinü* or *yitai hua* ("the one-child policy"), this ideal—one child per couple—has essentially been implemented in urban areas only, never universally, partly due to persistent resistance in various forms by many rural residents. From the beginning, the Chinese program had two interrelated goals: controlling the *quantity* and improving or enhancing the *quality* of the population. Its ultimate objective is to produce "fewer but healthier births," as tersely projected in the household slogan, *shaosheng yousheng*.

The Chinese state has been rigorously carrying out population control as the "long-term, fundamental, and strategic" national policy essential to the prosperity and strength of the nation as well as to the welfare of families, individuals, and future generations. The scheme has been advocated and designed by the elite and strongly supported by the educated stratum. Birth control has been enshrined in

Chinese law through major national legislation including the Marriage Law in 1980, the Constitution in 1982, and especially the first national Law on Birth Planning that came into effect in 2002. While changing social and political circumstances are likely to require modifications to the policy as its demographic implications become clearer and as the pressures for reform grow stronger, national leaders and official documents have made it crystal clear that restrictive national family planning policies will continue into the future in China.

The Chinese birth control program represents a giant and quintessential project of social engineering. It is the most ambitious, intrusive, and effective demographic initiative ever undertaken in human history. It has profoundly altered every dimension of Chinese society—personal, interpersonal, familial, institutional, political, economic, societal, and cultural. Just as the economic miracle has a heavy human, social, and environmental price, the extraordinary demographic success has been achieved at extraordinary human and social costs. The far-reaching consequences—positive and negative, intended and unintended—include the prevention of an estimated 200 million or more births (the official claim is more than 300 million) and a deficit of 40 million female babies (not merely due to the population policy).

China's birth control program has engendered positive and negative responses worldwide. On the one hand, the international community has highly commended the Chinese government's efforts at population control and offered financial support to China through various channels. As early as 1983, the United Nations granted the then commissioner of China's family-planning program its prestigious inaugural awards for population control. On the other hand, this program and especially the means employed to implement it have provoked serious concerns, intense criticism, and even straightforward condemnation in the West —as shown in extensive media coverage and parliamentary or congressional hearings. Western attention has been centered on reports of forced abortion and compulsory sterilization, viewed as an insult to human life and individual liberty. Outraged by the coercive nature and practice of the program, scholars and politicians have used such phrases as "the most draconian [program] since King Herod's slaughter of the innocents" (Aird 1990, 1) and "doubly dehumanizing" (Subcommittee on International Operations and Human Rights, 1998, 6). At the same time, the large number of demographic, medical (public health), anthropological, sociological, and historical studies are emblematic of the enduring academic interest in the subject in the West (for two comprehensive Western reviews, see Banister 1987 and Scharping 2003; for a more recent overview in English, see Zhao and Guo 2007).

Challenges for Ethics and Feminism

Surprisingly and disturbingly, there is a dearth of serious ethical studies of the Chinese program as applied to both quantitative control and qualitative improvement (eugenics) through addressing perennial human values and the moral quandaries surrounding human reproduction, and at the same time attending to *guoqing* (Chinese sociopolitical reality and cultural traditions). This is surprising because a high moral tone has often been adopted by both the Chinese government and its Western supporters and critics alike and because so many thorny moral and political issues are raised by such an immense social scheme. It is disturbing because as history has tragically illustrated again and again, without careful attention to their moral and social predicaments, large-scale state projects of social engineering have often resulted in massive destruction of life, property, institutions, values, and the natural environment, however good or noble their intentions may have been.

Both demography as a discipline and population control as a worldwide social enterprise have so far given no substantial attention to ethics. Two major comprehensive and updated references on population—*Encyclopedia of Population* (Demeny and McNicoll 2003) and *Handbook of Population* (Poston and Micklin 2006) reveal an absence of ethical concerns: neither work carries an article on moral issues in demography and population control. The former has dropped the article on ethics that originally appeared in its previous edition, *International Encyclopedia of Population*, although both have articles on gender and feminist perspectives.

The strongest and most insightful critical voice on population control, including the Chinese program, has come from women and men who see the realities of the issue and seek political change through the perspectives of gender. Reproduction has probably been the most prominent item on the agenda of international feminism, an increasingly influential political-cultural movement and a dynamic academic field. In theory, feminism has made gender into a significant, if not central, category of analysis in demography as a discipline over the past two decades or so (for a review, see Riley 2005). In practice, since the 1990s it has refocused global attention from population control to reproductive rights and women's well-being, as demonstrated in the landmark 1994 U.N. International Conference on Population and Development (ICPD) in Cairo and in the 1995 World Congress of Women in Beijing (Eager 2004).

Nevertheless, the Chinese population program has been a "vexed issue" for feminism, in the words of Susan Greenhalgh (2001, 847), a leading feminist anthropologist and population expert. Fifteen years ago, the authors of a publication on population and feminism in the global South, produced in association with the international network Development Alternatives with Women for a New Era (DAWN), found it "interesting" that "few feminists have evaluated the Chinese policy" (Corrêa and Reichmann 1994, 26). Although this deplorable situation has significantly improved following the appearance in the past decade of pioneering feminist studies of China's birth control program, today, at a time when the policy has been in effect for nearly three decades, substantial feminist ethical inquiries into the Chinese program are still lacking.

It is even more surprising and disturbing that feminist political and scholarly engagement with the Chinese program is far from adequate. For the program has impinged on the life of virtually every Chinese woman—more than one-fifth of the world's female population. This inadequacy is obviously a result of an array of political, intellectual, and practical obstacles. Among them is the ideological polarization and conflict aroused by the subject. As Greenhalgh pointed out, "Although the gender violence perpetrated in the name of urgent demographic goals marks the one-child policy as an important focus of feminist critique, the contradictory, highly ideological discourses circulating around the policy complicate and discourage feminist engagements with it." Feminists are "wedged between an antitotalitarian, China-demonizing discourse emerging from conservative forces in the United States and an anti-Western, U.S.-demonizing discourse emanating from some elements of the party in China" (2001, 847). The sociocultural and intellectual barriers to accessing information, especially from Chinese women, or the lived experiences and views of other involved parties, form formidable obstacles to adequate feminist engagement. Feminism, often treated as too radical in the West, has been seen as too Western—if not a part of Western cultural imperialism and thus irrelevant and reprehensible—in the non-Western world. In other words, like the powerful political and intellectual discourse of human rights, feminism is too often perceived as merely a Western invention—so feminist critiques of the Chinese population control program are readily disregarded as culturally alien to China. Despite the inclusive tendency of feminism, its Western dominance means that the voices of women in non-Western countries are far from well heeded by global feminism.

Mainstream bioethics has produced only scattered literature on population ethics and policy (e.g., Callahan 1971, Veatch 1977, Bok 1994, and the series of articles in the three editions of the *Encyclopedia of Bioethics*). Partly because of Western dominance, international bioethics has concentrated on research ethics and the moral concerns raised by the brave new life sciences and biotechnologies. The issues that matter for the great majority of the world's people—Chinese women included—such as population control and poverty, have often been marginalized or ignored. Even in international feminist bioethics, population issues are barely touched on by the major texts (e.g., Tong, Anderson, and Santos 2001; Tong, Donchin, and Dodds 2004; Donchin, Dodds, and Nie 2007).

This chapter is a part of an ongoing sociologically based normative study to identify and examine the dominant ideological doctrines and major ethical issues of China's birth control program, for instance, the relevance of reproductive liberty and rights in the Chinese context and the limits of state in regulating reproductive issues, including sex-selective abortion (Nie 2004, 2005a, 2005b, 2009). Here I attempt (1) to better understand and critically engage with the Chinese program by putting it under the lens of feminist ethics, and (2) to extend the intellectual and political horizons of feminist bioethics by embracing Chinese experiences of population control. To help develop a more adequate feminist normative account that is also attentive to the Chinese social reality and cultural traditions, I discuss the benefits and costs of the remarkable demographic achievement, the complexity of women's lived experiences, and the *raison d'état* of population control. I argue for the necessity of a women-centered population policy in China.

Along with the eminent feminist bioethicist Susan Sherwin (1999), I see moral theories, feminist moral theories in particular, not as foundations or frameworks but as lenses that can be used to identify and answer ethical questions. Another mother of feminist bioethics, Rosemarie Tong (1997), has shown how the power of feminist approaches to theoretical and practical issues in bioethics can be appreciated by comparing them with nonfeminist ones. Employing this method, I seek to illustrate that the lens of gender makes a significant difference to our ethical assessment of the Chinese population policy, magnifying issues that are often unnoticed or blurred in nonfeminist views.

A Demographic Miracle

China experienced a sharp drop in population growth from the 1970s onward, especially since the early 1990s. Since 1949, fertility rates (total births per woman across the lifespan) have fallen dramatically: 6.14 (1949), 5.81 (1950), 6.26 (1955), 4.02 (1960), 6.08 (1965), 5.81 (1970), 3.57 (1975), 2.24 (1980), 2.20 (1985), 2.17 (1990), 1.68 (1995), 1.55 (2000) (*China Statistical Yearbook 2002*, cited in Greenhalgh and Winckler 2005, 17–18). The annual birth rate (the number of births per 1,000 people in one year) has decreased as a general tendency: 18.21 (1980), 21.04 (1985),

21.06 (1990), 17.12 (1995), 14.03 (2000), 12.40 (2005). So has the annual natural growth rate (the number of births minus the number of deaths per 1,000 people over a given year): 11.87 (1980), 14.55 (1981), 14.26 (1985), 14.39 (1990), 10.55 (1995), 7.58 (2000), 5.89 (2005) (*China Statistical Yearbook 2006* by National Bureau of Statistics of China).

According to official Chinese pronouncements, the national birth planning program, "guided" by the policies of central government and participated in "voluntarily" by millions of Chinese people, has brought "excessive" population growth under "effective control." And the rapid decline in fertility rates, as emphasized by the State Council's 1995 white paper on family planning, has produced enormous positive economic and social benefits, including a major improvement in living standards. The State Council's 2000 white paper on population, similarly tailored for an overseas audience, proudly declares:

> China has accomplished a historic transition in population reproduction pattern from one featuring high birth rate, low death rate and high growth rate to one featuring low birth rate, low death rate and low growth rate in a relatively short period of time... Since the implementation of the family planning program, over 300 million births have been averted nationally, thus saving a great amount of payment for the upbringing of children for the society. This has alleviated the pressure of excessive population growth on the natural resources and environment, thus contributing to the economic development and the improvement of the people's living standard.

The dramatic improvement in the general living standards of Chinese people since the late 1970s has been universally acknowledged as probably the single most important social progress achieved by modern China. Between the establishment of the People's Republic in 1949 and the death of Mao in 1976, the rigidly planned economy of the Maoist dictatorship had led China to the brink of social collapse. It is indeed a socioeconomic miracle that, in the space of about twenty years, China has by and large rid itself of absolute poverty: *jiejue le wenbao wenti* (having solved the problems of insufficient food and clothing) is the often-used Chinese phrase. As a result of this Chinese phenomenon, the global population living in absolute poverty has significantly declined over the past three decades. In the 2000 white paper, the State Council of China asserts that "the Chinese people now live a relatively comfortable life," with the gross national product (GNP) increasing fourfold in the 1980s and 1990s. Most notably, "impoverished people in rural areas have generally secured adequate food and clothing," with a fall in the number of people living below the poverty line from more than 250 million in the late 1970s to 34 million—down from 33 percent to about 3 percent of the total rural population in 1999. Although poverty is still a serious problem in China—far more serious than officials are willing to admit publicly—and although the gap between rich and poor is growing, the significant improvement in general living standards achieved in a single generation, including much greater political freedom compared to Mao's era, should never be underestimated.

According to official statements, as we have seen, recent improvements in living standards are due to two main factors: the economic development initiated by state policies directed at constructing a "socialist market economy" and a more systematic intervention by the state in the reproductive dynamics of the population. However, while the positive causal relationship between economic development and living standards seems unquestionable, the extent to which the low fertility rate has contributed to economic development (and thus improved living standards) has been strenuously contested by demographers, economists, and other social scientists. One can argue that, as the modern history of developed countries and regions has demonstrated, it is economic and social development, together with changes in other aspects of the sociocultural environment, that has produced low fertility rates, rather than the other way around. Although the official Chinese view attributes the present low fertility rate mainly, if not solely, to the state birth control program, it is also questionable how effective this state policy—in particular its coercive aspect—has been. The sociological puzzle behind China's recent decades' major demographic transformation is the extent to which this decrease in fertility has been brought about by economic development or by population policy, or by both together acting in concert with other related sociocultural changes. The positive role played by the state birth planning program in controlling population growth and improving economic well-being is apparently crucial in this process—although probably not as significant as the official view claims.

The demographic miracle directly associated with, if not created by, the Chinese program is typically Pyrrhic in a modern Eastern context—that is, an extraordinary victory achieved at extraordinary human and social costs. Not surprisingly, the Chinese official documents often downplay, if not dismiss, most of these costs as well as the negative impact (whether anticipated or unintended) at the individual and collective levels. In the West, even enthusiastic supporters of the Chinese policy, such as the public health expert Malcom Potts (2006, 361), acknowledge that the policy that has changed not only China but the world has been "a source of great pain for one generation." Apparently, the pain will go beyond one generation, because the coming generations must deal with the ex-

tremely unbalanced sex ratio and other dramatic changes of population structure, including the care of the growing number of elderly people and the likely
shortage of labor. In the long run, the manmade demographic miracle is a mixed
blessing to say the least.

"Double Effects" on Women

The coexistence of remarkable socioeconomic benefits with huge collective and
individual costs, especially for women, makes it extremely challenging to evaluate China's birth control program in ethical terms. Although not always completely unnoticed, women and their interests are often marginalized in nonfeminist discourses, such as official Chinese and mainstream medical pronouncements
on the subject. A recent editorial in the *British Medical Journal* never once mentioned the word "women" while emphasizing that the one-child policy had undoubtedly caused both "important economic benefits" and "great individual
pain" (Potts 2006, 361). A report coauthored by Western and Chinese public
health specialists on the effects of the one-child policy and published in another
major medical periodical, the *New England Journal of Medicine* (Hesketh, Lu,
and Zhu 2005), focused on the problems of unbalanced sex ratios and the rapidly
increasing numbers of elderly people in China but failed to mention the impact
of the policy on Chinese women—let alone analyze the Chinese program through
the lens of gender.

According to official announcements, the population policy has greatly benefited Chinese women and helped improve the status of women. The 1995 white
paper expressed it thus:

> Family planning in China has extricated women from frequent birth after
> marriage and the heavy family burden, further liberated and expanded the so-
> cial productive forces latent in women, and provided them with more oppor-
> tunities to learn science and general knowledge and take part in economic and
> social development activities, hence greatly promoted the improvement of the
> Chinese women's status in economic and social affairs as well as in their families.
> In other words, having been freed to bear and raise a restricted number of chil-
> dren, women have gained important opportunities to receive a better education,
> pursue employment, and thus live better lives. (State Council of China 1995)

A group of Chinese scholars led by the outstanding family planning expert
Zhu Chuzhu has used the term "double effects" to encapsulate the consequences

of the family planning program for women. They acknowledged a number of benefits highlighted by the government, including the substantial reduction in the risks related to frequent pregnancies and childbearing and in the burden associated with housework, the better dissemination of reproductive health information and knowledge, and the significant improvement in accessing effective contraceptives, safe abortions, and other related medical services. For the Chinese scholars, all these have greatly contributed to help Chinese women "become the master of their lives," their reproductive lives in particular. At the same time, they have documented grave negative effects on women, including side effects of contraceptive use, mental and physical problems caused by uninformed selection of contraceptive methods, conflict between the people's birth desire and the population goals, and the lifetime distress of not having a male child (Zhu et al. 1997).

Feminist commentators show a clear appreciation of the positive consequences of China's birth control program. Anthropologist Vanessa Fong (2006) documented how the program has empowered the first generation of urban children, girls in particular, born under the one-child policy, despite problems in carrying out traditional duties such as caring for elderly parents, grandparents, and in-laws. Research by Chinese scholar Hong Zhang (2007) indicates that, even in the countryside where the majority of Chinese still live and where the one-child policy has been resisted (and families often have two children), female children enjoy an enhanced economic role and social status as a result of the reduced fertility rate. This is connected with the improved earning capacity that rural people, especially women, have gained through the development of the market economy.

Feminists have proven far more sensitive than other commentators to the physical, psychological, social, and moral suffering endured by Chinese women in reaching centrally planned demographic goals (e.g., Wolf 1985; Davin 1987; Anagnost 1988; Greenhalgh 1994). Greenhalgh hit the nail on the head: "By world-historical standards, China's birth control program has been exceptional in its hostility to women. It is women's bodies that have been made to bear the burden of contraception and abortion, and women's private and public selves that have been diminished by the policy's prescriptions and social sequelae" (1994, 3). She further pointed out the major pros and cons involved: "The post-Mao birth project helped to create a hard-edged, competitive Chinese modernity in which the new generation of 'quality,' cosmopolitan, and consumerist singletons exists in a large cultural sea of *peasant suffering and female sacrifice*" (Greenhalgh and Winckler 2005, 249, italics added). Perceptively, Greenhalgh and Winckler (2005) summarized the heavy costs of the Chinese demographic miracle:

> Even without precise measurement, it is clear that the human and bodily costs of rapid, essentially coerced fertility decline have been enormous, and unevenly distributed in such a way that it has been the most powerless member of Chinese society—rural women, infant girls, and the unborn—who have endured the most... the extent of social suffering and the scale of the costs incurred in the name of demographic modernization is staggering. Even the birth program's most vociferous Western critics have not added these up. Not only is the *scale* of the human problem imposed on China's people greater than has been appreciated—in China or the West—but the *scope* of those problems is broader as well. (247–48, italics in original)

Employing a Foucauldian theoretical perspective of power and biopolitics, Greenhalgh and Winckler (2005) documented and interpreted how China has placed population issues under strict state management, as well as the social and political consequences of its birth control polices—including how these policies have modified the local politics of birth norms and practice, restratified Chinese society, and redefined China's position in global politics.

Feminism offers a distinctive perspective on the notorious phenomenon of China's "40 million missing girls." While this is an issue of life and death for girls, from a nonfeminist viewpoint the extremely unbalanced sex ratio is alarming mainly because it will result in millions of men without wives. It is important to point out that the birth control program alone should not be blamed for the shocking shortage of girls in contemporary China. According to the official view, the problem may not be as serious as it appears, because it may be a result of the underreporting of girl children. And if there is a problem, it is the poverty and ignorance of rural people—and especially the "feudalist" notions that persist among them—along with the easy availability of modern technology such as prenatal ultrasound diagnosis, that lead them to favor boys over girls and that have caused large-scale sex-selective abortion and in some cases female infanticide. Nevertheless, as the demographer Judith Banister (2004) has shown, a careful analysis of Chinese survey, census, and historical data, taking account of other cultural, social, and technological issues, shows that compulsory family planning (and especially the one-child policy) has made the severe loss of girls "more extreme than it otherwise would be." Feminist anthropologist Laurel Bossen (2005) demonstrated that, together with the implementation of national family planning policies, the revival of patrilineal control over village land rights (women lack equal rights to land) during the reform period has significantly contributed to the extreme shortage of girls in rural China. As a series of serious ethical and practical problems are associated with the mainstream approach (i.e., coercive state intervention), in order to adequately address the problem of widespread sex-selective abortions, it is imperative to develop alternative social schemas that are women-centered, community-oriented, and voluntary in nature (Nie 2009).

It is essential to notice how intrusive birth control has been for women. The statistical data (cited in Hesketh, Lu, and Zhu 2005) speak for themselves: nearly half of married Chinese women are using an intrauterine device: 50 percent in 1982, 40 percent in 1988 and 1992, 43 percent in 1997, and 46 percent in 2001. Over one-third of married women have been sterilized: 25 percent in 1982, 37 percent in 1988, 42 percent in 1992, 40 percent in 1997, and 37 percent in 2001. In contrast, the rate of condom use is low and has fallen steadily: 8 percent in 1982, 5 percent in 1988, 4 percent in 1992, 2 percent in 1997, and 3 percent in 2001. And rates of male sterilization are also low: 10 percent in 1982, 13 percent in 1987, 12 percent in 1992, 9 percent in 1997, and 8 percent in 2001. In a large-scale Chinese survey of family planning and reproductive health conducted in 2001, the great majority of women (80 percent) reported that they had no choice about contraceptives and just accepted the recommended methods. In spite of the heavy reliance on long-term contraception, at least one-quarter of women of reproductive age (25 percent) have had one or more abortions. In my own study (Nie 2005a), 41 percent of 348 women from 13 sample groups said that they had had at least one abortion. Interviews with thirty women revealed that abortion in general, despite its social acceptance, is such a "bitter" experience that "no words can describe" the physical pain and emotional suffering caused by it. Of course, one should not attribute all these trends to the national birth policy alone, as many people would have recourse to various methods of contraception and abortion without the policy. Nevertheless, it is undeniable that the birth control policy has made many of these practices compulsory.

The Primacy and Complexity of Women's Lived Experiences

Notably different from traditional sociopolitical and ethical theories, feminism cherishes the enormous diversity and profound individuality of human experience as actually lived by women. To see the world, society, and life in general through the lens of gender means to see them through the lived experiences of women. Women's lived experiences constitute the lifeline of feminist intellectual exploration. In this feminist spirit, I want to recount a story narrated by a physician about a Chinese woman who had to terminate her pregnancy as a result of the birth control policy:

A young woman who looked to be in her early 20s told us that she was 29. We felt she was not telling the truth about her age. The man who accompanied her to the clinic was in his middle 40s. We thought the man was not her husband. We did not ask more questions. What we should do is to perform the abortion. The girl was far from calm. She was really not willing to have the abortion. She was not even willing to answer questions such as when her last menstrual period was. Then, the man came and answered questions about her medical history for her. When the man took a note from us to the cashier to pay, I asked her who this man was. The girl cried at once and told me he was her partner (*duixiang*, boyfriend or husband). I said to her: "The ages of you two are rather different." She replied: "He was re-married. But I am married for the first time. His wife died a couple of years ago." I guessed the girl might come from the small towns or countryside to work in this city. But she said that was not so. The present policy is that a couple cannot have a second child if one of them has already had a child. The girl was really miserable and very unhappy. When she first came to schedule an abortion several days before, she had been drinking very much.

She cried badly. I told her that she should not be like this. I said something to her like this: "Since you have married him, you must accept everything about him. He has had a child and you thus cannot have your own. You also must accept this." Sometimes, we will let the woman go home if we feel it is possible for her to continue the pregnancy. But in this case, it was impossible. If he was divorced and the court gave the child to his ex-wife, the man could have another child. But now the situation was that his wife had died. Therefore, the girl had to have an abortion no matter how much she was not willing to. Because it was impossible for her to carry the pregnancy to term, the sooner she had the abortion, the better. A late abortion would be more damaging for her. What we could do was just to persuade her to accept the fact. Actually, we could see that the man was very good and caring toward her. In face of this condition, even though we sympathized with her, we as doctors could not do anything. We have no other alternative [*meiyou biede banfa*]. We could only persuade her, try to comfort her, and be more careful in the abortion operation. She chose to use the abortion drug. But the drug abortion was not complete. Then, we had to perform vacuum suction. (Nie 2005a, 185)

This sad case raises a number of issues. It offers a window on how population control is operating in China and how it has affected women, including ob/gyn physicians and family-planning workers (almost all of whom are female). I will confine myself to these points. First, there is what can be called a paradox in the Chinese program—the coexistence of widespread acceptance with continuous resistance. Contrary to the common wisdom in the West and supporting official claims, the policy has been widely and "conscientiously" accepted as necessary by Chinese, especially urban people (Milwertz 1997). While this acceptance by Chinese is a result of heavy state propaganda and the lack of adequate public debate on the subject, acceptance and support for the policy have been overwhelming. One way of understanding the reasoning behind this is to compare the Chinese attitude to Westerners' views on taxation (Nie 2005a, chap. 7). At the same time, large numbers of individuals, especially in the vast rural hinterland, have engaged at great personal risk in persistent and even violent resistance to the population policy by strategies ranging from direct confrontation to evasion and accommodation (White 2006, chap. 7).

Second, just as in the West effective analysis of gender cannot be isolated from the analysis of class and race, in the Chinese context an adequate analysis of gender must be combined with "residency" as a category of analysis. As the doctor guessed, the patient probably came from the rural area. If this is the case, her denial indicates the long-rooted and widespread discrimination against rural residents in China. There is a caste-like social stratification in China in which people are divided into two birth-ascribed civil status groups: rural as the lower and urban as the higher. Social, economic, and cultural inequality between these two groups means that a rural woman who marries an urban man is "marrying up."

Third, feminist intellectual exploration should always attend to the complexities—often involving conflicting impulses—of women's lived experience. Given the diversity of feminist theory, one should not expect an overarching feminist interpretation of Chinese women's experiences of birth control. Feminist bioethics should make every effort to avoid falling under the spell that too long haunted international bioethics—overgeneralizing and oversimplifying the moral beliefs and reality of non-Western societies by dichotomizing East and West into such dualisms as individualism vs. collectivism (Nie 2007, forthcoming).

Questioning the Fundamental Rationales of Population Control

Official Chinese discourse has presented the practical and ethical issues involved in terms of stark alternatives: either a rigorous state population control program or the continuation of poverty and underdevelopment. This rationale for China's national population control policy has been well articulated in numerous propaganda documents. The initial expression of what later came to be called the "one child per couple" policy, the 1980 "Open Letter of the Central Committee of the Communist Party to the General Membership of the Communist Party and the Membership of the Communist Youth League on the Problem of Controlling Population Growth in Our Country," argues that, with the rapid growth of China's population, "we have to encounter increasingly severe problems in such areas as feeding the entire people, clothing them, housing them, providing adequate transportation, education, public health care, and employment for our people. This makes it difficult for the country as a whole to transform its state of poverty and backwardness over a short time." Overpopulation would "greatly increase the difficulty" of realizing the goals of modernization and "create a severe situation in which we could hardly expect to make any appreciable improvement in the lives of the people at large." Moreover, it would "increase excessively the consumption of natural resources, such as energy resources, water, and forests... aggravate the pollution of the environment and severely worsen the conditions for production and the people's living environment, making it difficult to improve these in the long run." For every couple to have no more than one child was thus proclaimed as "the most effective way" of solving these massive problems (White 1992, 11–16).

Following the reasoning of the 1980 Open Letter, the State Council of China's 2000 white paper identified population control as the key to national development: "China has a huge population, but a weak economic foundation with relatively inadequate per capita resources. These are its basic national conditions. Many contradictions and problems in China's economic and social development are closely associated with the issue of population, which has become *the key factor and primary problem restricting China's economic and social development*" (italics added).

Therefore, the logic of population control appears to be obviously straightforward. In the face of limited natural resources, overpopulation and rapid population growth must be contained. Otherwise, hunger and poverty will prevail. China thus has to formulate and implement a vigorous population policy simply for its people to survive and live better lives. According to this logic, the Chinese population, characterized as large in quantity and low in "quality," is the major obstacle to economic and social development.

In the same way that the establishment of socialist China was inspired by Marxism, which originated in the West and was part of a worldwide socialist movement, China's population control program has close links with dominant beliefs about population in the international community. Eight major approaches have dictated the population debate since the 1950s: the developmentalist perspective, the redistributionist perspective, the limited resources perspective, the sociobiological perspective, the people-as-a-source-of-instability perspective, the women's rights and human rights perspectives, the people-as-problem-solvers perspective, and the religious pronatalist perspective (Furedi 1997). As the most prominent and influential, the developmentalist perspective has two distinctive paradigms. The first argues that economic development is the solution to the identified overpopulation problem in the Third World. The second holds that population growth must be controlled for the economy to develop. Most state-run population control bodies, such as the Chinese program, are based on this second, developmentalist paradigm.

Feminists in general have been critical—skeptical at least—of the manipulative and coercive measures used against women by local, national, and international population control policies and bodies. Furthermore, they have also questioned the *raison d'état* of population policies. In a review paper, feminist sociologist Ines Smyth (1998) says that for many years a "feminism vs. population control" debate has been going on. Many important common grounds, such as promoting social and economic developments and improving women's status, exist between feminism and population control. However, there are always some essential tensions between the two. Feminists are legitimately concerned that "family planning programmes worldwide are developed and implemented with the stated or implicit aim of reducing fertility rates and population growth, rather than with the intention of promoting women's health and productive freedom" (Smyth 1998, 224). The governmental programs often reinforce Malthusian notions of population growth as a problem of socioeconomic development.

The fundamental moral concern of feminism about population control is the *instrumentalization* of women. Feminists thus advocate a genuinely women-centered population policy in which women are treated as ends in themselves rather than merely the means to achieve other social goals. They insist that any population control policy is ethically justifiable and politically acceptable only if it is women-centered. In other words, going beyond the monitoring of the actual and possible negative impacts of population control on women, feminist critics have challenged the popular justifications and fundamental assumptions in which women's well-being and interests have often been marginalized (at best) or used as a means for population control. Theoretically, feminism would endorse the well-known notions developed by economist Amartya Sen (1999) and philosopher Martha Nussbaum (2000)—an agent-centered and capabilities-oriented approach—and urge the expansion of these theories in the area of population policy.

Without denying that population control establishments have adopted many crucial feminist values such as reproductive rights and health, feminists are concerned that "it is not sufficient for the population establishment to display a notional adherence to such ideas, to advocate them only in the pursuit of ulterior aims, or simply to use their language without their substance" (Smyth 1998, 233). In a feminist classic on the global politics of population control written from the perspective of women's reproductive rights, Betsy Hartmann (1987/1995) powerfully argued against the basic philosophy of population control. Her feminist approach does not regard rapid population growth as the root cause of underdevelopment in the developing world but a symptom of those problems. It emphasizes that improvements in living standards and the position of women through more equitable social and economic development are the best ways to pursue the desirable demographic goals. Population control not only restricts reproductive choice and the rights of women but also "dangerously obscures the real causes of the earth's afflictions, helping to perpetuate poverty" and other social diseases (Hartmann 1987/1995, xxi). Practically, population control does not offer real solutions to the serious economic, political, and environmental problems humans face. Hartmann concludes: "Stripped of all the economic arguments, political justifications, and soft-sell marketing, population control at heart is a philosophy without a heart, in which human beings become objects to be manipulated... Population control profoundly distorts our world view, and negatively affects people in the most intimate areas of their lives. Instead of promoting ethics, empathy, and true reproductive choice, it encourages us to condone coercion" (Hartmann, 1987/1995, 309).

Some feminists have started to examine and question the fundamental rationales of China's birth control. For feminist anthropologist and sinologist Ann Anagnost (1997), in China the issue of population, the quality of population in particular "is not a self-evident problematic of political economy but is first and foremost a discursive category" (137). In a major book on the history and sociology of birth planning in the People's Republic up to 2005, feminist political scientist Tyrene White suggests that "China's longest campaign," the demographic engineering "born under Mao, perfected under Deng," "would be best left behind as a relic of the twentieth century." A major reason lies in that "one can completely reject the Chinese policy—state regulation of childbirth—without denying the problem it was intended to address" (White 2006, 265, 263).

Conclusion

In this chapter I have attempted to see and evaluate the Chinese family planning program through a feminist perspective. The policy and practice of the program challenge feminism in many ways and also can significantly extend its theoretical horizons and political commitments. Meanwhile, feminism has offered insights into and constructive criticism of China's birth control program, giving us a clearer view of the moral and social dilemmas involved in this massive project of social engineering, its benefits and costs for women, the many different dimensions of women's lived experiences, and the problems that arise from the fundamental philosophy of population control. To sum up, the heavy human costs for China's population initiatives have been paid mainly by Chinese women. While the birth control program has benefited women directly and indirectly, from a feminist perspective it can hardly be said that the program has empowered women in general or is intrinsically women-centered.

Feminism has been an important element in the Chinese social and cultural life since the early twentieth century. Gender equality and justice were central themes in the socialist revolution and the construction of a socialist society, even though these values have suffered a backlash along with the development of the market economy. Since the 1980s Chinese discourse has given more and more attention to the empowerment of women in population policy (Qiu 2006). More and more Chinese feminists are voicing their opinions on this topic, as about many other social issues. As documented in the insightful report by Susan Greenhalgh (2001), although the state and popular narratives of the perceived population problem often override the narratives of women's liberation and well-being, and although a genuinely independent Chinese feminist voice on population has yet to emerge, fresh feminist winds have indeed started stirring in China.

Elsewhere, I have argued that, despite its apparent Western origins, feminism and feminist ethics provide Chinese with useful lenses through which to view the marginalized, oppressed, and exploited condition of Chinese women. Feminism can also provide Chinese with powerful strategies and the political means to change their unjust environment. Moreover, as important as is it for Chinese bioethics to learn about and use Western feminist theories and perspectives, it is even more important and urgent for Chinese bioethicists to focus on native problems as articulated through the voices and experiences of Chinese women, especially those who are underprivileged and marginalized, and to develop a feminist language rooted in indigenous Chinese moral and political traditions such as Confucianism and Daoism (Taoism) (Nie 2004).

Examining China's population program through feminist lenses has reinforced these arguments on the mutual significance of feminism and Chinese society. I began this chapter by pointing out that the Chinese program requires a feminist ethical scrutiny that is simultaneously sensitive to the Chinese context. I hope that my preliminary effort has identified some of the moral issues essential in developing such an inquiry and will serve as a call for feminist scholarship, feminist bioethics in particular, to produce further studies of the subject.

ACKNOWLEDGMENTS

This chapter is a part of a larger research project, "Predicaments of Social Engineering: The Ideologies and Ethics of China's Birth Control Program," supported by a grant from the Marsden Fund of the Royal Society of New Zealand. It is developed from some materials initially presented at the Fifth International Congress on Feminist Approaches to Bioethics in Sydney in 2004. I am grateful to Dr. Paul Sorrell for his professional help with the English language and Dr. Ole Döring for his characteristically helpful comments.

REFERENCES

Aird, J. S. 1990. *Slaughter of the innocents: Coercive birth control in China.* Washington, D.C.: AEI Press.

Anagnost, A. S. 1988. Family violence and magical violence: The women as victim in China's one-child family policy. *Women and Language* 11 (2): 16–22.

———. 1997. *National past-times: Narrative, representation, and power in modern China.* Durham, N.C.: Duke University Press.

Banister, J. 1987. *China's changing population.* Stanford, Calif.: Stanford University Press.

———. 2004. Shortage of girls in China today. *Journal of Population Research* 27 (1): 19–45.

Bok, S. 1994. Population and ethics: Expanding the moral space. In *Population policies reconsidered: Health, empowerment, and rights,* ed. G. Sen, A. Germain, and L. C. Chen. Boston: Harvard University Press.

Bossen, L. 2005. Forty million missing girls: Land, population control and sex imbalance in rural China. *Asia-Pacific E-Journal: Japan Focus.* www.japanfocus.org/-Laurel-Bossen/1692.

Callahan, D. 1971. Ethics and population limitation. An occasional paper of the population council. New York: Population Council.

Corrêa, S., and R. Reichmann. 1994. *Population and reproductive rights: Feminist perspectives from the south.* London: Zed Books.

Davin, D. 1987. Gender and population in the People's Republic of China. In *Women, state, and ideology: Studies from Africa and Asia,* ed. H. Afshar, 111–29. New York: State University of New York Press.

Demeny, P. G., and G. McNicoll, eds. 2003. *Encyclopedia of population.* New York: Gale.

Dixon-Mueller, R. 1993. *Population policy and women's rights: Transforming reproductive choice.* Westport, Conn.: Praeger.

Donchin, A., S. Dodds, and J.-B. Nie. 2007. *Moving toward gender justice.* A special issue of *Bioethics* 21:6.

Eager, P. W. 2004. *Global population policy: From population control to reproductive rights.* Hants, U.K.: Ashgate.

Fong, V. L. 2006. *Only hope: Coming of age under China's one-child policy.* Stanford, Calif.: Stanford University Press.

Furedi, F. 1997. *Population and development: A critical introduction.* Cambridge, Mass.: Polity Press.

Greenhalgh, S. 1994. Controlling births and bodies in village China. *American Ethnologist* 21 (1): 3–30.

———. 2001. Fresh winds in Beijing: Chinese feminists speak out on the one-child policy and women's lives. *Signs: Journal of Women in Culture and Society* 26 (3): 843–86.

Greenhalgh, S., and J. Li. 1995. Engendering reproductive policy and practice in peasant China: For a feminist demography of reproduction. *Signs: Journal of Women in Culture and Society* 20 (3): 601–41.

Greenhalgh, S., and E. A. Winckler. 2005. *Governing China's population: From Leninist to neoliberal biopolitics.* Stanford, Calif.: Stanford University Press.

Hartmann, B. 1987/1995. *Reproductive rights and wrongs: The global politics of population control,* rev. ed. Boston: South End Press.

Hesketh, T., L. Lu, and W. X. Zhu. 2005. The effect of China's one-child family policy after 25 years. *New England Journal of Medicine* 353 (11): 1171–76.

Milwertz, C. N. 1997. *Accepting population control: Urban Chinese women and the one-child family policy.* Surrey, U.K.: Curzon Press.

National Bureaus of Statistics of China, 2006. *China statistics yearbook 2006.* Beijing: China Statistics Press.

Nie, J.-B. 2004. Feminist bioethics and its language of human rights in the Chinese context. In *Linking visions: Feminist bioethics, human rights, and the developing world,* ed. R. Tong, A. Donchin, and S. Dodds, 73–88. Lanham, Md.: Rowman & Littlefield.

———. 2005a. *Behind the silence: Chinese voices on abortion.* Lanham, Md.: Rowman & Littlefield.

————. 2005b. Reproductive rights matter in China. Keynote speech at the Second Nordic-China Women and Gender Studies Conference on Gender and Human Rights, Sweden, August 7–10.

————. 2007. The specious idea of an Asian bioethics: Beyond dichotomizing East and West. In *Principles of heath care ethics*, 2nd ed., ed. R. E. Ashcroft, A. Dawson, H. Draper, and J. R. McMillan, 143–49. London: John Wiley & Sons.

————. 2009. The limits of state intervention in sex-selective abortion: The case of China. *Culture, Health and Sexuality: An International Journal for Research, Intervention and Care.* In press (DOI# 10.1080/13691050903108431).

————. Forthcoming. *Medical ethics in China: A cross-cultural interpretation.* Washington, D.C.: Georgetown University Press.

Nussbaum, M. C. 2000. *Women and human development: The capabilities approach.* Cambridge: Cambridge University Press.

Poston, D. L., and M. Micklin, eds. 2006. *Handbook of population.* New York: Springer.

Potts, M. 2006. China's one-child policy: The policy that changed the world. *British Medical Journal* 333:361–62.

Qiu, R. 1996/2006. *Shengyu jiankang yu lunlixue* (reproductive health and ethics). Beijing: Beijing Medical University and Peking Union Medical University.

Riley, N. E. 2006. Demography of gender. In *Handbook of population,* ed. Dudley L. Poston and Michael Micklin, 109–42. New York: Springer.

Scharping, T. 2003. *Birth control in China, 1949–2000: Population policy and demographic development.* London: Routledge Curzon.

Sen, A. 1999. *Development as freedom.* New York: Anchor Books.

Sherwin, S. 1999. Foundations, frameworks, lenses: The role of theories in bioethics. *Bioethics* 13:198–205.

Smyth, I. 1998. Gender analysis of family planning: Beyond the "feminist vs. population control" debate. In *Feminist visions of development: Gender analysis and policy,* ed. R. Pearson and C. Jackson, 217–38. London: Routledge.

State Council of China. 1995. *White paper on family planning.* www.china.org.cn/e-white/familypanning/index.htm.

————. 2000. *China's population and development in the twenty-first century: White paper on population in China* (official English version). www.gov.cn/english/official/2005-07/27/content_17640.htm.

Subcommittee on International Operations and Human Rights of the Committee on International Relations, U.S. House of Representatives. 1998. *Forced abortion and sterilization in China: The view from the inside: Hearing before the Subcommittee.* Washington, D.C.: U.S. Government Printing Office.

Tong, R. 1997. *Feminist approaches to bioethics.* Boulder, Colo.: Westview Press.

Tong, R., G. Anderson, and A. Santos, eds. 2001. *Globalizing feminist bioethics: Cross-cultural perspectives.* Boulder, Colo.: Westview Press.

Tong, R., A. Donchin, and S. Dodds, eds. 2004. *Linking visions: Feminist bioethics, human rights, and the developing world.* Lanham, Md.: Rowman & Littlefield.

Veatch, R. M., ed. 1977. *Population policy and ethics: The American experience.* New York: Irvington.

White, T., guest ed. 1992. Special issue on family planning in China. *Chinese Sociology and Anthropology* 24:3.

———. 1994. The origins of China's birth planning policy. In *Engendering China: Women, culture, and the state,* ed. C. Gilmartin, G. Hershatter, L. Rofel, and T. White, 250–78. Cambridge, Mass.: Harvard University Press.

———. 2006. *China's longest campaign: Birth planning in the People's Republic, 1949–2005.* Ithaca, N.Y.: Cornell University Press.

Wolf. M. 1985. *Revolution postponed: Women in contemporary China.* Stanford, Calif.: Stanford University Press.

Zhang, H. 2007. China's new rural daughters coming of age: Downsizing the family and firing up cash-earning power in the new economy. *Signs: Journal of women in culture and society* 32 (3): 671–698.

Zhao, Z., and F. Guo. 2007. *Transition and challenge: China's population at the beginning of the twenty-first century.* Oxford: Oxford University Press.

Zhu, C., S. Li, C. Qiu, P. Hu, and A. Jin. 1997. *The double effects of the family planning program on Chinese women.* Xi'an: Xi'an Jiaotong University Press. (Published bilingually in Chinese and English).

CHAPTER FOURTEEN

A Feminist Standpoint on Disability

Our Bodies, Ourselves

MARY B. MAHOWALD, PH.D.

Anyone familiar with the literature of feminism is well aware of the philosophical diversity that feminism embraces.[1] Rosemarie Tong, for example, identifies eight versions of feminism: liberal feminism, radical feminism, Marxist and socialist feminism, psychoanalytic and gender feminism, existentialist feminism, postmodern feminism, multicultural and global feminism, and ecofeminism. As she acknowledges, however, using these categorizations may have the undesired effect of endorsing "the fathers' labels" (Tong 1998, 1). Moreover, while (probably) pedagogically useful, these labels do not adequately capture the uniqueness of feminism or the range of philosophical orientations within its diverse interpretations. Among radical feminists, for example, some favor androgyny while others reject it, and some support reproductive technologies while others oppose them (Tong 1998, 2).

The philosophical diversity of feminism is also expressed within various specializations, such as esthetics, epistemology, ethics, philosophy of science, linguistics, social and political philosophy, and the history of philosophy. In ethics as well as social and political philosophy, some endorse a liberal theory while others develop a socialist version of feminism. Susan Okin (1989), for example, defends a liberal version of feminism in her critique of Rawls's theory of justice, while Alison Jaggar (1983) articulates a socialist version of feminism. In previous writings, I have characterized the feminism to which I am committed as "egalitarian" (see, for example, Mahowald 2000, 69–81). The theory of justice that is most congenial to my view is that of Amartya Sen (1992), on whom Martha Nussbaum (2000) draws in her delineation of basic human capabilities to be facilitated by a just society. This approach differs from a Rawlsian account of justice, which, while calling for "fair equality of opportunity," pays insufficient attention to the social causes of inequality (e.g., Rawls 1971, 83–90; 1996, 363–68).

The commonality that exists among feminist philosophers, despite their diversity, arises from agreement about the following:

1. women have been oppressed throughout history through subordination of their interests to those of men;
2. this state of affairs is morally wrong because it constitutes gender injustice;
3. resistance to this wrongness, and efforts to correct it, are moral and political imperatives; and
4. women's experience and input is remedially relevant to all areas of philosophy.

Empirical data compellingly support the first (descriptive) claim by documenting the oppression of women and overall exclusion of women's input in determining policies that affect us. Women in general are nondominant, whereas men in general are dominant. The second (prescriptive) point of agreement arises from recognition of justice as a cardinal principle of ethics and gender justice as a necessary subset of justice. The third common claim links ethics as moral philosophy, a theoretical enterprise, with morality as the lived behavior of individuals who choose or refuse to act in a manner that is consistent with the conclusions of ethics.

Regarding the fourth point of agreement, the input of women in decisions that affect all human beings expands the knowledge base on which policy decisions are predominantly made by men. When such decisions affect women only, men are even more likely to be insufficiently knowledgeable because they lack experiences that women alone have had or can have. Unfortunately, however, women are seldom included among the dominant decision makers. By outlining a strategy to reduce or overcome this deficiency, feminist standpoint theory offers a means by which feminism's third (behavioral) claim can be implemented.

Because the dominant decision makers of society are not only male but also physically and cognitively able, middle class or affluent, heterosexual, and mainly white, the strategy recommended by feminist standpoint theory is applicable also to other nondominant groups whose voices are seldom heard by those in positions of power. Among others, these include people who are impaired, the poor, homosexuals, and people of color.

Women, while nondominant by gender, may be dominant in other ways, and men, though dominant by gender, may be nondominant in other ways. White, affluent women, for example, are dominant vis-à-vis women of color and economically impoverished women. Even within nondominant groups, some individuals may be dominant in relation to others within the group. Among people of color, for example, those who have lighter skin than others may be dominant over those whose complexion is darker; and among people with impairments, those who are cognitively able but physically impaired may be dominant over those who are cognitively impaired. Ironically, differences within nondominant groups tend to reinforce the dominance of characteristics attributed to the dominant group.

The term *disability* is prevalently used for conditions that reduce the capabilities of some nondominant members of society. Interestingly, it is not used for conditions that reduce capabilities based solely on social arrangements, such as poverty and minority status. Instead, disabilities are commonly viewed as impairments that are unrelated to societal arrangements. Some, such as blindness or lameness, are limitations that social arrangements cannot wholly overcome. But some impairments, such as myopia, do not constitute disabilities because social arrangements are readily available to avoid any impediment to capabilities.

In what follows, I offer a brief interpretation of feminist standpoint theory[2] and the egalitarian feminism that underlies it. The strategy proposed through this theory is doubly applicable to women with disabilities because they are nondominant not only in relation to men but also in relation to people who are currently able. To illustrate this strategy, I focus on people with cognitive impairments who, in comparison with those who have physical but not cognitive impairments, are less able to articulate their interests or needs. I recommend a human flourishing standard, which is applicable to other nondominant groups as well as women, as the norm to be met with regard to the second claim of feminism. While defending this standard as preferable to a function-based norm, I leave to others the explicit characterization of what these norms entail.[3] My argument supports the function-based standard only if resources are inadequate for promoting the flourishing standard for everyone.[4]

An Egalitarian Feminism and Feminist Standpoint Theory

An egalitarian account of justice starts with recognition that every person has the same value as every other, regardless of differences between them. The differences by which individuals and groups are distinguishable from one another entail (but are not limited to) different capabilities for human flourishing. This concept of equality as "same value" is at odds with a construal of equality as "sameness." Construing equality as sameness rather than as same value ignores the fact that every human being has a unique set of capabilities that may or may not be fostered by social circumstances. If all individuals or groups are regarded and treated as the same, disregarding their differences, disparities between the capability for flourishing of some and the capability for flourishing of others are inevitably exacerbated. Thankfully, this exacerbation is only partially achieved through the liberal theory of justice that prevails in the United States. Liberal theory, while less egalitarian than capabilities theory, is nonetheless preferable to a libertarian approach, which would exacerbate the disparities even more.

Because women and men have the same value despite their biological and social differences, an egalitarian account of justice necessarily supports an egalitarian version of feminism. Normative implications of this view are applicable to differences between men and women only if they are associated with inequality of capability; other differences may not only be acceptable but desirable. With regard to differences associated with unequal capabilities, the ethical imperative is to facilitate the capabilities of those for whom capabilities are unnecessarily limited—either by altering circumstances or social arrangements or, if these are unchangeable, by introducing measures that reduce the impediments, as required by the Americans with Disabilities Act of 1990. Such measures may entail reduction of capabilities in those for whom they have been unlimited, or less limited, by social arrangements. Taxing the affluent to provide capabilities that poor people cannot otherwise enjoy is an obvious example in this regard.

On grounds of feminism's first claim, that women have generally been oppressed throughout history, feminist standpoint theory delineates a strategy of privileged inclusion through which to fulfill the behavioral implication of the third claim: that we exert practical efforts to reduce gender inequality so that women as women can flourish as fully as men can flourish. Ironically, a capability that men lack, namely, the ability to conceive, gestate, bear, and nurse children, tends to reduce rather than promote the flourishing of women with regard to other capabilities (cf. Firestone 1970). Other gender or sex differences in capabilities are socially triggered, changeable, and generally disadvantageous to women.

According to Nancy Hartsock, privileging women's participation in decisions that affect them is necessary to reduce or overcome the inevitable limitations of the dominant group, who lack the experience of women as women (Hartsock 2004, 35–50). Nondominant groups, she maintains, are capable of seeing beneath the surface of the social relations they experience, and the standpoint thus achieved allows them to see beyond present structures to possibilities that members of the dominant group, who designed the structures according to their lights, are unable to envision. Both groups are advantaged through the reversal of privilege: members of the dominant group are empowered to correct and expand their vision; members of the nondominant group are empowered to liberate themselves from limitations imposed through the decisions of those who are dominant.

The epistemological justification for feminist standpoint theory is based on two factors: recognition that the experiences on which knowledge depends are incomplete and partial, and desire to reduce this limitation through collaborative inquiry. Implementation of the theory cannot totally overcome epistemological limitations or liabilities because nondominant individuals are also subject to distortive influences on their perspectives (for example, socialization and cultural pressures). However, imputing privileged status to them does not imply that their views are immune to critique by the dominant groups or by others who are nondominant. The input of nondominant others as well as the dominant group remains necessary to minimize epistemological limitations. Moreover, the perspective of those who have not directly or personally had the experiences that individuals from nondominant groups have had can facilitate knowledge that is otherwise unavailable to them especially if this perspective is based on long-term relationships and interactions with nondominant others. Family members or friends of those who are cognitively impaired, for example, often provide relevant information about the interests and capabilities of those who are unable to voice them for themselves.

The ethical warrant for feminist standpoint theory stems from recognition that all persons have the same value regardless of differences by which they are distinguishable. This recognition implies a *prima facie* obligation to respect the autonomy of, and practice beneficence toward, those who are nondominant as well as those who are dominant. While the liberating potential of feminist standpoint theory is morally desirable, its potential for reducing inequality is just as desirable and is crucial to flourishing for nondominant members of society. An additional warrant for privileging the standpoint of those who are nondominant is the rationale that participation, or at least representation, of all members of society is required for a genuinely democratic system of government.

A Human Flourishing Standard

Feminist standpoint theory and an egalitarian account of justice apply to people with impairments as well as women because bodily differences between both groups and their dominant counterparts are associated with unequal capabilities that impede function or flourishing. Identifying these unequal capabilities is ethically incumbent on those who are dominant because the capacity to live as human beings is inseparable from our bodies. We cannot think or choose or fulfill any other capability of human beings except through our bodies.

The terms *function* and *flourishing* have both been used in recent discussions of disability, but with different implications. A function-based definition implies a narrower extension than a flourishing-based definition. Consistent with Rawlsian justice, it sets a standard that defines the obligations of those who are more fortunate to attend to the needs or rights of those less fortunate. In contrast, a flourishing-based definition accords with an Aristotelian conception of justice as virtue, attributing to each individual a *prima facie* right to flourish as who she is, and a *prima facie* duty to assist others to flourish as who they are.[5]

From an egalitarian feminist standpoint, I subscribe to the broader, flourishing-based definition of disability, which encompasses the narrower, function-based definition as a standard for government-funded interventions. Both definitions raise problems of ambiguity and possible arbitrariness. The ambiguity occurs because conceptions of functioning or flourishing proper to humans vary. The arbitrariness occurs because criteria for selecting among different conceptions, and for determining who may justifiably make such selection, are either lacking or questionable.

More precisely, the narrow conception of disability that I consider inadequate is the Rawlsian one developed by Norman Daniels and applied by him and his colleagues to issues in bioethics: lack of ability to function in a species-typical or "normal" manner (cf. Daniels 1985; Buchanan et al. 2000). The broader conception, supported in different ways by Alasdair MacIntyre, Sen, and Nussbaum, defines disability as lack of ability to flourish as a human being (cf. MacIntyre 1981, chap. 16; Sen 1992, chap. 3; Nussbaum 2000, 4–14, 78–80). Both conceptions rely on a particular view of what constitutes a human being as such; in one case, this is defined as a norm; in the other, as a universal.

For Daniels, "normal function" in human beings is the set of functions that *most* humans are able to perform; these are determined quantitatively in a way that excludes people who have more or fewer abilities compared with most members of the human species. Specification of normal functions is apparently determined by statistical averaging, but just what range counts as normal on either side of the precise average is disputable. In contrast, human flourishing is based on each individual's different mix of abilities and disabilities, the capabilities that emerge from that combination, and external circumstances that may promote or hinder expression of these capabilities. Specification of what counts as human flourishing can only be done qualitatively—by examining the potential of each individual *qua* individual rather than as belonging to a group on either side of what is "normal." Both accounts include consideration of social factors in the determination of disability, and both attempt to promote equality as well as individual autonomy. However, a flourishing-based conception of disability puts greater emphasis on equality because it applies to everyone's capability instead of limiting its application to those who do not rise to the level of "normal species function"; this makes it more egalitarian than the function-based definition.

A flourishing-based definition of disability is epistemologically preferable because it takes into account the fact that human beings experience a greater range of disabilities and abilities than the range defined as that of "normal-species functioning."[6] Even those who cannot meet the latter standard are often capable of flourishing. A flourishing-based definition may also be construed as more democratic than a function-based definition because it pays attention to the needs and preferences of all individuals as individuals. Ethically, a flourishing-based definition of disability is preferable to a normal function–based definition because it requires more respectful and supportive attitudes and behavior toward all individuals, who have the same value despite their differences. The flourishing model thus promotes the ideal of social equality more than the function-based model does.

Admittedly, a broad or flourishing-based definition of disability has some limitations or liabilities. First among these is the possibility that it communicates little or nothing explicit about the individuals to whom it applies; second, it may be unrealistically demanding in its implications for social measures that promote equality; and third, it is subject to the ambiguity and possible arbitrariness mentioned above with regard to both definitions of disability.

With regard to the first limitation, a broad definition of disability does not leave us in the dark about those to whom it applies unless "human flourishing" is defined as the optimal capability achievable by *any* human being or human beings *in general*, taking no account of the unique mix of abilities and disabilities that characterize each embodied individual. The definition I support starts with recognition of this wide empirical variability and defines flourishing not as a generic ideal but as an ideal specific to each embodied person. It thus eschews the averaging or generalizing on which a normal-function definition is based. A flourishing-based definition requires maximal input about all of the variables associated with the disabilities that people experience as individuals. This is provided through the strategy proposed by feminist standpoint theory.

With regard to the second limitation, a human-flourishing definition is not actually unrealistically demanding of measures to reduce inequality unless it is impossible to introduce or implement such measures. But it isn't. A broad definition of disability is *more* demanding than the function-based definition, but it is not unrealistically demanding because the participation of all those whose ability to flourish exceeds the limitations associated with their impairments can be enlisted on behalf of those for whom the opposite situation exists. Moral suasion as well as governmental measures, including laws, can and should be introduced to secure their participation, and if moral suasion fails, the "haves" (those whose abilities are proportionately greater than their disabilities) should be "taxed" for the sake of the "have-nots." This means that the autonomy of some may be curtailed for the sake of others; from an egalitarian perspective, curtailment of some people's liberty for the sake of others is not only justified but also obligatory.

The third limitation involves two questions: who is to decide, and by what criteria? The first question is procedural and the second question is substantive, but the answer to the first is a means of determining the answer to the second. Feminist standpoint theory provides the strategy by which to answer the procedural question; implementation of this strategy reduces the ambiguity and arbitrariness of a flourishing-based definition of disability.

Disability and Feminist Standpoint Theory

An egalitarian feminism views every person as a unique collection of abilities and disabilities that determine her capability for functioning or flourishing as a human being. Ignoring these differences risks injustice through neglect of factors associated with but not necessarily caused by them. Some differences are disabling for some people or in some circumstances but not for others or in other circumstances. Some disabilities are different from others in that they do not impede, or only minimally impede, the capability for flourishing (because the ability that is lacking is not one that the person needs or wants to use or because social accommodations have already reduced or eliminated the burden of the impairment). Other disabilities require drastic and costly interventions or societal changes to facilitate human flourishing. The social arrangements that make some conditions disabling are least likely when the condition occurs in individuals who simultaneously have a capability that others lack, namely, a position of power or dominance within society. People whose disabilities outweigh their abilities or whose disabilities are not shared across the power spectrum are unlikely to be part of that group. Consideration of differences such as these reduces controversiality and lack of clarity regarding the meaning of human flourishing and determination of who should decide whether a condition meets that standard in particular individuals or groups.

Admittedly, my insistence that differences be considered to determine whether or to what extent a specific condition impedes human flourishing and therefore should be regarded as a disability is at odds with the view that justice is blind. Justice cannot be blind if its charge is to treat every individual as a unique assemblage of capabilities (abilities and disabilities) and support that uniqueness to the point of human flourishing. Justice must be not only sighted but also as acutely sighted as possible, if it is to impute the same value to every person as a unique embodiment of capabilities. In fact, however, justice as practiced is usually neither blind nor perfectly sighted. Instead, it is nearsighted. Those whose role is to articulate what justice means for everyone are inevitably myopic because they cannot see beyond their own experience or knowledge base. Although all of us have this disability, the nearsightedness of those in power is, as we have seen, ethically and epistemologically more problematic than that of those not in power because nondominant people do not determine policies that affect either themselves or others.[7] Moreover, those in power are more likely than those not in power to think and act as if their vision is unimpaired. They thus assume an ability to universalize based solely on their limited vision of the whole.

As an example of how feminist standpoint theory may reduce the injustice or discrimination associated with disabilities, consider one specific disability: cognitive impairment. While *cognitive*, this impairment should not be understood as separable from the body of the individual because it is in fact an expression of bodily function. Sensory (bodily) experiences are indispensable to the acquisition of knowledge, and higher brain function is only possible through a bodily organ whose capability for thought may be impeded through physical anomaly or trauma.

Cognitive impairment may be profound, severe, moderate, or mild (cf. Grossman 1983, 11), and it may affect one or more kinds of cognitive function (e.g., long- or short-term memory, abstract reasoning, quantitative or spatial reasoning, etc.). Many people with cognitive impairments are able to flourish in ways that people with unimpaired cognitive function cannot or do not flourish. Some, for example, are happier or more satisfied in their lives than some people who are cognitively unimpaired. People with cognitive impairments may have special talents or physical skills that are lacking in those who are cognitively able. Some with cognitive impairments live in loving homes where they thrive maximally because of that love, while some who are cognitively unimpaired are cut off from the love that is crucial to their thriving. Affluence may buy opportunities to flourish, regardless of a person's cognitive capacity, while poverty impedes flourishing, at times even impeding those who are cognitively able from meeting a normal human functioning standard.

Support for flourishing of people who are cognitively impaired requires efforts to recognize and address those areas of their lives in which they can flourish. To determine what those areas are and how to address them effectively requires eliciting their standpoint as much as possible. This is obviously difficult because of the specific nature of their impairment. Those who are physically but not cognitively impaired can usually inform others of their standpoint regarding their needs for flourishing. Those with cognitive impairments cannot do that as well, and some cannot do it at all.

Applying feminist standpoint theory to determination of policies that promote flourishing in people who are cognitively impaired thus requires greater efforts than are required for those who are cognitively able or physically rather than cognitively impaired. To the extent that an individual is able to articulate her own standpoint on matters that affect her, this should be accorded privileged status. When this is not possible, input from caregivers or from those who are impaired in other ways should be sought, because they are more likely than others to have a sense of what facilitates flourishing for the affected individual. Their standpoint on behalf of the cognitively impaired person is privileged also, but less so than that of the individual herself, and only to the extent that the proxy attempts to articulate the standpoint of the cognitively impaired person rather than the proxy's own standpoint. The question to be asked of proxies or representatives of those who are cognitively impaired in order to discover the standpoint of the cognitively impaired individual is not the Golden Rule question "what would *I* want done or not done if I were in this person's situation," but "what would this person, as a different embodied self, want done or not done?"

As already suggested, the extent to which cognitive impairment impedes human functioning or human flourishing depends in part on the socioeconomic status of the affected individual. Unfortunately, some parents or caregivers are unable to provide optimal care because they lack the financial or psychological resources for doing so; they are socioeconomically nondominant, which makes them deserving, by feminist standpoint theory, of a privileged status in the development of policies that affect them and those for whom they care.[8] In a sense, these caregivers, most of whom are women, also have a disability that impedes their function or flourishing: they are unable to fulfill their caregiving function adequately, let alone flourish as caregiving human beings.

Support from government programs or private agencies may reduce the socioeconomic causes of disability, but rarely if ever do they offer adequate means for doing so. As a result, cognitively impaired individuals whose caregivers are socioeconomically nondominant are impeded from functioning or flourishing to the same degree available to those whose caregivers are socioeconomically dominant. Even when individuals have the same base line of cognitive impairment, therefore, some are more impeded than others in fulfillment of their capabilities. Those who are more impeded because of their socioeconomic nondominance should be attributed a privileged status in relation to those who are socioeconomically dominant, because their socioeconomic nondominance adds a perspective that is otherwise missing in those who are socioeconomically dominant—even if they have the same impairment. Moreover, when a flourishing standard cannot be met for everyone, efforts to meet at least a function-based standard for everyone take priority over efforts to meet a flourishing standard for some—because social inequality is thus reduced even if it isn't eliminated.

Conclusion

I have briefly described an egalitarian conception of feminism and an understanding of feminist standpoint theory that it supports. An egalitarian feminism imputes the same value to every person, regardless of differences among them, and argues for a standard of justice that maximally promotes the flourishing of all individuals. Feminist standpoint theory is not only applicable to women but also to people with disabilities, and it is doubly applicable to women with disabilities. Both groups tend to be nondominant vis-à-vis their male or able counterparts, who comprise the majority of those who make policies affecting everyone.

To reduce the inevitable nearsightedness of the dominant group in formulating policies affecting those who are nondominant, feminist standpoint theory argues for imputing privileged status to the nondominant groups. This argument also applies to people who are nondominant within nondominant groups, such as people with cognitive impairments who are unable to articulate their needs or interests to those who are physically but not cognitively impaired.

The goal of human flourishing that an egalitarian feminism supports is different from and more demanding than the narrower goal of normal human functioning that a liberal theory of justice supports. However, when resources are limited, a normal functioning standard is an acceptable standard by which to distinguish between those to whom resources should be offered and those who may be denied them. Unfortunately, what constitutes normality remains, even then, debatable.

NOTES

1. The most recent collections that explain and illustrate the philosophical diversity of feminism are Alcoff and Kittay 2006; and Jaggar and Young 1998. Websites that list publications by philosophically diverse feminist authors are www.cddc.vt.edu/feminism/phi.html and www.cddc.vt.edu/feminism/enin.html; the former website divides the material according to the historical period of philosophy the authors present and critique, whereas the second lists feminist works in three categories: fields, national and ethnic groups, and individual feminists.

2. My interpretation of feminist standpoint theory relies mainly on the work of Nancy Hartsock and Donna Haraway (cf. Hartsock 1985; 1998, 105–32; Haraway 2004, 81–101). The collection edited by Harding offers an excellent sampling of philosophical diversity within feminism and feminist standpoint theory.

3. For example, Norman Daniels maintains that "species-typical normal functioning" requires fulfillment of "course-of-life needs" such as food, clothing, shelter, exercise, rest, and companionship (1985, 26), and Martha Nussbaum lists the capabilities that she considers necessary to human flourishing in *Women and Human Development* (2000, 78–80).

4. I have also developed this argument in "Our Bodies Ourselves: Disability and Standpoint Theory" (Mahowald 2005, 237–46).

5. On virtue theory in an Aristotelian context, see MacIntyre (1981) and Hursthouse (1999).

6. This is the term commonly used by Daniels and colleagues as the normative standard for just distribution of health care services. For a critique of their usage, see Silvers 1998, 64–74. Ethically relevant differences among disabilities are identified and examined from an egalitarian perspective in Silvers 1998, 217–27.

7. Nondominant people are sometimes invited to join the dominant group who develop policies, but their representation is often mere tokenism. Their presence and input is rarely motivated by the desire of the dominant group to overcome their limitations.

8. This point is convincingly made by Eva Kittay (1999), who argues, on grounds of justice, that people with profound mental disabilities and their caregivers are particularly deserving of social supports.

REFERENCES

Alcoff, L. M., and E. F. Kittay. 2006. *Blackwell guide to feminist philosophy*. Oxford: Blackwell.

Buchanan, A., D. Brock, N. Daniels, and D. Wikler. 2000. *From chance to choice*. Cambridge: Cambridge University Press.

Daniels, N. 1985. *Just health care*. New York: Cambridge University Press.

Firestone, S. 1970. *The dialectic of sex.* New York: Bantam Books.

Grossman, H. J., ed. 1983. *Classification in mental retardation.* Washington, D.C.: American Association on Mental Deficiency.

Haraway, D. 2004. Situated knowledges: The science question in feminism and the privilege of partial perspective. In *The feminist standpoint reader,* ed. S. Harding, 81–101. New York: Routledge.

Hartsock, N. 1985. *Money, sex, and power.* Boston: Northeastern University Press.

———. 1998. *The feminist standpoint revisited and other essays.* Boulder, Colo.: Westview Press.

———. 2004. The feminist standpoint: Developing the ground for a specifically feminist historical materialism. In *The feminist standpoint reader,* ed. S. Harding, 35–50. New York: Routledge.

Hursthouse, R. 1999. *On virtue ethics.* Oxford: Oxford University Press.

Jaggar, A. 1983. *Feminist politics and human nature.* Totowa, N.J.: Rowman & Allanheld.

Jaggar, A., and I. Young. 1998. *A companion to feminist philosophy.* Oxford: Blackwell.

Kittay, E. F. 1999. *Love's labor: Essays on women, equality, and dependency.* New York: Routledge.

MacIntyre, A. 1981. *After virtue.* Cambridge: Cambridge University Press.

Mahowald, M. B. 2000. *Genes, women, equality.* New York: Oxford University Press.

———. 2005. Our bodies ourselves: Disability and standpoint theory. In *Social philosophy today: Human rights, religion, and democracy,* ed. J. R. Rowan, 237–46. Charlottesville, Va.: Philosophy Documentation Center.

Nussbaum, M. 2000. *Women and human development.* New York: Cambridge University Press.

Okin, S. M. 1989. *Justice, gender, and the family.* New York: Basic Books.

Rawls, J. 1971. *A theory of justice.* Cambridge, Mass.: Harvard University Press.

———. 1996. *Political liberalism.* New York: Columbia University Press.

Sen, A. 1992. *Inequality reexamined.* Cambridge, Mass.: Harvard University Press.

Silvers, A., D. Wasserman, and M. Mahowald. 1998. *Disability, difference, discrimination.* Boulder, Colo.: Rowman & Littlefield.

Tong, R. 1998. *Feminist thought,* 2nd ed. Boulder, Colo.: Westview Press.

Reassessment and Renewal

JACKIE LEACH SCULLY, PH.D.

Feminist Bioethics and the Mainstream

Putting this book together presented us, as editors and as feminist bioethicists looking at our own field, with many more ambiguities of *both/and* than clear-cut cases of *either/or*. Bioethics is an interdisciplinary area of growing international substance and influence, and yet at the same time it is still unknown territory for many people outside philosophy or medicine. Bioethics is interdisciplinary and diverse—as Richard Twine says in his chapter, what someone thinks bioethics *is* depends a lot on the form of bioethics they have been exposed to at conferences— and yet it remains so dominated by the approaches of traditional moral philosophy and of the pragmatic principlism introduced by Beauchamp and Childress in 1979 that it still makes sense to talk of a mainstream (or streams, as contributors have often done in this book). From one perspective, feminist bioethics is a minor specialty within a larger disciplinary area; and yet a solid and coherent body of feminist theory, predating the birth of bioethics itself, has enabled some aspects of feminist thought to influence the infant field.

When the idea of this book first arose, we as editors felt that feminist bioethics was at a decisive point in its development. We still hold that view. But it has become clearer to us that it is next to impossible to say anything certain and straightforward about where *exactly* that point is in relation to the development of mainstream bioethics. The contributions by Anne Donchin, Jessica Prata Miller, and Christoph Rehmann-Sutter all highlight the contradictions and complexities of feminist influences on mainstream bioethics. This is not a simple case of a margin gradually shrinking as its arguments become recognized by the center. Hence, it is not a contradiction to acknowledge that feminist bioethics has had some success in its project to change the way that bioethics is done, while simultaneously saying that its overall impact on bioethics has been limited.

Where its methodological and theoretical insights have been taken up by the mainstream, they tend not to be labeled as "feminist." Rehmann-Sutter notes that bioethics generally presents feminist arguments as minor variants of the main show, and for a discipline to present marginal perspectives *as* marginal, as in his example of the *Encyclopedia of Bioethics*, is not the same as their becoming part of the mainstream. Genuine integration would require bioethics to allow feminist influences not just to alter the scope of the topics addressed or the amount of attention paid to the gendered nature of morally troubling situations, although both of these shifts are important. Bioethics would also have to alter its *moral perspective*: that is, to change the kind of issues that are identified as morally troubling in the first place, and the questions that are asked about them in bioethical analyses. Jessica Prata Miller gives one example in her examination of how the same problem (the "crisis of trust" in medicine) is viewed quite differently by feminist and by mainstream bioethics. A feminist perspective provides an account of the way relationships of trust in clinical settings are gendered and is therefore able to detect the potential distortion of such relationships through inequalities of authority that mean trust may be misplaced, with personally and politically harmful consequences.

This is most apparent where mainstream bioethics adopts approaches that are standard feminist practice and presents them as innovative in the field. Here we can point to the so-called empirical turn (Borry, Dierickx, and Schotsmans, 2005; De Vries et al. 2006) in mainstream bioethics. The effective use of empirical and experiential data to inform normative reflection is based on the argument that ethics needs information about "actual moral and social orders" (Walker 1998), an argument that is foundational to feminist moral epistemology. The same can be said of bioethics' recent calls for greater inclusion of public health issues (Brock 2000), or for a more critical scrutiny of the social arrangements by which certain questions are identified as relevant to bioethics and how they determine the epistemic and moral resources drawn on by academics and policy makers (Haimes 2002; Hedgecoe 2004). This routine disclosure of social and political privilege's capacity to skew ethical perspectives, including our own, is part of feminism's stock in trade.

Still, it would be a mistake to overstate the case for feminist bioethics and to imagine it is now on the descending arc of its trajectory, having done its job. Not even the most optimistic contributor in this collection suggests that the assimilation of feminist insight by the bioethical mainstream is anything more than partial. In fact, the evidence points to a highly selective uptake. The most notable exclusion is the bulk of feminism's fundamental commitment to social and political change. Having grown out of an emancipatory social movement, the academic enterprise of feminism retains the broad goal of improving the lives of women (feminism's argument is that this will ultimately improve the lives of everyone, but women are of primary concern). Although for individual scholars feminism's overt political agenda may take second place to the analytic or methodological tools it provides, feminist effort in academia is still nourished by a strong undercurrent of transformative commitment. Thus while mainstream bioethics has been able to assimilate some of feminist bioethics' *theoretical* insights and its *methodologies* (although more than one of the contributions here traces the limits of that assimilation), its specific *political* goals remain outside.

It's not clear whether we should take a pessimistic or optimistic view of this state of affairs. One response is to find it regrettable but inevitable, a part of the process familiar to the history of radicalism whereby a transformative political or intellectual movement is never fully acknowledged by the institutions it tries to change, because institutionalized authority will always have a vested interest in maintaining the status quo. Richard Twine points to one of the potential consequences when he asks whether the desire to be accepted by mainstream bioethics determines the kind of feminism that is put forward—in effect, whether "extreme" or radical views are suppressed as a strategy to greater acceptance. "Strategic moderation" of this sort is familiar to most of us in other contexts, and it represents a real danger for feminists working in mainstream philosophy. An alternative, more optimistic explanation is that feminist bioethics' lack of political impact reflects what might be considered an appropriate division of labor, in which the supposedly neutral mainstream is preserved from political partisanship, leaving the margins of the discipline free to indulge in it. The problem with that model is its implicit acceptance of two ideas: first, that neutrality and objectivity are necessarily at the heart of intellectual inquiry; and second, that the epistemic and ethical mainstream of a discipline is *not* already politicized. Feminist epistemology, and in fact critical epistemology as a whole, would find both of these suppositions questionable. The more pessimistic diagnosis, then, is that feminist bioethics' relative lack of impact on the political consciousness of the field means that it has so far failed to complete its job. If that is the case, then even as we celebrate the uptake of feminist methodological and theoretical insights by mainstream bioethics, the absence of its radical edge should not go unremarked.

Feminist Bioethics and the Margins

Let's turn now from the relationship between feminist bioethics and the mainstream and consider how feminist bioethics and other marginalities interact.

Within mainstream bioethics, most attention so far has been focused on ethnic and geographical margins. Over the last decade or so there has been a growth of interest in the bioethics being played out in societies beyond those of the familiar Euro–North American–Australasian axis, an interest illustrated by the launch of the journal *Developing World Bioethics* in 2000. Although the bioethical literature remains dominated by work from the United Kingdom and Europe, North America, Australia, and New Zealand, the bioethics of the future will be more global, and inevitably more socially, culturally, and ethnically diverse than it has been so far. And there is no escaping the fact that genuine cross-cultural bioethical engagement presents formidable practical as well as intellectual barriers. At the best of times bioethical debate is complex and contentious. It becomes exponentially more tricky as diversity increases in language (with a concomitant need for accurate translation) and in ethical terminology, in the status given to ethical concepts such as the relationship of the individual to larger collectives, or the prioritization of key goods, or in expectations about the proper format of debate or of public involvement.

Feminist bioethics has an advantage here, because both intellectually and practically it has taken a global perspective for far longer. As Donna Dickenson has noted, "The debates that now exercise mainstream philosophy, international relations, and political theory so vigorously concerning universalism, particularism, and global ethics, have been going on in feminist philosophy for at least 20 years, largely unobserved by canonical philosophers." (Dickenson 2004, 21) And Anne Donchin recalls in her chapter that earlier FAB collections (Tong, Anderson, and Santos 2001; Tong, Donchin, and Dodds 2004) took a global tack, with contributions that took into consideration features, such as the "economic, social and political effects of globalized capitalism," that affect global bioethical problems but rarely appear in mainstream bioethical writing. Similarly, throughout its history feminist bioethics has been confronted by and learned to cope with the realities and responsibilities of the disciplinary heterogeneity that resulted from the inclusion of diverse perspectives. While there are many contested analyses of the crisis of political identity and fragmentation that feminism endured in the 1980s and '90s, some scholars argue that precisely these fault lines of dissent and disagreement were the strongest growing points of intellectual activity. As a result, contemporary feminist theory tries to maximize the benefit of the diversity in women's experiences and in women's understanding of what "feminist" means in the globalized twenty-first century, while being acutely conscious of the need to avoid sweeping assumptions about sameness and otherness.

Feminism not only has a track record of experience in managing these tensions, but it has also learned from experience that the perspectives of geographically and economically privileged philosophers or policy makers are not universally valid. They are certainly not the perspectives of the majority of people in the developing world, just as the perspectives of Western women philosophers are not coterminous with women elsewhere. So to speak of developing world bioethics does not (or should not) just meant the bioethics emerging as those countries engage with Western bioethics on the international regulatory or research stage. Developing world bioethics also needs to come to grips with the forms of thinking about good lives and right acts, health and wholeness, that are indigenous to those societies, although they may be unfamiliar and at first sight have little relevance to the issues that preoccupy international bioethical debate.

As bioethics becomes more and more global, the longstanding principles of feminist theory and methodology, some of which we saw in this collection, increase rather than decrease in relevance. Globalization takes feminist thought to parts of the world where such analyses are innovative, stimulating new lines of thinking and exciting a new generation of scholars and activists. The chapters by Jennifer Baker, Terry Dunbar, and Margaret Scrimgeour; Ruth Groenhout; Jing-Bao Nie; and Mary Mahowald all demonstrate feminist bioethics' capacity to reexamine the ethical implications of social groupings and stratification—not just by gender but also by race, culture, class, and disability—by mobilizing a feminist sensitivity to the effect of power differentials that mainstream bioethics generally neglects. Within its relatively short tradition, feminist bioethics has developed unique theoretical and methodological tools to share with the more recent bioethics of Asia, Southeast Asia, Africa, and elsewhere. An example in this collection is Jing-Bao Nie's subtle and nuanced application of feminist ethics to the culture of mainland China.

However, it would be misleading to think that feminist bioethics and the bioethics of other marginalities go together unproblematically simply by virtue of being "other" to mainstream bioethics. Baker, Dunbar, and Scrimgeour explore the tensions inherent in forming strategic alliances between feminist bioethics and Indigenous communities in Australia. They suggest that, while beneficial in principle, especially in giving severely marginalized groups like these access to international forums through the feminist presence there, formal engagement in Australia and elsewhere has been less common and less successful than predicted. In part, this is because Indigenous men and women (and other racial minorities) have tended to see feminism as a distraction from their more pressing issues of racism and colonialism.

The quasicolonialist trap is to think solely in terms of what feminist bioethics has to offer to those marginal others. As the work of Baker, Dunbar, and Scrim-geour and of Nie shows, the traffic between feminist bioethics and other "others" is far from one-way. It is true that the (still rather few) bioethicists working from within ethnic, cultural, or religious minorities or within disability often draw on feminist theory and methodology; but their use of it is not uncritical. Their critique, and the modifications they are obliged to make to correct for the epistemic and ethical assumptions of a bioethics crafted by white, Western, able-bodied women, presents feminists with challenging negotiations of power and perspective. Dealing with this critique is not always comfortable, but it produces a richer feminist bioethics. In the engagement between feminist bioethics and other social margins, feminism gains just as much as the other marginalities or bioethics itself. So it may be argued that the interactions with other "others" is one way in which feminist bioethics retains, or is reminded of, its critical and self-critical responsibilities.

Bioethics and the Future

Given that feminist bioethics seems to be not only heterogeneous but also simultaneously assimilating into the central mainstream(s) *and* allying itself with some newer margins, it's reasonable to ask whether anything remains that is coherent and distinctive enough to be identified as feminist bioethics at all. In the academy, the plurality of feminist bioethics means that a poststructuralist feminist might well find more in common with a mainstream colleague using poststructuralist language and concepts than with a feminist colleague working from within the analytic tradition. But having said that, in practice, feminist contributions to bioethics are almost always immediately recognizable as such. There is an irreducible minimum, which Alison Jaggar defined as an agreement that "the subordination of women is morally wrong and that the moral experience of women is worthy of respect" (Jaggar 1991, 95). Hilde Lindemann called these the two normative legs on which feminist ethics stands (Lindemann 2006, 14). These are the commitments that give consistency to the feminist handling of bioethical issues.

What of the future? Lindemann has elsewhere suggested two directions in which bioethics and feminist bioethics could go (Lindemann 2007). One is to apply feminist methodology and theoretical frameworks to *cutting-edge topics*: in 2010, these could be stem cell technology and neuroethics, but "cutting-edge" will undoubtedly mean something different in a few years' time. The other direction sees feminist bioethics contributing to the development of new *bioethical theory.* The contributions in the second section of this collection demonstrate the results of such engagement for theorizing around the concepts of autonomy, equality, and choice, for example. What is distinctive about the feminist engagement with theory is its strategy of starting with specific concrete examples— donation of eggs and embryos, market in body parts—and working outward from there toward a consideration of the implications for canonical bioethical theory. Lori d'Agincourt-Canning, for example, shows us how a study of individuals from families with hereditary breast cancer not only generates empirically based understanding of what these lives are like and the choices that may be made by those living them but also acts as a springboard for deeper theoretical engagement with the epistemological significance of the "lived experience" that is frequently evoked in feminist and other writing, yet too rarely subjected to rigorous scrutiny. Additional empirically rooted theorizing of this sort would be especially welcome in bioethics, which has long been criticized for its instrumentality and more recently for its distance from everyday social and political realities.

In addition to new topics and new theory, we would warn against assuming that central feminist insights are so familiar that they do not bear repeating. As the chapters by Catriona Mackenzie, Mary Rawlinson, Janice McLaughlin, and Fiona Utley illustrate, expanding moral perception is an ongoing process. Mackenzie acknowledges that the questions of redistributive justice and autonomy have been extensively discussed in the areas of genetics and reproductive technologies but goes on to note that the discussions "tend to take the standard conception of individual autonomy [which many feminist philosophers find problematic] for granted." The key to her reframing of the debate over tissue donation is her use of the feminist concept of relational autonomy (Mackenzie and Stoljar 2000). In a similar vein, Rawlinson makes an argument for a feminist-inspired scrutiny of the origins of familiar ethical concepts, such as equality and human personhood, that are mobilized in the contemporary discourse of universal human rights. McLaughlin again restructures a familiar bioethical debate, this time about choice, by considering the possible use of prenatal selection for sexual orientation, and so her analysis creates a shift in moral perception of familiar (possibly even over-familiar) issues and arguments. And Fiona Utley's chapter is one example of how a subject that is not normally considered to concern bioethics at all (in this case, rape) can be placed within a feminist ethical analysis and as a result can generate new insights of not just theoretical but also practical significance. Utley sees feminist bioethics as necessary here because the "cultural narratives of illness...can ascribe undue responsibility to the individual and evade the political problem of women's need to experience the world as safe," an evasion that a feminist consciousness does not allow.

Over and above the existing diversity of approaches, the bidirectional dynamic we have described—where feminist bioethics is taking a place at the center of bioethical scholarship and simultaneously building alliances with activists of the margins—introduces another dimension of possibilities for the future. In some respects, bridge building between activism and scholarship is nothing new for feminist bioethics. In her chapter, Anne Donchin mentions that from its earliest days, feminists in bioethics have tended to straddle the activist and academic communities, forming a variety of professional and cross-disciplinary links. Joint projects of different kinds were to everyone's advantage, for strategic political as much as intellectual reasons. In this collection, the chapter by Al-Yasha Ilhaam and Ina May Gaskin exemplifies this tradition: they take as their starting point empirical observation of women's experience, in this case the experience of pregnancy and birth; they bring critique and self-critique into play as they examine the dynamics of the physician-philosopher collaboration; and they write from the perspective of a practicing midwife and a bioethicist with a conscious desire to strengthen the bond between bioethics discourse and the women's health movement.

While many of the contributors to this volume would wholeheartedly identify themselves as feminist bioethicists, others might be reluctant to claim to be doing more than drawing on some of its tools. Still others would be happier to claim some kind of hyphenated identity as bioethicists plus something else. Nevertheless, on reading these chapters, we as editors were struck by the common factor that all of them are clear that what they are doing, or what they describe, is a *different* kind of bioethics—one that differs from the mainstream in theory, methodology, and subject matter. Moreover, all the contributions convey a strong sense of the vitality of thought that feminist approaches bring to bioethics and the novel avenues its practitioners continue to open up.

REFERENCES

Borry, P., K. Dierickx, and P. Schotsmans. 2005. The birth of the empirical turn in bioethics. *Bioethics* 19:49–71.
Brock, D. W. 2000. Broadening the bioethics agenda. *Kennedy Institute of Ethics Journal* 10:21–38.
De Vries, R., C. Bosk, L. Turner, and K. Orfali, eds. 2006. *The view from here: Social science and bioethics.* London: Blackwell.

Dickenson, D. 2004. What feminism can teach global ethics. In *Linking visions: Feminist bioethics, human rights, and the developing world,* ed. R. Tong, A. Donchin, and S. Dodds, 15–30. Lanham, Md.: Rowman & Littlefield.

Haimes, E. 2002. What can the social sciences contribute to the study of ethics? Theoretical, empirical and substantive considerations. *Bioethics* 16:89–113.

Hedgecoe, A. 2004. Critical bioethics: Beyond the social science critique of applied ethics. *Bioethics* 18:120–43.

Jaggar, A. M. 1991. Feminist ethics: Problems, prospects. In *Feminist ethics,* ed. C. Card, 78–106. Lawrence: University of Kansas Press.

Lindemann, H. 2006. *An invitation to feminist ethics.* New York: McGraw-Hill.

———. 2007. Feminist bioethics: Where we've been, where we're going. In *The Blackwell guide to feminist philosophy,* ed. L. M. Alcoff and E. F. Kittay, 116–30. Oxford: Oxford University Press.

Tong, R., G. Anderson, and A. Santos, eds. 2001. *Globalizing feminist bioethics: Women's health concerns worldwide.* Boulder, Colo.: Westview Press.

Tong, R., A. Donchin, and S. Dodds, eds. 2004. *Linking visions: Feminist bioethics, human rights, and the developing world.* Lanham, Md.: Rowman & Littlefield.

Walker, M. U. 1998. *Moral understandings: A feminist study in ethics.* New York: Routledge.